A Clinician's Guide to Newborn Screening

A Clinician's Guide to Newborn Screening

Editor: Elizabeth Curling

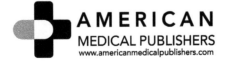

AMERICAN
MEDICAL PUBLISHERS
www.americanmedicalpublishers.com

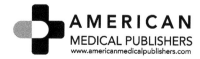

AMERICAN
MEDICAL PUBLISHERS
www.americanmedicalpublishers.com

Cataloging-in-Publication Data

A clinician's guide to newborn screening / edited by Elizabeth Curling.
    p. cm.
Includes bibliographical references and index.
ISBN 978-1-63927-576-2
1. Newborn screening. 2. Newborn infants--Medical examinations.
3. Newborn infants--Diseases--Diagnosis. I. Curling, Elizabeth.
RJ255.5 .C55 2023
618.920 1--dc23

American Medical Publishers,
41 Flatbush Avenue,
1st Floor, New York,
NY 11217, USA

ISBN 978-1-63927-576-2 (Hardback)

Contents

Preface

Over the recent decade, advancements and applications have progressed exponentially. This has led to the increased interest in this field and projects are being conducted to enhance knowledge. The main objective of this book is to present some of the critical challenges and provide insights into possible solutions. This book will answer the varied questions that arise in the field and also provide an increased scope for furthering studies.

Newborn screening involves a specialized collection of point-of-care tests and laboratory assessments that are conducted on newborn infants for discovering clinically occult but potentially serious illnesses, which requires immediate intervention. Furthermore, newborn screening can also consist of skin-to-skin contact between the newborn and the mother, newborn examination, safe-sleep principles, newborn mental health issues, etc. It encompasses various processes, such as diagnostic testing, parental education, disease management, follow-up and continuous assessment. The most important aspect of newborn screening is collecting a blood sample to test for hematologic, inheritable, metabolic, and endocrine disorders. The targets of newborn screening usually comprise of those medical conditions, which will result in significant intellectual disability, mortality and morbidity without clinical intervention. This book aims to understand the clinical perspectives of newborn screening. Researchers and students in the field of neonatal care will be assisted by it.

I hope that this book, with its visionary approach, will be a valuable addition and will promote interest among readers. Each of the authors has provided their extraordinary competence in their specific fields by providing different perspectives as they come from diverse nations and regions. I thank them for their contributions.

Editor

Evaluation of Outcomes and Quality of Care in Children with Sickle Cell Disease Diagnosed by Newborn Screening

Valentine Brousse [1,*], Cécile Arnaud [2], Emmanuelle Lesprit [3], Béatrice Quinet [3], Marie-Hélène Odièvre [4], Maryse Etienne-Julan [5], Cécile Guillaumat [6], Gisèle Elana [7], Marie Belloy [8], Nathalie Garnier [9], Abdourahim Chamouine [10], Cécile Dumesnil [11], Mariane De Montalembert [1], Corinne Pondarre [2,9], Françoise Bernaudin [2], Nathalie Couque [12], Emmanuelle Boutin [13], Josiane Bardakjian [14], Fatiha Djennaoui [15], Ghislaine Ithier [16], Malika Benkerrou [16] and Isabelle Thuret [17]

[1] Department of General Pediatrics and Pediatric Infectious Diseases, Sickle Cell Disease Reference Center, Necker-Enfants Malades Hospital, Assistance Publique-Hôpitaux de Paris (AP-HP), Université de Paris, 75005 Paris, France; mariane.demontal@aphp.fr

[2] Department of Pediatrics, Sickle Cell Disease Reference Center, CHIC Hospital, Université de Paris-Est Créteil, 94000 Créteil, France; cecile.arnaud@chicreteil.fr (C.A.); corinne.pondarre@chicreteil.fr (C.P.); francoise.bernaudin@chicreteil.fr (F.B.)

[3] Department of Pediatrics, Sickle Cell Disease Reference Center, Trousseau Hospital, Assistance Publique-Hôpitaux de Paris (AP-HP), 75012 Paris, France; emmanuelle.lesprit@efs.fr (E.L.); quinetlaos@aol.com (B.Q.)

[4] Department of Pediatrics, Louis Mourier Hospital, Assistance Publique-Hôpitaux de Paris (AP-HP), 92700 Colombes, France; marie-helene.odievre@aphp.fr

[5] Sickle Cell Disease Unit, Sickle Cell Disease Reference Center, University Hospital of Pointe-à-Pitre/Abymes, BP 465 Pointe-à-Pitre, Guadeloupe, France; maryse.etienne-julan@chu-guadeloupe.fr

[6] Department of Pediatrics, Centre Hospitalier Sud Francilien, 91100 Corbeil-Essonne, France; cecile.guillaumat@chsf.fr

[7] Sickle Cell Disease Unit, Sickle Cell Disease Reference Center, University Hospital of Martinique, 97261 Fort De France, Martinique, France; gisele.elana@chu-fortdefrance.fr

[8] Department of Pediatrics, Robert Ballanger Hospital, 93600 Aulnay Sous Bois, France; marie.belloy@ch-aulnay.fr

[9] Department of Pediatric Onco-Hematology, Institut d'Hématologie et d'Oncologie Pédiatrique, 69008 Lyon, France; nathalie.garnier@ihope.fr

[10] Department of Pediatrics, Mamoudzou Hospital, 97600 Mayotte, France; a.chamouine1@chmayotte.fr

[11] Department of Pediatric Onco-Hematology, Charles Nicolle Hospital, 76600 Rouen, France; Cecile.Dumesnil@chu-rouen.fr

[12] Biochemistry and Molecular Biology Laboratory, Robert Debré Hospital, Assistance Publique-Hôpitaux de Paris (AP-HP), 75019 Paris, France; nathalie.couque@aphp.fr

[13] Department of Public Health And Biostatistics, Henri Mondor Hospital, Assistance Publique-Hôpitaux de Paris (AP-HP), 94010 Créteil, France; emmanuelle.boutin@aphp.fr

[14] Department of Biochemistry and Genetics, Henri Mondor Hospital, Assistance Publique-Hôpitaux de Paris (AP-HP), 94010 Créteil, France; bardakdjian@wanadoo.fr

[15] Clinical Research Unit, Albert Chenevier Hospital, 94010 Créteil, France; fatiha.djennaoui@aphp.fr

[16] Sickle Cell Disease Reference Center, Robert Debré Hospital, Assistance Publique-Hôpitaux de Paris (AP-HP), 75019 Paris, France; ghislaine.ithier@aphp.fr (G.I.); malika.benkerrou@aphp.fr (M.B.)

[17] Department of Pediatric Onco-Hematology, Thalassemia Reference Center, Timone Enfant Hospital, Assistance Publique-Hôpitaux de Marseille (AP-HM), 13005 Marseille, France; Isabelle.thuret@ap-hm.fr

* Correspondence: valentine.brousse@gmail.com

Abstract: This study's objective was to assess, on a national scale, residual risks of death, major disease-related events, and quality of care during the first five years in children diagnosed at birth with sickle cell disease (SCD). Data were retrospectively collected from medical files of all children with SCD born between 2006–2010 in France. Out of 1792 eligible subjects, 1620 patients (71.8% SS or S/beta°-thalassemia -SB°-) had available follow-up data, across 69 centers. Overall probability of survival by five years was 98.9%, with 12/18 deaths related to SCD. Probability of overt stroke by five years in SS/SB° patients was 1.1%, while transcranial Doppler (TCD) was performed in 81% before three years of age. A total of 26 patients had meningitis/septicemia (pneumococcal in eight cases). Prophylactic penicillin was started at a median age of 2.2 months and 87% of children had received appropriate conjugate pneumococcal vaccination at one year. By five years, the probability of survival without SCD-related events was 10.7% for SS/SB° patients. In contrast, hydroxyurea was prescribed in 13.7% and bone marrow transplant performed in nine patients only. In this study, residual risks of severe complications were low, probably resulting from a good national TCD, vaccination, and healthcare system coverage. Nonetheless, burden of disease remained high, stressing the need for disease-modifying or curative therapy.

Keywords: sickle cell disease; newborn screening; mortality; morbidity; transcranial Doppler; vaccination coverage

---

1. Introduction

Newborn screening (NBS) programs for sickle cell disease (SCD) aim to reduce early mortality and morbidity by introducing preventive measures directed towards major disease-related identified risks: Pneumococcal infection, acute splenic sequestration, and neurovascular injury. Prophylactic intervention such as penicillin and pneumococcal vaccination, parental education, and neurological screening by transcranial Doppler (TCD) have demonstrated significant efficacy in reducing these risks in children [1–4]. Recent studies from either monocentric reference centers [5,6] or regional multicenter hospital-based network [7] or performed on a national scale [8] in different high-income settings (USA, England, and France) have consistently shown low childhood mortality and an improved survival into adulthood of 94%–100% for SCD children diagnosed at birth and who benefitted from such measures.

Only very few nation-wide data are available, however, regarding both medical care and residual early morbidity and mortality in countries where newborn screening and prophylactic measures are implemented. Only such studies may in fact address disparities across regions, centers, or countries and provide a true-to-life evaluation.

A SCD NBS program was fully implemented since 2000 in France, targeting newborns identified at risk in mainland France and all newborns in French overseas territories. More specifically, regarding the targeted SCD NBS program, newborns are screened when parents originate from a country where SCD is endemic (an official list is available) and/or in case of family history of SCD and/or in case of uncertainty regarding both previous issues, in accordance with national guidelines [9]. Following confirmed diagnosis, children with SCD have free medical care regarding all SCD-related specific prophylactic or therapeutic measures, consultation, and hospitalization. A specialized follow-up is offered in the closest hospital with expertise in SCD, in relation to a tertiary reference center for additional expertise if needed. In addition, free medical surveillance and immunization is offered in France to all children aged less than six years.

The main objective of this retrospective study was to assess, on a national scale and during the first five years of life, residual risks of death, overt stroke, and bacterial meningitis/septicemia resulting from current transcranial Doppler (TCD) and pneumococcal prophylactic utilization in SCD children diagnosed at birth. The secondary objective was to evaluate in these young children the frequency of other main SCD-related events and the use of disease-modifying or curative therapy (hydroxyurea (HU), transfusion (TF) programs, and hematopoietic stem cell transplantation (HSCT)).

2. Experimental Section

2.1. Study Population

We retrospectively identified all patients born between 1 January 2006 and 31 December 2010 diagnosed with SCD through the national NBS program in mainland France, French West Indies (Guadeloupe, Martinique), and Réunion-Mayotte. Results of NBS indicating SCD were fed back to a referral sickle cell center where confirmatory tests were performed, and results were explained to parents. The follow-up was thereafter organized in the closest sickle cell center according to the child's residence. Sickle cell centers were formally identified in a national network in 2004. Patients diagnosed in French Guyana were not included in the study because at the time of data collection, cross identification of patients following NBS was not possible in that region.

2.2. Data Collection

Data were collected in 2014/2015 from the patients' medical files up to the age of 5 years regarding age at first prescription of penicillin prophylactic therapy, occurrence of death/overt, stroke/bacterial meningitis or septicemia, first event of acute splenic sequestration, acute chest syndrome/pneumonia, vaso-occlusive crisis (VOC), age at first transfusion, as well as use of pneumococcal vaccines/first chronic TF program/hydroxyurea/hematopoietic stem cell transplantation and TCD results.

Patients were considered lost to follow-up when no data were available during the 2-year period of data collection i.e., 2014/2015 in any center in France. In addition, patients residing abroad and who were seen only occasionally in France were excluded from analysis.

2.3. Outcomes

Fatal cases were analyzed in detail and the numbers were checked with the National French Death Registry for exhaustivity purpose.

TCD velocities were considered abnormal when ≥ 2 m/s and conditional when ≥ 1.7 m/s but <2 m/s (according to the STOP criteria [10]), as recorded in the medical files.

Other clinical outcomes were collected as reported in the medical file and no further verification was performed. However, the following definitions are consensual in France:

- Vaso-occlusive crisis (including dactylitis) was defined as an acute non-infectious, non-traumatic pain requiring analgesics for more than 12 h and/or hospital admission.
- Acute chest syndrome (ACS) was defined as a new pulmonary infiltrate on chest X-ray, with or without pain, cough, fever (≥ 38.5 °C), or hypoxemia. Given the overlapping definition of pneumoniae in young children, the latter events were pooled with ACS.
- Acute anemic events were defined by reductions in hemoglobin $\geq 20\%$ versus steady state.
- Acute splenic sequestration (ASS) was defined as splenic enlargement increased ≥ 2 cm from baseline associated with acute anemia.
- Stroke was defined as an ischemic or hemorrhagic event lasting >24 h and resulting in focal neurologic deficit.

During the study period, national guidelines recommended prophylactic penicillin to all children with SCD at least until the age of 5, pneumococcal vaccinations using conjugate vaccines (3 injections of 7 valent pneumococcal conjugated vaccine (PCV7) in the first year of life (replaced by 13 valent pneumococcal conjugated vaccine (PCV13) from April 2010) followed by a boost during 2nd year, and a dose of polysaccharidic 23 valent pneumococcal vaccine (P23) at 2 years. Annual TCD screening was recommended from 2 to 16 years in patients with SS or SB°-thalassemia (SB°) disease only [11] and was performed with the same methodology across centers.

Chronic transfusion program was defined as any transfusion program that lasted >3 months. Hydroxyurea was recommended by national guidelines in 2005 for adults and children over 2 years with recurrent vaso-occlusive crises and/or acute chest syndrome but was specifically licensed with adapted pediatric dosage for patients with SCD in 2007 only.

2.4. Ethics

This study (NCT 03119922) was approved by the Inserm Ethics Committee/Institutional Review board (13–118), the French National Committee for Computerized Databases (CNIL-127020), and by EC/CCTIRS (13–118/12319). In accordance with the French regulation authorities, given the observational retrospective nature of the study, families were informed about the study by their physician including the possibility to decline participation but were not required to give written informed consent.

2.5. Statistical Analysis

The results are expressed as numbers and percentages for categorical variables and as median (25th quartile; 75th quartile) for continuous variables. The distribution of variables was analyzed using the chi-square test for categorical variables and the Mann–Whitney test for continuous variables.

Entry into the study cohort was defined by the date of the birth. Data were censored at the date of 5 years or last follow-up in 2014/2015 or death. Assessment of overall survival and survival without specific SCD-related complications were generated by the time to first event. Kaplan–Meier survival estimates and the 95% confidence interval (95% CI) were calculated for all SCD-related complications. Given that patients with SS or SB° tend to have a more severe clinical course than those with SC or S-beta$^+$thalassemia (SB$^+$), we stratified the analysis into two groups, SS/SB° (including SDPundjab) and SC/SB$^+$ (including HbSE) patients, whenever appropriate. Survival curves were compared using the log-rank test. Statistical analyses were performed using STATA version 14.1 (College Station, TX 77845, USA). Overall and age-specific rates of mortality and stroke were calculated as the number of deaths/strokes divided by total person–years at risk.

3. Results

3.1. General Results

Between 01/01/2006 and 31/12/2010, 1801 consecutive newborns with SCD were identified by the National NBS program (Figure 1). Nine families declined participation and 20 patients did not reside in France (their follow-up was occasionally performed in France). Out of the 1772 remaining patients, 152 (8.5%) were lost to follow-up at the time of data collection (from January 2014 to December 2015), of whom 44 were known to have returned to their country of origin. Among the 152 children lost to follow-up, 43 (28.3%) were lost to follow up following NBS and 109 (71.7%) later on. Finally, a total of 1620 patients with available follow-up data during 2014/2015 or deceased before five years were thereafter analyzed and constituted the EVADREP cohort. Subsequently, at the time of data analysis, 100% of living patients in the cohort had reached at least three years of age while 77% had reached five years.

Of note, the targeted nature of the NBS program in mainland France during our study period most likely did not leave out a significant number of SCD cases: A large retrospective study over the period ranging from 2005–2017 found 24 missed cases, representing 0.6% of the screened cohort during that same period (Pluchart and Remion, personal communication, manuscript in revision). In addition, during our study period (2006–2010), the mean national proportion of babies targeted for SCD at birth in mainland France was 30%, a rather large proportion.

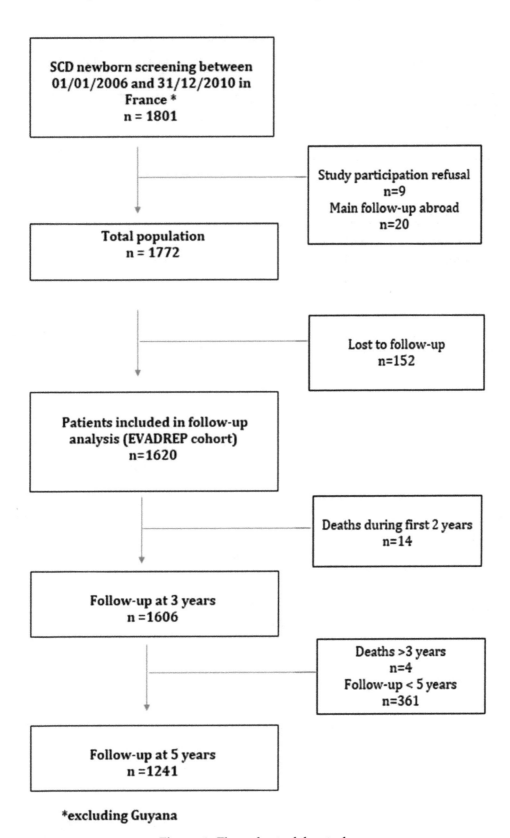

*excluding Guyana

Figure 1. Flow-chart of the study.

A majority of children (71.8%) was diagnosed with SS or SB° and 20.3% with SC or SB⁺ disease. Main characteristics of the cohort are shown in Table 1.

Table 1. General characteristics of the population.

	Total	Paris Area	Province	French West Antilles	Mayotte-Réunion
n (%)	1620 (100)	967 (59.6)	443 (27.3)	152 (9.4)	58 (4.4)
SS/SB°/SDPunjab	1164 (71.8)	703 (72.7)	336 (75.8)	74 (48.7)	51 (87.9)
SC/SB$^+$/Other *	456 (28.2)	264 (27.3)	107 (24.2)	78 (51.3)	7 (12.1)
Sex ratio (M/F)	824 (50.9)	-	-	-	-

* SO-Arab/SE/S-Lepore.

Follow up was performed in 69 centers across four main French regions: Paris area, province, French West Indies (Martinique-Guadeloupe-St Martin), and Réunion-Mayotte. Over a half of patients (59.6%) were residents in the greater Paris area, while 9.4% resided in the French West Indies where a substantially greater fraction of patients had SC disease (42%).

Among the 69 centers, a majority (42; 60.8%) followed less than 20 patients included in the study: 17 (24.6%) centers followed between 20–50 patients; 10 centers (14.5%) followed more than 50 patients (between 50–100 and >100 patients in 8 and 2 centers, respectively).

3.2. Follow-up Results

Altogether, among the patients included in EVADREP cohort, 1540 (95.1%) had a regular follow-up while 80 (4.9%) were temporarily lost to follow-up at some point during the study period—during the first 6 months in 31(1.9%) or later during at least a 2 year period in 49 (3%). These figures did not change significantly across regions of birth, but did according to the size of the centers, the largest centers having the lowest percentage of patients lost to follow up, both following NBS or thereafter (Table 2). In addition to a hospital-based follow-up in the 69 centers, a vast majority of these children (1151, 83.6%) had a community-based follow up by the French primary care system and 1396 (91.8%) had also an identified general practitioner or pediatrician.

Table 2. Outcomes and coverage rates by five years of age according to center size.

Size of Center †	Total	<10	(10–20)	(20–50)	(50–100)	≥100	*p* Value *
Nb. of centers	69	24	18	17	8	2	-
Nb. of patients	1620	125	258	452	516	269	-
Nb of patients with continued follow-up, *n* (%)	1540 (95.1)	116 (92.8)	247 (95.7)	421 (93.2)	490 (94.9)	266 (98.9)	0.009
No TCD screening *N*, (%) **	81 (7.0)	15 (16.0)	18 (9.4)	25 (7.1)	18 (5.6)	5 (2.4)	<0.001
Complete pneumococcal coverage # *N*, (%)	768 (47.4)	31 (24.8)	89 (34.5)	206 (45.6)	230 (44.6)	212 (78.8)	<0.001
Probability of HU treatment ** *n*, %	145 13.7% (11.7–15.9)	14 16.5% (10.1–26.4)	28 16.5% (11.7–23.1)	27 8.4% (5.8–12)	35 12.1% (8.8–16.4)	41 21.2% (16–27.7)	<0.001
Probability of TF program ** *n*, %	204 18.4% (7.2–20.8)	10 11.2% (6.2–19.8)	27 15.0% (10.5–21.2)	39 11.6% (8.6–15.6)	56 18.2% (14.3–23)	72 36.3% (30–43.5)	<0.001
Probability of abnormal TCD ** *n*, %	105 10.4% (8.6–12.4)	8 10.5% (5.4–20.0)	19 11.5% (7.5–17.4)	21 6.8% (4.5–10.3)	19 7.0% (4.5–10.8)	38 20.0% (15–26.5)	<0.001

† Size of center according to the number of patients enrolled in the study * Log-rank test or chi-squared test; ** only for SS/SB° patients # defined by ≥4 doses of pneumococcal conjugated vaccine (either PCV7 or PCV13) and 1 polysacchardic dose at 3 years; TCD: Transcranial Doppler; TF: Transfusion.

3.3. Outcomes

3.3.1. Major Severe Outcomes and Prophylactic Coverage

- Survival and mortality rates and causes

Probability of survival for all children at five years was 98.9% (95%CI: 98.2–99.3) and was 98.6% (97.7–99.1) and 99.6% (98.2–99.9) in SS/SB° and SC/SB+ patients, respectively (Figure 2).

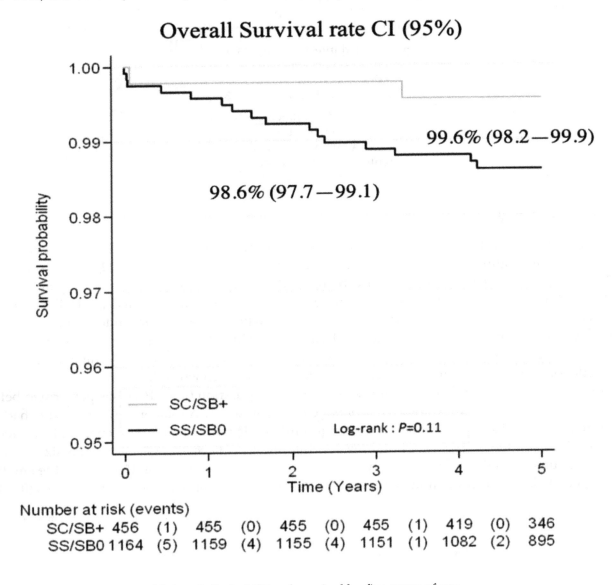

Figure 2. Probability of survival by five years of age.

Mortality rate for all patients was 0.31/100 person–years (0.17–0.58) and 0.23/100 person–years (0.15–0.37) at two years and at five years, respectively. When analyzing by disease severity, mortality rate was 0.29/100 person–years (0.18–0.47) at 5 years in children with SS/SB° as opposed to 0.09/100 person–years (0.02–0.36) in SC/SB+ children.

A total of 18 patients died at a median age of 1.6 years (range: 0.01–4.2) with 10 of these deaths occurring before age 2. Among all deaths, 12 (66.7%) were SCD-related, all but one in patients with SS/SB° (Table 3). Over half of those (7/12) were from infection (four of which from pneumococcal infection). Survival at three years and probability of survival at five years excluding SCD-unrelated cause were 99.7% (95%CI: 99.3–99.9) and 99.2% (95%CI: 98.7–99.4). There was no additional death reported by the National Death Registry during the study period.

Table 3. Overall causes of death.

Causes of death (*n* = 18)
Unrelated causes: *n* = 6
Pulmonary dysplasia
Spinal muscular atrophy
Neonatal herpes
Premature birth
Mitochondriopathy
Neonatal Streptococcus B meningitis
SCD-related infectious causes: *n* = 7
Pneumococcal septicemia (*n* = 3)
Pneumococcal meningitis
Undocumented sepsis (*n* = 3)
Miscellaneous SCD-related causes: *n* = 5
Dehydration
Acute pancreatitis
Acute cardiorespiratory failure
Acute splenic sequestration *n* = 2

- Stroke and TCD coverage

Probability of overt stroke by five years of age was 1.1% (0.6%–1.9%) in SS/SB° patients only, as illustrated in Figure 3a and incidence rate of stroke at five years was 0.22/100 person–years (0.12–0.38). Twelve patients experienced overt stroke at a median age of 3.1 years (interquartile range (IQR), 2.2–4.3). All had an SS genotype and six had never been investigated by TCD before the occurrence of stroke. Among the remaining six patients who had undergone at least one prior TCD examination (performed at a median age of 2.1 years (1.8–2.2)), four patients had at least one normal TCD, one had a conditional TCD, and one had twice had an inconclusive TCD examination (the child was restless). Following stroke, all 12 patients were chronically transfused.

Overall, the very first TCD screening in the SS/SB° population (*n* = 1164) was performed before two and three years of age in 56% and 81% of patients, respectively. A total of 81 (7%) children had not benefitted from TCD screening at five years, with comparable numbers of unscreened children across regions. However, the proportion of unscreened children varied according to the center size with the lowest% of unscreened children in the two largest centers (5 (2.4%) versus 15 (16%) in the smallest centers) (Table 2). The median number of annual TCD in children above the age of 2 was 0.8 (0.5–1).

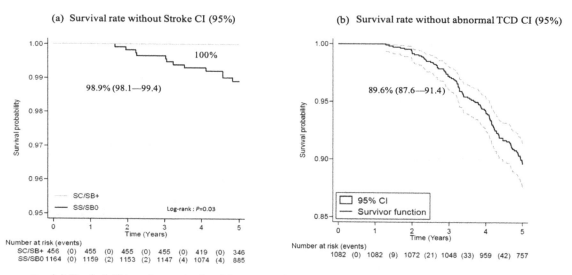

Figure 3. (**a**) Probability of survival without stroke; (**b**) probability of survival without abnormal transcranial Doppler (TCD) in children with SS/SB° disease.

The overall probability of abnormal TCD (velocities ≥200 cm/s) at five years of age was 10.4% (8.6–12.4). This probability varied across regions with the highest probability in the Paris area (13.3% (10.8–16.2)) and was significantly higher in the two largest centers (20.0% (15.0–26.5)) (Table 2). The probability of abnormal TCD did not vary significantly during the study period. Probability of survival without abnormal TCD is shown in Figure 3b.

- Severe Infection and infection prophylaxis coverage

A severe infection (meningitis or septicemia) developed in 26 patients at a median age of 2.3 years (1.3–2.6), in all but two patients with SS/SB° disease. Bacteria was identified in 21 patients, with Streptococcus pneumoniae in nine patients (including one patient with SC disease). Of them, 8/9 had been fully vaccinated with PCV7 and 3/5 aged over two years with 23-valent pneumococcal polysaccharide vaccine (P23).

The outcome of severe infection was fatal in eight cases (30.8%), following pneumococcal infection in half the cases.

Overall probability of severe infection at five years was 1.6% (1.1%–2.4%) in children with SS/SB° while it was significantly lower 0.4% (0.1–1.8) in patients with SC/SB+.

- Penicillin prophylaxis and vaccination coverage

Over 99% of all SCD patients had been prescribed prophylactic penicillin, which started at a median age of 2.2 months of life (1.7–3.0). Regarding vaccination, 87% of children received at least three doses of either PCV7 or PCV13 during their first year of life. However, only 768 (47.4%) children had been fully vaccinated before age 3, i.e., had received at least four PCV and one P23. P23 was administered in 65% of patients before three years and the probability of receiving P23 was of 90% at five years. The pneumococcal immunization coverage increased according to the size of the center, ranging from 24.8% to 78.8% in centers with <10 patients to centers >100 patients (Table 2). Conversely, this coverage did not vary according to SCD genotype (data not shown).

3.3.2. Other SCD-Related Events:

At three years, 42.9% of the EVADREP cohort had experienced a first VOC and the probability of survival without VOC was 37.6% (35.2–40.0) at five years. Expectedly, this probability differed significantly according to genotypes and was 29.0% (26.3–31.7) and 59.6% (54.8–64.1) in SS/SB° and SC/SB[+], respectively, illustrated in Figure 4a.

A total of 549 children developed at least one episode of either pneumonia or ACS or both leading to a five-years probability of survival without experiencing a first episode of pneumonia/ACS of 64.8% (62.4–67.2). This probability was significantly higher for patients with SC/SB+ genotype than for those with for SS/SB° (p < 0.001); see also Figure 4b.

Among SS/SB° patients, 16.9% had experienced a first episode of acute splenic sequestration at three years and their probability of survival without SSA at five years was 77.3% (74.7–79.6). This complication was fatal in two cases. This probability differed significantly (97.1% (95–98.3)) in patients with SC/SB[+] disease, as shown in Figure 4c.

When pooling all SCD-related events (death, stroke, severe infection, VOC, acute anemia, as well as abnormal TCD, pneumonia, and/or ACS and transfusion), 58.6% of children had experienced at least one event at three years. The probability of survival without SCD-related events at five years was 10.7% (8.9–12.6) for SS/SB° patients versus 46.3% (41.5–51) for SC/SB+.

At three years, 78.1% of all children had experienced a first hospitalization and the probability rose to 89.9% (88.3–91.3) by five years of age.

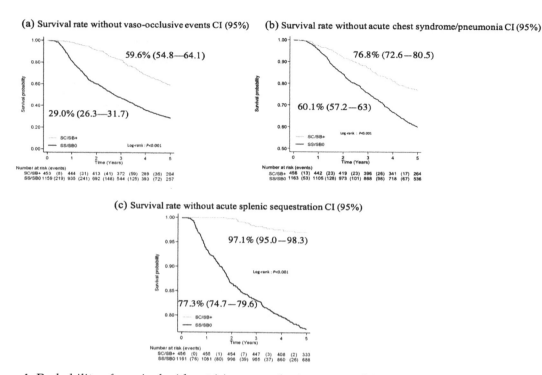

Figure 4. Probability of survival without (**a**) vaso-occlusive events, (**b**) acute chest syndrome/pneumonia, (**c**) acute splenic sequestration.

3.3.3. Disease Modifying Therapy and Other Therapeutic Measures

- Transfusion

The probability of being transfused at least once at five years was 65.2% (62.3–68.0) in SS/SB° patients and 11.8% (9.1–15.2) in patients with SC/SB$^+$ genotypes (Table 4). Splenectomy/cholecystectomy: In SS/SB° children, the probability of splenectomy was 7.0% (5.6–8.7) by five years as opposed to 0.3% (0.04–1.9) by five years in children with other genotypes (no children with SC/SB$^+$ disease was splenectomized at three years). Cholecystectomy concerned only children with SS/SB° with a probability of 3.7% (2.7–5.1) by five years of age.

Table 4. Proportion of therapeutic intervention or disease modifying therapy initiation by three years of age and probability by five years of age.

	All	SS/SB°	SC/SB$^+$	P Value †
First transfusion				
by 3 years	32.8% (30.6–35.2)	43.8% (41.0–46.2)	4.8% (3.2–7.3)	
by 5 years	50.1% (47.6–52.6)	65.2% (62.3–68.0)	1.8% (9.1–15.2)	<0.001
Splenectomy				
by 3 years	1.9% (1.4–2.7)	2.7% (1.9–3.8)	0	
by 5 years	5.1% (4.1–6.3)	7.0% (5.6–8.7)	0.3% (0.04–1.9)	<0.001
Cholecystectomy				
by 3 years	0.1% (0.03–0.5)	0.2% (0.04–0.7)	0	
by 5 years	2.7% (2.0–3.7)	3.7% (2.7–5.1)	0	<0.001
Chronic Transfusion program *				
by 3 years	7.0% (5.9–8.4)	9.7% (8.1–11.6)	0.2% (0.03–1.6)	
by 5 years	13.2% (11.6–15.0)	18.4% (16.2–20.8)	0.2% (0.03–1.6)	<0.001
Hydroxyurea				
by 3 years	1.4% (0.9–2.1)	1.9% (1.3–2.9)	0	
by 5 years	9.8% (8.4–11.5)	13.7% (11.7–15.9)	0	<0.001

* A chronic transfusion program was defined by a duration > 3 months, † log-rank test for comparison of SS/SB° versus SC/SB+ patients at 5 years.

- Chronic transfusion:

Overall, the probability by five years of age to have benefitted from a chronic TF program was 13.2% (11.6–15) and concerned a total of 204 patients, all but one with SS/SB°. Indication for initiation of the first TF program in SCA patients was stroke in 10 cases (4.9%); acute splenic sequestration in 75 (36.8%); abnormal TCD in 76 (37.2%), and other reasons in 42 (20.6%), including vaso-occlusive events in 22 cases, additional neurovascular reasons in 14, and severe anemia in 6. At the time of data collection, the TF program was ongoing in 101 (49.5%) patients and had been halted for the remaining 103 children. Out of 60 children who were initially transfused for acute splenic sequestration and discontinued, 39 (65%) were thereafter splenectomized; among 23 children who discontinued TF initiated for abnormal TCD, 12 were thereafter switched to HU, 4 underwent HSCT, and 5 had no specified subsequent treatment. Among 15 who stopped TF initiated for ACS/VOC, 14 were switched to HU, while the last patient had no subsequent treatment. The remaining five children had miscellaneous indications for both initiating and stopping TF. The mean duration for those in whom the program was discontinued was 1.1 year (0.7–1.9). Probability of receiving a first transfusion program by five years of age was significantly increased in Paris area versus other regions and significantly increased in the largest centers (Tables 2 and 4).

- Hydroxyurea (HU):

In children with SS/SB°, the proportion of treated patients by three years of age was 1.9% (1.3–2.9) and the probability was 13.7% (11.7–15.9) at five years. No patient with SC/SB⁺ disease was treated with HU. At five years, among the 145 children who were initiated on HU, 137 (94.5%) were still on treatment. There was no major difference in the proportion of treated children according to regions, but there was a significant difference according to the size of the centers, with an increased probability in the largest centers (Tables 2 and 4).

- Hematopoietic stem cell transplantation (HSCT):

Only nine patients with SS/SB° underwent HSCT before the age of five, at a median age of 4.1 (4.0–4.4). Indication for HSCT was alloimmunization in one case, VOC despite HU in one case, acute splenic sequestrations in one case, and cerebral vasculopathy in six cases (abnormal TCD in five patients).

4. Discussion

This study allows for the first time, to the best of our knowledge, a "real world" analysis on a national scale of both the early burden and mortality of sickle cell disease in a high-income country where up-to-date standard of care is easily available. Outcomes regarding 1620 children born between 2006 and 2010 and evaluated at five years show a very low SCD-related mortality and demonstrates that frequency of serious SCD-related complications such as severe infection and stroke have drastically declined. In contrast, the overall burden of the disease remained very high with a sustained elevated proportion of abnormal TCD results, VOC, ASS, ACS, transfusion requirement, hospital admissions, and chronic transfusion programs, contrasting sharply with a very low fraction of children benefitting from disease modifying or curative therapy, namely hydroxyurea and HSCT. Overall, 8.5% of the children identified following NBS were lost to follow-up at the time of data collection, with a fraction of them known as not residing in France. In this study, overall mortality rate for all patients was 0.23/100 person–years during the first five years of life and overall probability of survival was of 98.9%. Although the rate of death between 1–4 years of age remained higher than in the French general population for this age-group during the same period (0.19 versus 0.03/100), [12] these results align with a recent UK national study [8] that showed a reduced mortality in children under five (death rate of 0.17/100 person–years of follow-up for all sickle cell disorders and 0.26 per 100 person–years in homozygous children) or older reports from pediatric cohorts in similar high-income settings (Dallas cohort, 1983–2007, 0.52/100 patient–years [6], New York, 2000–2008, 0.38/100 person–years in the first two years of life) [13], East London (1982–2005, no deaths at five years) [5] or regional French cohorts (0.25 and 0.32/100 patient–years, respectively in North East Paris area and Créteil) [4,7]. Arguably, our study differs by focusing on the first five years of life only, but in SCD these are the most vulnerable years, along with young adulthood when a second peak of mortality occurs after transitioning [14]. Residual risks of stroke by five years of age was low (1.1%) in the range found in children benefitting from early TCD screening (0.7%–1.9%) [4]. Likewise, probability of severe infection (meningitis or septicemia) was low (1.6%), despite a known persistent increased risk of invasive pneumococcal infection with a high mortality rate in SCA patients [15,16]. This low rate probably reflects the effectiveness of pneumococcal vaccination and penicillin prophylaxis, as reported consistently in other settings [17]. Indeed, vaccination coverage regarding conjugated vaccine was 87% during first year of life, although this percentage fell to 47.4% by age three regarding full pneumococcal vaccination including P23 at two years, mainly because P23 was generally administered later i.e., during the fourth or fifth year of life. In comparison, vaccination coverage, which included both PCV and P23, was 64.3% at five years in a state study in children benefitting from Medicaid in the US [18]. Almost all infants in the EVADREP cohort benefited from early prophylactic penicillin initiated within three months of NBS, a figure comparable to a nation-wide report in England, [8] although there was no further information on compliance issues in either studies. Regarding TCD screening, a vast majority of children at risk (80.5%) were investigated with TCD before three years of age and the probability rose to 93% by age 5, contrasting sharply with cross sectional reports of TCD annual screening rates ranging from 22% to 44% in the US [19].

In addition to the known beneficial effect of current management guidelines, these results also reflect a real-life efficient access to medical care for patients in the French healthcare system, including "vulnerable" populations like patients with SCD who are, for the majority, children of recently immigrated families with significant socio-economic difficulties [7]. In France, access to care for children under six is highly facilitated through a network of primary medical care where free follow-up and immunization is offered. Additional specific prophylactic and therapeutic measures for SCD children are free of charge once the diagnosis is confirmed, regardless of age or the region of follow-up. Centers are organized in a national network where patients may easily access emergency departments and may be addressed to tertiary hospitals for expertise if necessary. In these conditions that actually allow for the practical application of guidelines, there was indeed an overall very good implementation of recommendations.

Despite these favorable conditions, it is noteworthy to mention that 6 of the 12 strokes occurred in children who had not been screened. Likewise, severe infections (including pneumococcal) still accounted for the main cause of death. Although severe pneumococcal infections most often occurred in patients fully vaccinated with PVC as previously reported, [17] further improvement can be achieved by increasing P23 vaccination coverage. One striking and recurrent result was the somewhat counter intuitive finding of decreased TCD and vaccination coverage in smaller centers, along with higher rates of patients lost to follow-up. It could indeed be hypothesized that with fewer patients, the coverage would be better. In fact, it is probable that not only do larger centers have specialized staff to ensure standard of care surveillance, but also dedicated time to track down non-attenders and reschedule missed appointments. Smaller centers, conversely, deal with pediatric patients with much more variable medical conditions, are probably less focused on specific needs, and are not staff-equipped to follow-up on compliance or educational issues. In addition, TCD screening requires specialized trained physicians and is generally performed in larger centers at farther distance from the patient's residence, a factor that was shown to negatively influence TCD utilization rates [20].

This study showed that 8.4% of children screened at birth were lost to follow-up in their first five years of life at the time of data collection. While there is no possibility of speculating on the outcomes, because this a nation-wide study, it is probable that none of these children died nor had a severe event such as stroke or severe infection in France. While such events may still have occurred abroad, it is probable that mortality and severe morbidity rates were not significantly biased by this missing data.

Although the rate of patients lost to follow-up is similar on a national scale to results from regional or single center European cohorts, which range from 6%–11% [4,7], the figure remains significant and calls for further improvement in order to decrease the number of non-attenders.

Results on less severe outcomes such as abnormal TCD, VOC, ASS, ACS, and hospitalization rates showed a very high burden of the disease with no improvement in their frequency when compared to cohorts in the previous decade [5]. The overall probability of abnormal TCD at five years was 10.4%, comparable to 7% in the East London cohort but lower than in regional French cohorts from tertiary centers (around 20%), [4,5] a difference that may reflect the "large center effect" with presumably a higher proportion of severe patients referred for tertiary expertise and/or monitored more intensively. Nearly 2/3 of children had experienced a VOC by five years and the same proportion (65.2%) was transfused at least once before age 5. The probability of an SCD-related event and the rate of first hospitalization were very high (79.3% and 89.9%, respectively, at five years). In sharp contrast, disease-modifying or curative therapies were only given to a small fraction of patients: HSCT was performed in only nine children while hydroxyurea therapy was prescribed in only 10%. More classical therapy like chronic transfusion programs was, on the other hand, widely used since 13% of the cohort was treated at least temporarily with a chronic transfusion program before five years. Arguably, this cohort was born in 2006–2010, i.e., before the publication of HU trials in infants [21] and the extension of indication as in the US to all children above nine months regardless of clinical severity [22] or as an alternative to transfusion in selected children with abnormal TCD [4,23]. In addition, HU was and still is licensed in France for children over two years with severe vaso-occlusive symptoms. It is likely that in the upcoming years, the proportion of young children treated with HU (or additional drugs) will increase. Likewise, the very small number of children who benefitted from HSCT during the study period probably reflects the relative reluctance of SCD physicians in addressing very young patients to transplant if they have not experienced severe complications, particularly without prior HU treatment. Recent studies have shown significant improvement with time of long-term results following matched-sibling-donor stem cell transplantation offering 97.8% event-free survival at five years post-transplant among 190 patients transplanted after year 2000 [24]. In addition, outcomes are improved when HSCT is performed at a younger age [25]. This should further encourage HSCT in SCD, given the high burden of the disease.

5. Conclusions

In conclusion, this study shows, on a national scale, the benefits of NBS and preventive measures, confirms the good implementation of these measures, and does not reveal major disparity across regions or centers, although the proportion of severe patients is highest in larger centers, most often located in the Paris area. Notwithstanding, this study underscores the importance of referral of patients to tertiary centers where systematic annual specialized work-up may be more readily performed and general educational or immunization issues double-checked by dedicated healthcare providers in order to further improve vaccination and TCD coverage, notably. In addition, this study reveals a very low proportion of children treated with HU or HSCT despite a sustained burden of the disease. Predictably, future studies will demonstrate an increase in disease modifying therapy use. In addition, given the ongoing progress in HSCT outcomes, indications will broaden so that altogether curative treatments (potentially including gene therapy [26]) will hopefully benefit more children.

Author Contributions: Conceptualization, I.T., M.D.M., and F.D.; methodology, E.B., M.B., C.A., and I.T.; validation, I.T., E.B., M.B., G.I., N.C., C.P., M.B., G.E., C.G., M.E.-J., E.L., B.Q., M.-H.O., N.G., A.C., and C.D.; formal analysis, V.B., E.B., F.D., and IT.; resources, I.T.; data curation, E.B., N.C., F.B., J.B., and M.B.; investigation, F.D.; methodology, C.A., F.B., N.C., E.B., J.B., M.B., and I.T.; writing—original draft preparation, V.B.; writing—review and editing, V.B. and I.T.; supervision, C.A., M.E.-J., M.B., C.P., and I.T.; project administration and funding acquisition, I.T.

Acknowledgments: The authors would like to acknowledge the important contribution of Zineddine Haouari, in charge of the database in Robert Debré Hospital and Cédric Viallette, data manager in Henri Mondor Hospital. The authors would like to thank the following additional physicians who collaborated in the study: R Akil (Neuilly Sur Seine); S Allali (Paris Necker) E Akodjeno (Chartres); B Ali (Auxerre); R Amira, A Malric (St Denis); C Armari (Grenoble); C Badens; G Michel (Marseille) C Barrey (Bry Sur Marne); J Bassil (Laval); P Benhaim (Bondy); M Benemou (Gonesse); P Bensaid (Argenteuil); D Bodet (Caen); R Campagni (Mulhouse); L Carausu (Brest); MP Castex, JM Pattier (Toulouse); F Cazassus (St-Martin); D Celicourt, G Elana, Y Hatchuel, AC Isidore, (Martinique); O Charara (Versailles); ML Couec, C Thomas (Nantes); G Couillault (Dijon); JP Diara, L Doumdo, M Petras, G Sibille (Guadeloupe); C De Gennes, L Le Carrer (Orsay); A Desbree (St Etienne); B Koehl, F Missud, L Holvoet (Paris R. Debré); A Gauthier (Lyon); JP Vannier (Rouen); A Duval, Z Osman (Creil); P Ferre, L Krayem, H See (Montreuil); J Furioli (Mantes La Jolie); V Gajdos (Clamart); N Garrec (Lagny); S Gatineau (Le Havre); V Giaccobi (Le Mans); E Georget (Villeneuve Saint Georges); F Gouraud, M Monfort (Meaux); C Guitton (Paris Kremlin Bicêtre); RM Herbigneaux (Chambery); N Houaime (Dunkerque); M Jehanne, P Nyombe (St Denis de la Réunion); A Kamdem (Centre Intercommunal de Créteil); T Khalifeh (Poitiers); M Lallande (Montpellier); A Lambilliotte (Lille); JM Perini (Lille); O Le Jars (Tours); V Li Thiao Te (Amiens); L Lutz (Strasbourg); L Mangyanda (Beaumont); C Manteau (Valence); A May (Evry); S Mensah (ROFSED); E Merlin (Clermont-Ferrand); F Monpoux (Nice); B Monnier (Eaubonne); G Mousset (Vannes); S Muller (Rambouillet); J Nzonzila (Melun); S Roullaud (Angoulême); S Ndizeye (Orléans); B Pellegrino (Poissy); I Pellier (Angers); MH Pierre (Roubaix); C Piguet (Limoges); C Pluchard (Reims); C Stoven (St Pierre De La Réunion); B Retali (Cergy Pontoise); C Runel (Bordeaux); P Simon (Besançon); O Sindihebura (Blois); V Soussan (Ambroise Pare); D Steschenko (Nancy); F Toutain (Rennes), A Vareliette (St Brieuc); L Vordonis, S Ducrocq (Longjumeau); A Zakaria (Aulnay); A Zelinsky (Niort); B Zimmermann (Troyes).

References

1. Gaston, M.H.; Verter, J.I.; Woods, G.; Pegelow, C.; Presbury, G.; Zarkowsky, H.; Iyer, R.; Lobel, J.S.; Gill, F.M.; Ritchey, K.; et al. Prophylaxis with Oral Penicillin in Children with Sickle Cell Anemia. *N. Engl. J. Med.* **1986**, *314*, 1593–1599. [CrossRef] [PubMed]

2. Adamkiewicz, T.V.; Silk, B.J.; Howgate, J.; Baughman, W.; Strayhorn, G.; Sullivan, K.; Farley, M.M. Effectiveness of the 7-Valent Pneumococcal Conjugate Vaccine in Children with Sickle Cell Disease in the First Decade of Life. *Pediatric* **2008**, *121*, 562–569. [CrossRef] [PubMed]

3. McCarville, M.B.; Goodin, G.S.; Fortner, G.; Li, C.S.; Smeltzer, M.P.; Adams, R.; Wang, W. Evaluation of a comprehensive transcranial doppler screening program for children with sickle cell anemia. *Pediatr. Blood Cancer* **2008**, *50*, 818–821. [CrossRef] [PubMed]

4. Bernaudin, F.; Verlhac, S.; Arnaud, C.; Kamdem, A.; Chevret, S.; Hau, I.; Coïc, L.; Leveillé, E.; Lemarchand, E.; Lesprit, E.; et al. Impact of early transcranial Doppler screening and intensive therapy on cerebral vasculopathy outcome in a newborn sickle cell anemia cohort. *Blood* **2011**, *117*, 1130–1140. [CrossRef] [PubMed]

5. Telfer, P.; Coen, P.; Chakravorty, S.; Wilkey, O.; Evans, J.; Newell, H.; Smalling, B.; Amos, R.; Stephens, A.; Rogers, D.; et al. Clinical outcomes in children with sickle cell disease living in England: A neonatal cohort in East London. *Haematologica* **2007**, *92*, 905–912. [CrossRef] [PubMed]

6. Quinn, C.T.; Rogers, Z.R.; McCavit, T.L.; Buchanan, G.R. Improved survival of children and adolescents with sickle cell disease. *Blood* **2010**, *115*, 3447–3452. [CrossRef] [PubMed]

7. Couque, N.; Girard, D.; Ducrocq, R.; Boizeau, P.; Haouari, Z.; Missud, F.; Holvoet, L.; Ithier, G.; Belloy, M.; Odièvre, M.-H.; et al. Improvement of medical care in a cohort of newborns with sickle-cell disease in North Paris: Impact of national guidelines. *Br. J. Haematol.* **2016**, *173*, 927–937. [CrossRef] [PubMed]

8. Streetly, A.; Sisodia, R.; Dick, M.; Latinovic, R.; Hounsell, K.; Dormandy, E. Evaluation of newborn sickle cell screening programme in England: 2010–2016. *Arch. Dis. Child.* **2018**, *103*, 648–653. [CrossRef]

9. *Dépistage Néonatal de la Drépanocytose en France, Rapport D'orientation*; Haute Autorité de Santé: Saint-Denis, France, 2013.

10. Adams, R.; McKie, V.; Nichols, F.; Carl, E.; Zhang, D.-L.; McKie, K.; Figueroa, R.; Litaker, M.; Thompson, W.; Hess, D. The Use of Transcranial Ultrasonography to Predict Stroke in Sickle Cell Disease. *N. Engl. J. Med.* **1992**, *326*, 605–610. [CrossRef]

11. ALD n° 10—Syndromes Drépanocytaires Majeurs de L'enfant et de L'adolescent. Haute Autorité de Santé. Available online: https://www.has-sante.fr/jcms/c_938890/fr/ald-n-10-syndromes-drepanocytaires-majeurs-de-l-enfant-et-de-l-adolescent (accessed on 18 September 2019).

12. La Mortalité Infantile est Stable Depuis dix ans Après des Décennies de Baisse—Insee Focus–117. Available online: https://www.insee.fr/fr/statistiques/3560308 (accessed on 24 July 2019).

13. Wang, Y.; Liu, G.; Caggana, M.; Kennedy, J.; Zimmerman, R.; Oyeku, S.O.; Werner, E.M.; Grant, A.M.; Green, N.S.; Grosse, S.D. Mortality of New York children with sickle cell disease identified through newborn screening. *Genet. Med.* **2015**, *17*, 452–459. [CrossRef]

14. Hamideh, D.; Alvarez, O. Sickle cell disease related mortality in the United States (1999–2009). *Pediatr. Blood Cancer* **2013**, *60*, 1482–1486. [CrossRef] [PubMed]

15. Payne, A.B.; Link-Gelles, R.; Azonobi, I.; Hooper, W.C.; Beall, B.W.; Jorgensen, J.H.; Juni, B.; Moore, M. Invasive Pneumococcal Disease among Children with and without Sickle Cell Disease in the United States, 1998–2009. *Pediatr. Infect. Dis. J.* **2013**, *32*, 1308. [CrossRef] [PubMed]

16. Oligbu, G.; Collins, S.; Sheppard, C.; Fry, N.; Dick, M.; Streetly, A.; Ladhani, S. Risk of Invasive Pneumococcal Disease in Children with Sickle Cell Disease in England: A National Observational Cohort Study, 2010–2015. *Arch. Dis. Child.* **2018**, *103*, 643–647. [PubMed]

17. Oligbu, G.; Fallaha, M.; Pay, L.; Ladhani, S. Risk of invasive pneumococcal disease in children with sickle cell disease in the era of conjugate vaccines: A systematic review of the literature. *Br. J. Haematol.* **2019**, *185*, 743–751. [CrossRef] [PubMed]

18. Reeves, S.L.; Jary, H.K.; Gondhi, J.P.; Kleyn, M.; Wagner, A.L.; Dombkowski, K.J. Pneumococcal vaccination coverage among children with sickle cell anemia, sickle cell trait, and normal hemoglobin. *Pediatr. Blood Cancer* **2018**, *65*, e27282. [CrossRef] [PubMed]

19. Reeves, S.L.; Madden, B.; Freed, G.L.; Dombkowski, K.J. Transcranial Doppler Screening Among Children and Adolescents with Sickle Cell Anemia. *JAMA Pediatr.* **2016**, *170*, 550–556. [CrossRef] [PubMed]

20. Armstrong-Wells, J.; Grimes, B.; Sidney, S.; Kronish, D.; Shiboski, S.C.; Adams, R.J.; Fullerton, H.J. Utilization of TCD screening for primary stroke prevention in children with sickle cell disease. *Neurology* **2009**, *72*, 1316–1321. [CrossRef] [PubMed]

21. Wang, W.C.; Ware, R.E.; Miller, S.T.; Iyer, R.V.; Casella, J.F.; Minniti, C.P.; Rana, S.; Thornburg, C.D.; Rogers, Z.R.; Kalpatthi, R.V.; et al. Hydroxycarbamide in very young children with sickle-cell anaemia: A multicentre, randomised, controlled trial (BABY HUG). *Lancet* **2011**, *377*, 1663–1672. [CrossRef]

22. Yawn, B.P.; Buchanan, G.R.; Afenyi-Annan, A.N.; Ballas, S.K.; Hassell, K.L.; James, A.H.; Jordan, L.; Lanzkron, S.M.; Lottenberg, R.; Savage, W.J.; et al. Management of sickle cell disease: Summary of the 2014 evidence-based report by expert panel members. *JAMA* **2014**, *312*, 1033–1048. [CrossRef]

23. Ware, R.E.; Davis, B.R.; Schultz, W.H.; Brown, R.C.; Aygun, B.; Sarnaik, S.; Odame, I.; Fuh, B.; George, A.; Owen, W.; et al. Hydroxycarbamide versus chronic transfusion for maintenance of transcranial doppler flow velocities in children with sickle cell anaemia-TCD With Transfusions Changing to Hydroxyurea (TWiTCH): A multicentre, open-label, phase 3, non-inferiority trial. *Lancet* **2016**, *387*, 661–670. [CrossRef]

24. Bernaudin, F.; Dalle, J.H.; Bories, D.; De Latour, R.P.; Robin, M.; Bertrand, Y.; Pondarre, C.; Vannier, J.P.; Neven, B.; Kuentz, M.; et al. Long-term event-free survival, chimerism and fertility outcomes in 234 patients with sickle-cell anemia younger than 30 years after myeloablative conditioning and matched-sibling transplantation in France. *Haematologica* **2019**, *104*. [CrossRef] [PubMed]

25. Gluckman, E.; Cappelli, B.; Bernaudin, F.; Labopin, M.; Volt, F.; Carreras, J.; Simões, B.P.; Ferster, A.; Dupont, S.; De La Fuente, J.; et al. Sickle cell disease: An international survey of results of HLA-identical sibling hematopoietic stem cell transplantation. *Blood* **2017**, *129*, 1548–1556. [CrossRef] [PubMed]

26. Hacein-Bey-Abina, S.; Magrin, E.; Caccavelli, L.; Bourget, P.; Bartolucci, P.; Weber, L.; Beuzard, Y.; De Montalembert, M.; Blanche, S.; Leboulch, P.; et al. Gene Therapy in a Patient with Sickle Cell Disease. *N. Engl. J. Med.* **2017**, *376*, 848–855.

2

Pulse Oximetry Screening in Germany—Historical Aspects and Future Perspectives

Frank-Thomas Riede [1,*], Christian Paech [1] and Thorsten Orlikowsky [2]

[1]   Department of Paediatric Cardiology, Heart Centre, University of Leipzig, 04289 Leipzig, Strümpellstr. 39, Germany; christian.paech@medizin.uni-leipzig.de

[2]   Department of Neonatology, University Childrens Hospital Aachen, 52072 Aachen, Pauwelsstr. 30, Germany; torlikowsky@ukaachen.de

*   Correspondence: frank-thomas.riede@medizin.uni-leipzig.de

Abstract: In January 2017, pulse oximetry screening was legally implemented in routine neonatal care in Germany. The preceding developments, which were the prerequisite for this step, are described in the specific context of Germany's health care system. Continued evaluation of the method is imperative and may lead to modifications in the screening protocol, ideally in accordance with the efforts in other countries.

Keywords: critical congenital heart disease; pulse oximetry screening; Germany

1. Historical Aspects: From Clinical Data

The most severe, life-threatening forms of congenital heart disease (CHD) requiring intervention very early in life are termed critical (CCHD). During the last decades of the past century, advances in surgical techniques, as well as in perioperative intensive care medicine, led to an improved survival of neonates with CCHD but further progress is likely to be limited.

Delayed diagnosis of CCHD with its potential of cardiac collapse and even death has long been recognized, but its relative importance increased only with the above-mentioned developments. In Germany, Prof. P. Schneider, the former head of the department of Paediatric Cardiology at the Leipzig Heart Centre, described addressing the postnatal diagnostic gap in CCHD as a challenge not only for paediatric cardiologists but for all involved in perinatal care, thus requiring an interdisciplinary and collaborative approach [1].

The first step was to increase the awareness of the problem by establishing and participating in regional educational programs for paediatricians, neonatologists and midwives, starting in the first years of the last decade. Although data from the literature at that time was very limited, using pulse oximetry screening to reduce the diagnostic gap in CCHD has been informally proposed in light of its well-known advantages (availability, ease of use, non-invasiveness, and low cost) [1–4].

A survey in Saxony (the federal state in which the Leipzig Heart Centre is situated) revealed that in January 2006, 62% (n = 29) of all responding perinatal and neonatal units (n = 47; response rate 92%) used pulse oximetry screening regularly. Thus, the prerequisites were ideal to perform a prospective multicentre study on pulse oximetry screening. In the study population, the prenatal detection rate of CCHD was comparatively high (60%). However, there was still a diagnostic gap of 20%, which could be reduced to 4.4% by pulse oximetry screening [5]. Based on the data from this study, the working Groups for Perinatology and Neonatology of the Saxonian Medical Association recommended the implementation of pulse oximetry screening in routine care in October 2009. At around the same time, Tautz et al. published their experience with pulse oximetry screening paralleled by the large series from Norway and Sweden [6–8].

In December 2009, a nationwide survey on pulse oximetry screening in Germany was conducted. A questionnaire was sent to all 890 perinatal and neonatal units; the response rate was 29% ($n = 255$). In 46% of the responding units, pulse oximetry screening had already been established. Although, in the majority of cases, it had only been established in the last three years. However, the percentage of units performing pulse oximetry screening showed remarkable regional differences, possibly at least in part related to the regional effects of the activities in Saxony (Figure 1).

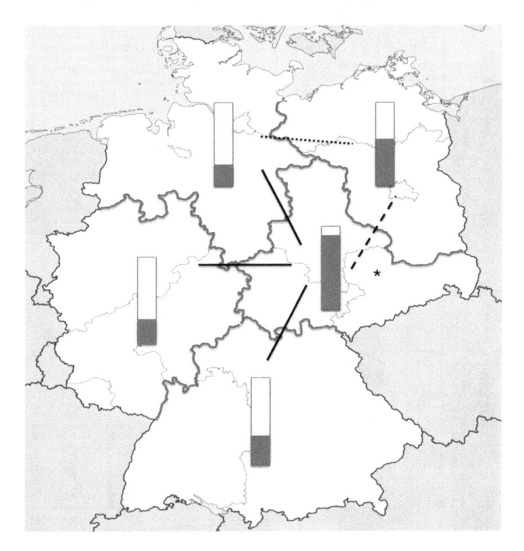

Figure 1. Pulse oximetry screening in Germany in December 2009. Green bars indicate the percentage of perinatal and neonatal units performing pulse oximetry screening as per December 2009 in five regions in Germany. The black lines indicate the level of significance (dotted line: $p < 0.05$, dashed line: $p < 0.01$, solid line, $p < 0.001$). The asterisk indicates the federal state of Saxony. Source of the map: adaptation from svg/2000px-Germany_location_map.svg.png; author: NordNordWest; http://creativecommons.org/licenses/by-sa/3.0/de/legalcode.

Another interesting finding was to reveal of differences in the use of pulse oximetry screening depending on the level of perinatal care. The latter had been defined in Germany in 2006 in an attempt to centralize the management of risk pregnancies and extreme prematurity (Table 1). Pulse oximetry screening was used less in obstetrical clinics (Figure 2). This may, in part, be explained by the expected low risk profile for pregnancies and neonates in these units. Yet, as existing strategies failed to completely predict CCHD, pulse oximetry screening may be especially useful in these settings.

Table 1. Levels of neonatal care in Germany (modified after [9,10]).

Level of Care	Admission Criteria
Perinatal centre level 1	Expected prematurity with a birth weight of <1250 g or a gestational age of <29 weeks triplet pregnancy and gestational age <33 weeks; multiple pregnancy Prenatal diagnosis of any fetal or maternal condition necessitating immediate postnatal intensive care (critical congenital heart disease, diaphragmatic hernia, myelomeningocele, gastroschisis)
Perinatal centre level 2	Expected prematurity with a birth weight of 1250–1499 g or a gestational age of ≥29 to <32 weeks HELLP syndrome Intrauterine growth restriction <3rd percentile Insulin-dependent gestational diabetes with elevated risk for the fetus/newborn
Perinatal clinic	Expected prematurity with a birth weight of ≥1500 g or a gestational age of ≥32 to <36 weeks Intrauterine growth restriction between third and tenth percentile Insulin-dependent gestational diabetes without elevated risk for the fetus/newborn
Obstetrical clinic	Gestational age ≥36 weeks, uncomplicated delivery expected

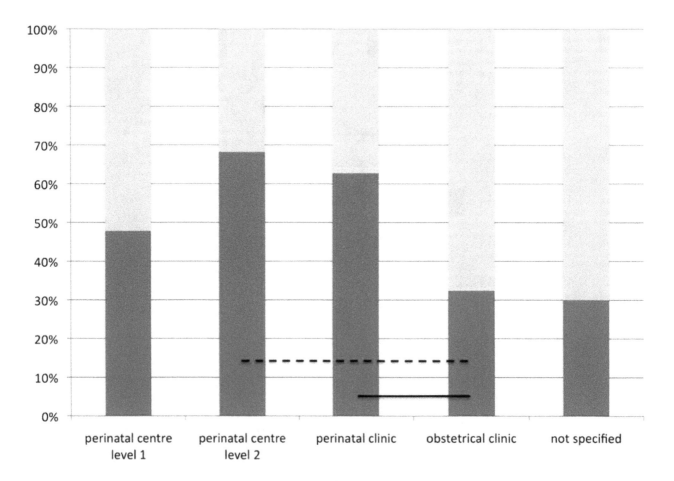

Figure 2. Pulse oximetry screening and level of neonatal care. Green bars indicate percentage of units using pulse oximetry screening as per December 2009 in Germany. Black lines indicate level of significance (dashed line: $p < 0.01$, solid line, $p < 0.001$).

In light of the increasing body of evidence on the benefits of pulse oximetry screening [11,12], the German Society for Paediatric Cardiology supported the use of pulse oximetry screening in 2011 and formulated a statement with recommendations for practical aspects of its implementation in 2013 [13,14]. Likewise, the German Society for Neonatology and Paediatric intensive care (GNPI) recommended the use of pulse oximetry screening in its guidelines for neonatal care in 2012 [15]. However, the effects of these nonbinding recommendations remained unknown.

2. To Legal Regulation

In the nationwide survey of 2009 only 26% of perinatal and neonatal units considered it necessary to have legal regulations in place, in case pulse oximetry screening should be implemented. However, patient representatives had a different view. A group led by the "Bundesverband herzkranke Kinder" (BVHK) initiated the development of a legal regulation.

Germany's national health care insurance system, introduced in 1883, has been highly regulated. Since 1975, more than 90% of the population have been enrolled in the statutory health insurance, the remaining 10% have been nearly completely covered by private or other health insurance [16]. Thus, regulations concerning the scope of health care services provided by insurers affect almost the entire population.

The regulation of medical care and the implementation of legal requirements on new drugs and methods of treatment by directives are the central tasks of a federal committee (Gemeinsamer Bundesausschuss, G-BA). It was established in January 2004 as the highest decision-making body of the joint self-administration of physicians, dentists, psychotherapists, hospitals and health insurance providers.

Preventive examinations and screening tests in neonates are regulated in the Directive on Early Detection of Diseases in Children up to the age of six years. Currently, each newborn is entitled to three examinations immediately after birth (U1), between the third and tenth day of life (U2), and at the end of (or early after) the neonatal period (fourth to fifth week of life, U3). Extended metabolic screening, hearing screening (since 2009), an ultrasound of the hips and the Brückner test (fundoscopy, since 2016) are also included.

The implementation of a new method requires a formal consultation process and a subsequent positive resolution by the G-BA. The initiation of such a process may be requested by independent members of the G-BA, by health insurers, the Association of Statutory Health Insurance Physicians, the corresponding association of dentists, the German Hospital Society and patient representatives, but not by physicians or medical professional societies.

In September 2012, the group of patient representatives mentioned above submitted an application at the G-BA to initiate a consultation process on pulse oximetry screening, which was granted in November 2012. In June 2013, an independent scientific organisation, the Institute for Quality and Cost Effectiveness in Health Care (Institut für Qualität und Wirtschaftlichkeit im Gesundheitswesen, IQWiG), was commissioned with a detailed analysis of the possible effects of pulse oximetry screening in the current setting of peri- and neonatal care in Germany. The evaluation was mainly based on available data from the literature, but statements from experts, national medical professional associations, and patient representatives were also included. In its final report, published in May 2015, the IQWiG concluded that current evidence suggests a benefit of pulse oximetry screening as an adjunct to the pre-existing diagnostic standard (U1 and U2) with respect to the timely diagnosis of CCHD in neonates [17].

In January 2017, after an internal evaluation of the IQWiG's report, statements from experts and medical professional associations, a decree of the G-BA was published, announcing the implementation of pulse oximetry screening in routine neonatal care in Germany [18].

The algorithm for pulse oximetry screening, as recommended by the G-BA, is shown in Figure 3. In most aspects, it is similar to the one used in the German multicentre study, published by one of the authors in 2010 [5]. However, an important difference lies in the role of echocardiography. According to the current recommendations, echocardiography may be omitted if another cause of hypoxia is found. This approach may be reasonable especially when a positive pulse oximetry screening draws attention to clinical signs suggesting other neonatal pathologies such as pneumonia or sepsis, cases in which echocardiography would only delay appropriate diagnosis and treatment.

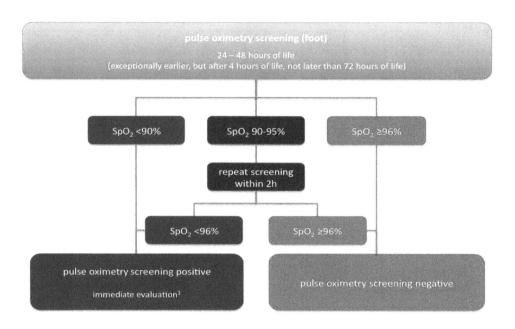

Figure 3. Algorithm for pulse oximetry screening in Germany as recommended by the Common Federal Committee (Gemeinsamer Bundesausschuss, G-BA), modified after [19] by a specialist in paediatrics, ideally with subspecialty training in neonatology/paediatric cardiology.

3. Future Perspectives

As per the decree of the G-BA, the quality and efficacy of pulse oximetry screening in Germany are going to be evaluated after its implementation. By no later than 31 December 2018, an independent scientific institution will be assigned to perform an analysis on the basis of a representative sample to answer a defined set of target parameters (Table 2). However, further aspects might also prove relevant and be included (Table 3).

Table 2. Target parameters for the evaluation of pulse oximetry screening after its implementation in Germany as defined by the G-BA [18].

Number and Percentage of Newborns
-      having received pulse oximetry screening   -   with a negative screening result on the first measurement ($SpO_2 \geq 96\%$)   -   with a positive screening result on the first measurement ($SpO_2 < 90\%$)   -   with an abnormal result on the first measurement with the need to repeat the test (SpO_2 90–95%)   -   with a negative screening result on the second measurement ($SpO_2 \geq 96\%$)   -   with a positive screening result on the second measurement ($SpO_2 < 96\%$)   -   referred to a paediatrician/neonatologist
False positive results   Number of newborns with CCHD detected by pulse oximetry screening   Timing of diagnostic and therapeutic procedures in newborns with CCHD

Table 3. Possible additional target parameters for the evaluation of pulse oximetry screening after its implementation in Germany.

Number and Percentage of Newborns
-      with a prenatal diagnosis of CCHD   -   with diagnosis of CCHD based on clinical signs/physical examination before pulse oximetry screening
False negative results   Detection of neonatal diseases in newborns with false positive screening results (with respect to CCHD)   Reasons for not performing pulse oximetry screening in eligible newborns

Screening is definitely better than no screening, and despite the fact that the national screening program will hopefully increase the early detection of CCHD systematically, several controversies will remain with respect to the time of screening, cut off-values, and the follow-up algorithm.

In comparison to the algorithm in the UK, suggesting an early screening before 24 h of age [11], the German, as well as the American algorithm, recommend screening between 24 h and 48 h of age as the "best screening window" [19,20]. The G-BA states that screening may be performed "in exceptional cases at the earliest of four hours after birth" to account for infants discharged from hospital within 24 h after birth. In most published data on screening before 24 h of age, the rate of false positives was up to 10 times higher (0.8% vs. 0.05%) [21]. In this respect, "false positive" means, "false test positive", i.e., no CCHD detectable in the follow-up. Nevertheless, early screening before 24 h identified more non-cardiac diseases (sepsis, persistent pulmonary hypertension of the newborn) at an early stage before newborns were symptomatic. In the German study, 18 of the 36 newborns with CCHD (50%) showed symptoms before screening [5], which is the very situation that screening aims to prevent. Thus, earlier screening might be desirable from both the neonatologist's and the paediatric cardiologist's perspective. However, the impact of pulse oximetry screening on the detection of noncardiac disease has not been evaluated systematically yet. Expanding the spectrum of target parameters for analysis of efficacy of pulse oximetry screening, as determined by the G-BA (Table 2) by additional parameters (Table 3), might provide appropriate data and allow for evidence-based modifications of the screening algorithm so that early screening and a timely diagnosis can be counterbalanced with the false positive rate. Nevertheless, one has to bear in mind that the problem of severe cardiovascular compromise related to CCHD cannot be completely avoided, neither by thorough clinical examination, nor by pulse oximetry, and not even by prenatal diagnosis. This is because for example, in neonates with hypoplastic left heart syndrome or transposition of the great arteries with restrictive or closed foramen ovale, symptoms may occur despite immediate and appropriate treatment.

Modification of the upper time limit for screening might also become necessary. The German algorithm specifies, that the screening may be performed no later than after the 2nd check-up by the paediatrician. Newborns who have already been discharged at that age, receive their standard investigation (U2) from a paediatrician either in his office or at home. This check-up has to be performed between the third and the tenth day of life. In these cases, if early screening has not been performed, substantial risk for falling into a diagnostic gap remains. Furthermore, it would be necessary for all paediatricians to use portable saturation devices for their outpatient visits (U2). For newborns born at home, midwives would have to be trained systematically.

It would be desirable that pulse oximetry screening for the detection of CCHD is recommended for all European countries. A consensus statement on its implementation includes that it should be performed with new-generation equipment that is motion tolerant, after 6 h of life or before discharge from the birthing centre (preferably within 24 h after birth), and should be done in two extremities, the right hand and either foot [22].

The majority of studies used saturations from one post ductal site—either foot. Recently, studies have employed saturations from two sites—the right hand and one foot—giving both pre- and post-ductal saturations. Therefore, rather than a single absolute saturation leading to the test result, two individual values, and also the difference between the two, contribute to the result. Although a systematic review did not identify a significant difference in sensitivity between the two methods [21], this may be explained by the preponderance of single measurement, and further analyses are necessary.

Post hoc analysis of the raw data revealed that post ductal only measurement would miss a small but significant proportion of babies that dual testing would identify [23]. This may become important in Germany considering the birth rate of approximately 800,000 per year.

In contrast to many other studies from the UK and the USA, the cut-off value was chosen to be 96%, following the experiences of the German trial [5]. Other rather big one-step screening studies used 95%. Whether this single point of saturation difference really makes a difference in specificity or false positives remains to be evaluated. However, combining regional or national studies in Europe in meta-analyses, maybe resulting in a common algorithm, is hampered by different thresholds and procedures. For example, all authors recommending a two-site screening use different combinations of thresholds and differences between measurement sites for definition of a positive screening result [7,9,20].

Prenatal echocardiography has the potential to detect virtually all forms of CCHD up to the point where, in single institutions, pulse oximetry screening for CCHD becomes ineffective [24]. Being highly dependent on operator experience and appropriate technical equipment, which are neither widely available, nor will be in the near future, prenatal detection rates in larger regions or countries remain substantially lower [25]. In Germany, the rate of prenatal diagnoses for all CHD has been 12%, ranging from approximately 5 to 68% in CCHD, depending on the type of lesion [26]. In 2013, completion of a four-chamber view has been implemented in routine pregnancy care by the G-BA. It has been estimated that this may ameliorate the prenatal detection rate up to 30–40%, concluding that pulse oximetry screening will be able to substantially contribute to a timely diagnosis of CCDH in the years to come [17].

A recent U.S. study has shown a substantial reduction of mortality from undiagnosed CCHD after the implementation of pulse oximetry screening [27]. In populations where mortality from undiagnosed CCHD was low before the introduction of pulse oximetry screening, a comparable effect might be expected on the reduction of severe morbidity in affected neonates [5,28].

4. Conclusions

In the past decade, pulse oximetry screening in Germany has made its way from clinical trials to the statutory introduction into clinical routine as an adjunct to prenatal diagnosis and clinical examination. This will hopefully further improve the prognosis of infants with CCHD. Continuing evaluation of its effectiveness is necessary to allow for modifications of the screening protocol when appropriate.

Author Contributions: F.-T.R. and T.O. conceived and designed the work. C.P. thoroughly revised the manuscript.

Acknowledgments: We thank Andy Ewer for his advice on creating the manuscript. We are grateful to Franziska Wagner for language editing of the manuscript. There is no funding to be disclosed.

References

1. Schneider, P.; Kostelka, M.; Kändler, L.; Möckel, A.; Riede, F.T.; Dähnert, I. Die diagnostische Lücke bei neonatalen Herzerkrankungen—Herausforderung für Neonatologie und Kinderkardiologie. *Kinder und Jugendmed.* **2004**, *4*, 188–193. [CrossRef]
2. Bakr, A.F.; Habib, H.S. Combining Pulse Oximetry and Clinical Examination in Screening for Congenital Heart Disease. *Pediatr. Cardiol.* **2005**, *26*, 832–835. [CrossRef] [PubMed]
3. Hoke, T.R.; Donohue, P.K.; Bawa, P.K.; Mitchell, R.D.; Pathak, A.; Rowe, P.C.; Byrne, B.J. Oxygen Saturation as a Screening Test for Critical Congenital Heart Disease: A Preliminary Study. *Pediatr. Cardiol.* **2002**, *23*, 403–409. [CrossRef] [PubMed]
4. Koppel, R.I.; Druschel, C.M.; Carter, T.; Goldberg, B.E.; Mehta, P.N.; Talwar, R.; Bierman, F.Z. Effectiveness of Pulse Oximetry Screening for Congenital Heart Disease in Asymptomatic Newborns. *Pediatrics* **2003**, *111*, 451–455. [CrossRef] [PubMed]
5. Riede, F.T.; Wörner, C.; Dähnert, I.; Möckel, A.; Kostelka, M.; Schneider, P. Effectiveness of neonatal pulse oximetry screening for detection of critical congenital heart disease in daily clinical routine—Results from a prospective multicenter study. *Eur J. Pediatr.* **2010**, *169*, 975–981. [CrossRef] [PubMed]
6. Meberg, A.; Brügmann-Pieper, S.; Due, R., Jr.; Eskedal, L.; Fagerli, I.; Farstad, T.; Frøisland, D.H.; Sannes, C.H.; Johansen, O.J.; Keljalic, J.; et al. First Day of Life Pulse Oximetry Screening to Detect Congenital Heart Defects. *J. Pediatr.* **2008**, *152*, 761–765. [CrossRef] [PubMed]

7. De-Wahl Granelli, A.; Wennergren, M.; Sandberg, K.; Mellander, M.; Bejlum, C.; Inganäs, L.; Eriksson, M.; Segerdahl, N.; Agren, A.; Ekman-Joelsson, B.M.; et al. Impact of pulse oximetry screening on the detection of duct dependent congenital heart disease: A Swedish prospective screening study in 39,821 newborns. *BMJ* **2009**, *338*, a3037. [CrossRef] [PubMed]

8. Tautz, J.; Merkel, C.; Loersch, F.; Egen, O.; Hägele, F.; Thon, H.M.; Schaible, T. Implication of pulse oxymetry screening for detection of congenital heart defects. *Klin. Padiatr.* **2010**, *222*, 291–295. [CrossRef] [PubMed]

9. Bekanntmachung eines Beschlusses des Gemeinsamen Bundesausschusses nach §91 Abs. 7 des Fünften Buches Sozialgesetzbuch (SGB V) zur Vereinbarung über Maßnahmen zur Qualitätssicherung der Versorgung von Früh- und Neugeborenen nach §137 Abs. 1 Satz 3 Nr. 2 SGB V. Gemeinsamer Bundesausschuss. Available online: https://www.g-ba.de/downloads/39-261-229/2005-09-20-Vereinbarung-Frueh_Neu.pdf (accessed on 31 March 2018).

10. Richtlinie des Gemeinsamen Bundesausschusses über Maßnahmen zur Qualitätssicherung der Versorgung von Früh- und Reifgeborenen. Gemeinsamer Bundesausschuss. Available online: https://www.g-ba.de/downloads/62-492-1487/QFR-RL_2017-10-19_iK-2018-01-01.pdf (accessed on 20 March 2018).

11. Ewer, A.K.; Middleton, L.J.; Furmston, A.T.; Bhoyar, A.; Daniels, J.P.; Thangaratinam, S.; Deeks, J.J.; Khan, K.S. Pulse oximetry screening for congenital heart defects in newborn infants (PulseOx): A test accuracy study. *Lancet* **2011**, *378*, 785–794. [CrossRef]

12. Turska Kmieć, A.; Borszewska Kornacka, M.K.; Błaż, W.; Kawalec, W.; Zuk, M. Early screening for critical congenital heart defects in asymptomatic newborns in Mazovia province: Experience of the POLKARD pulse oximetry programme 2006–2008 in Poland. *Kardiol. Pol.* **2012**, *70*, 370–376. [PubMed]

13. Abdul-Khaliq, H.; Berger, F. Die Diagnose wird häufig zu spät gestellt. *Dtsch. Arztebl.* **2011**, *108*, A1684.

14. Lindinger, A.; Dähnert, I.; Riede, F.T. Stellungnahme zum Pulsoximetrie-Screening zur Erfassung von Kritischen Angeborenen Herzfehlern im Neugeborenenalter. Available online: http://www.kinderkardiologie.org/fileadmin/user_upload/Stellungnahmen/POS%20Stellungsnahme%20DGPK%2011%2013%20final.pdf (accessed on 20 March 2018).

15. Herting, E.; Vetter, K.; Gonser, M.; Bassler, D.; Hentschel, R.; Groneck, P. Betreuung von Gesunden Reifen Neugeborenen in der Geburtsklinik. Available online: http://www.awmf.org/uploads/tx_szleitlinien/024-005l_S2k_Betreuung_von_gesunden_reifen_Neugeborenen_2012-10-abgelaufen.pdf (accessed on 20 March 2018).

16. Bärnighausen, T.; Sauerborn, R. One hundred and eighteen years of the German health insurance system: Are there any lessons for middle- and low-income countries? *Soc. Sci. Med.* **2002**, *54*, 1559–1587. [CrossRef]

17. Screening auf Kritische Angeborene Herzfehler Mittels Pulsoxymetrie bei Neugeborenen. Institut für Qualität und Wirtschaftlichkeit im Gesundheitswesen (IQWiG). Available online: https://www.iqwig.de/download/S13-01_Abschlussbericht_Pulsoxymetrie.pdf (accessed on 20 March 2018).

18. Beschluss des Gemeinsamen Bundesausschusses über eine Änderung der Richtlinie über die Früherkennung von Krankheiten bei Kindern bis zur Vollendung des 6. Lebensjahres (Kinder-Richtlinie): Screening auf Kritische Angeborene Herzfehler Mittels Pulsoxymetrie bei Neugeborenen. Available online: https://www.g-ba.de/downloads/39-261-2762/2016-11-24_Kinder-RL_Pulsoxymetrie-Screening-Neugeborene_BAnz.pdf (accessed on 20 March 2018).

19. Screening auf Kritische Angeborene Herzfehler Mittels Pulsoxymetrie bei Neugeborenen–Zusammenfassende Dokumentation. Available online: https://www.g-ba.de/downloads/40-268-4066/2016-11-24_Kinder-RL_Pulsoxymetrie-Screening-Neugeborene_ZD.pdf (accessed on 20 March 2018).

20. Kemper, A.R.; Mahle, W.T.; Martin, G.R.; Cooley, W.C.; Kumar, P.; Morrow, W.R.; Kelm, K.; Pearson, G.D.; Glidewell, J.; Grosse, S.D.; et al. Strategies for Implementing Screening for Critical Congenital Heart Disease. *Pediatrics* **2011**, *128*, e1259–e1267. [CrossRef] [PubMed]

21. Thangaratinam, S.; Brown, K.; Zamora, J.; Khan, K.S.; Ewer, A.K. Pulse oximetry screening for critical congenital heart defects in asymptomatic newborn babies: A systematic review and meta-analysis. *Lancet* **2012**, *379*, 2459–2464. [CrossRef]

22. Manzoni, P.; Martin, G.R.; Luna, M.S.; Mestrovic, J.; Simeoni, U.; Zimmermann, L.; Ewer, A.K.; Manzoni, P.; Martin, G.R.; Granelli, A.D.W.; et al. Pulse oximetry screening for critical congenital heart defects: A European consensus statement. *Lancet Child. Adolesc. Health* **2017**, *1*, 88–90. [CrossRef]

23. Narayen, I.C.; Blom, N.A.; Ewer, A.K.; Vento, M.; Manzoni, P.; te Pas, A.B. Aspects of pulse oximetry screening for critical congenital heart defects: When, how and why? *Arch. Dis. Child. Fetal Neonatal Ed.* **2016**, *101*, F162–F167. [CrossRef] [PubMed]

24. Johnson, L.C.; Lieberman, E.; O'Leary, E.; Geggel, R.L. Prenatal and newborn screening for critical congenital heart disease: Findings from a nursery. *Pediatrics* **2014**, *134*, 916–922. [CrossRef] [PubMed]

25. Quartermain, M.D.; Pasquali, S.K.; Hill, K.D.; Goldberg, D.J.; Huhta, J.C.; Jacobs, J.P.; Jacobs, M.L.; Kim, S.; Ungerleider, R.M. Variation in Prenatal Diagnosis of Congenital Heart Disease in Infants. *Pediatrics* **2015**, *136*, e378–e385. [CrossRef] [PubMed]

26. Lindinger, A.; Schwedler, G.; Hense, H.W. Prevalence of Congenital Heart Defects in Newborns in Germany: Results of the First Registration Year of the PAN Study (July 2006 to June 2007). *Klin. Padiatr.* **2010**, *222*, 321–326. [CrossRef] [PubMed]

27. Abouk, R.; Grosse, S.D.; Ailes, E.C.; Oster, M.E. Association of US State Implementation of Newborn Screening Policies for Critical Congenital Heart Disease With Early Infant Cardiac Deaths. *JAMA* **2017**, *318*, 2111–2118. [CrossRef] [PubMed]

28. Wren, C.; Reinhardt, Z.; Khawaja, K. Twenty-year trends in diagnosis of life-threatening neonatal cardiovascular malformations. *Arch. Dis. Child. Fetal Neonatal Ed.* **2008**, *93*, F33–F35. [CrossRef] [PubMed]

3

A Single-Extremity Staged Approach for Critical Congenital Heart Disease Screening: Results from Tennessee

William Walsh [1,*] and Jean A. Ballweg [2]

[1]   Department of Pediatrics, Vanderbilt University Medical Center, Nashville, TN 37232, USA
[2]   Department of Pediatrics, University of Nebraska Medical Center, Nashville, TN 37232, USA;
      jballweg@childrensomaha.org
*   Correspondence: bill.walsh@vandbilt.edu

Abstract: Tennessee initiated single-extremity staged screening by pulse oximetry for undetected CCHD in 2012. The algorithm begins with a saturation reading in the foot and allows an automatic pass if the foot pulse oximetry is 97% or greater. This was based on the principle that it is not possible to have a greater than 4% difference in the pulse oximetry between upper and lower extremities if the lower extremity is equal to or greater than 97%. This approach eliminates over 75,000 "unnecessary" pulse oximetry determinations in Tennessee each year without affecting the ability to detect CCHD before hospital discharge.

Keywords: pulse oximetry screening; screening algorithm; critical congenital heart disease; state screening; coarctation of aorta

---

1. Introduction

Congenital heart disease is present in approximately one in every one hundred live births in the United States. Critical congenital heart disease (CCHD) comprises a significant percentage of heart lesions. The Center for Disease Control (CDC) has identified seven congenital heart lesions that are deemed critical diseases. These seven lesions include hypoplastic left heart syndrome, pulmonary atresia, tetralogy of Fallot, total anomalous venous return, transposition of the great arteries, tricuspid atresia and truncus arteriosus.

Until pulse oximetry screening in the United States was begun, about 30% of infants with CCHD—or 6 per 10,000 babies—with the seven critical congenital heart disease lesions identified by the CDC were not diagnosed until after initial hospital discharge [1].

With the recommendation for screening in 2011, the USA Secretary of Health and Human Services recommended routine newborn pulse oximetry screening be performed prior to hospital discharge. As of 2015, 46 states and the District of Columbia require hospitals to screen newborns for critical CCHDs [2].

The protocol recommended by the AHA and CDC for screening was based on extensive review of evidence from major European trials [3–6].

In 2011, the AHA and the CDC decided upon a protocol that evaluates the pulse oximetry reading of the infant on a hand and foot after 24 h of age. To avoid the problem of multiple false positives, it was decided to repeat the screen twice prior to declaring the infant a failure [7].

Seven key lesions which would be expected to have a low saturation were targeted by the AHA and comprise the group of lesions referred to as CCHD as defined above. In addition to the 7 identified CCHDs, the CDC has targeted an additional five lesions when studying CCHD screening.

These five lesions include coarctation of the aorta, double outlet right ventricle, Ebstein's anomaly, interrupted aortic arch and single ventricle lesions other than HLHS.

This protocol for screening two extremities was based on the possibility that a baby with secondary targets such as coarctation may have decreased saturations in the lower extremity compared to the upper, and therefore a persistent difference greater than 3% between upper and lower extremity was considered an indication for further evaluation. Using this protocol, it was estimated that about half the infants with CCHD who would have been missed by lack of prenatal diagnosis and absence of signs in the newborn nursery would be identified by a failed pulse oximetry screening test [8].

It was estimated that, each year, about 875 more newborns with a CCHD could be identified at birth hospitals using pulse oximetry newborn screening, but an equal number (880 babies) might still be missed each year in the United States. Lesions that were of concern for being missed and significant included truncus arteriosus, coarctation of the aorta and interrupted aortic arch.

The state of Tennessee had been evaluating the possibility of screening since 2006 [9]. We and the state reported on the incidence of missed CCHD, and identified that a diagnostic gap existed in Tennessee prior to the beginning of state-wide screening [10].

Based on our experience and the literature, it was estimated that pulse oximetry would detect CCHD in 5 to 7 Tennessee infants who would otherwise be missed. It was also suggested that the upper extremity pulse oximetry reading would be unnecessary if an initial foot pulse oximetry reading was 97% or higher, since it would be impossible to have a difference of greater than 3%. Therefore, the Genetics Advisory Committee of the state of Tennessee presented to the Commissioner of Health a modified Tennessee algorithm with an initial assessment of a single lower extremity reading, which, if 97% or higher a second, upper extremity, test was not required. Figure 1 The two-year results of this screening algorithm are presented in this report.

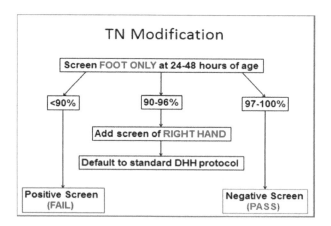

Figure 1. Foot only screen, if the pulse oximetry level is 97% or higher, the test is a pass and no upper extremity result is obtained, if the level is less than 90% the infant fails and is referred for further evaluation. A measurement of 90–96% results in a default to the AHA, CDC algorithm.

2. Materials and Methods

The State of Tennessee Health Department collected data on pulse oximetry screening as part of the State Genetics screening program on all live births. The State established a separate CCHD screening task force to monitor and assess newborn pulse oximetry screening. The pulse oximetry data are gathered from the pulse oximetry screening form on each metabolic screening blood spot test.

Surveillance for missed cases of CCHD was done through reports from the separate State of Tennessee Birth Defects Registry and the TIPQC missed-CCHD database as previously reported [10].

De-identified information collected by the TIPQC registry of missed cases included the neonate's diagnosis, age at diagnosis, presenting symptoms, and outcome. For the purpose of the registry, CCHD was defined as severe and life-threatening CHD requiring either surgical or catheter-based intervention in the first month of life. Reportable lesions included the 12 CDC targeted lesion which were ductal dependent lesions and lesions resulting in hypoxia. Acyanotic and non-ductal-dependent congenital heart defects requiring semi-elective surgical repair (tetralogy of Fallot without cyanosis, atrioventricular septal defect, atrial septal defect, ventricular septal defect, and patent ductus arteriosus) were excluded from the study.

3. Results

In 2013, there were 84,964 births, and in 2014 there were 87,184 births, for a total of 172,148 births in 2013–2014. During that time 95% (163,699) submitted pulse oximetry screening data. From that cohort, 96% passed with foot only evaluations. This eliminated the need for a second pulse oximetry reading in 156,948 infants.

For these 2 years, 232 infants failed the screen, with 51 true positives, or 22%. Eight babies had no prenatal suspicion or clinical signs, and were picked up solely by the screening tool. During the same period, there were 13 infants with CCHD not picked up by the screen. Ten of these had left-sided obstruction, which subsequently presented with clinical signs between day of life 3 and 30. Two infants were found to have TAPVR, one of whom was found on autopsy review after unexplained death at 14 days of age. One baby with no recorded screen presented with Tetralogy of Fallot and one with coactation presented at 9 days of age.

4. Discussion

Pulse oximetry screening for CCHD is a valuable adjunct to physical exam and clearly worth the effort. Even in the false positive cases, there are a significant number of infants with other disorders who benefit from evaluation and treatment. We did not systematically track all the babies who failed and who did not have CCHD, but we found a case of intracranial hemorrhage with apnea, a nasal lacrimal tumor, several babies with pneumonia and sepsis. It is clear that no baby should be discharged with a saturation of less than 95% without a clinical diagnosis [11].

The Tennessee algorithm saved 150,000 unnecessary pulse oximetry readings and still detected the predicted number of CCHD cases.

Using the cost data from Peterson et al. [12], and assuming the pulse oximeter probe is not changed between sites, the time necessary for screening would be reduced from 9 to 5 min; based on the Peterson approximation of average hourly nursing salary, the labor cost would be reduced from $6.68 to $3.71 per screen; it would therefore cost approximately $3.00 per baby, or over $240,000 per year, in Tennessee to obtain a pulse oximetry reading in the upper extremity, which could not be more than 3% greater than the foot reading. In addition to this financial cost, nursing time is valuable and better-used counseling families on newborn care, including Safe Sleep teaching or feeding.

In discussion with physician heath care leaders in other states, the major objection to using the Tennessee approach is the lack of endorsement by the CDC, and the concern that it is "too complicated". However, in discussion with nursing leaders, it is almost instantaneously understood that if the foot saturation is 97% or higher, it is not possible for the hand to be over 3% higher, and thus an upper extremity saturation is unnecessary. Thangaratinam et al., in their meta-analysis [13], actually showed no benefit from additional two-extremity testing. However, it is clear from the data reported that, although they are rare, babies with a true differences in saturation due to right to left ductal shunting can be identified, and the two-extremity test should be used whenever there is a possibility of an abnormal result. In the future, new technology may also allow two-site pulse oximetry to detect coarctation of the aorta by using pulsatility information [14].

The possibility of a reversal of saturations due to a TGA is not uncommon, but this condition would also have to be associated with a saturation of over 97% in the foot. To date, there have been no actual reports of such a condition. To require an additional 150,000 pulse oximetry readings each year looking for such a rare condition would not be cost-effective.

The 13 babies over two years with false negative results are particularly concerning. It is difficult to identify false negative cases, and we were fortunate in developing a state-wide voluntary reporting system. No screen result was found on 2 infants, one baby with Tetralogy had no screen recorded, and was found to be a home birth without pulse oximetry available. The other baby with coarctation presented at 9 days, and had no screen reported; this was during the first month of establishing the screening program. We have subsequently worked with our mid-wives in TN, and all have portable pulse oximetry capability and education. In addition, through the state genetics quality improvement program, there is now documented screening on over 97% of all infants. Tennessee does not require the actual saturation levels to be reported, just pass or fail, and whether one or two extremities were tested. The 11 false negatives that were screened passed with a single lower extremity test of over 97%. Nine of these infants were left-sided obstructed lesions, and upon final presentation had saturations ranging from 92 to 100%. There was one TAPVR who presented with respiratory distress, and there was one death of a baby with TAPVR who presented at 2 weeks of age in arrest; both had passed the screen. Without prospective saturation data, it is not possible to know whether some of these babies would have been diagnosed by the CDC algorithm.

Extrapolating the savings from using the Tennessee approach nationwide would result in 3.8 million fewer pulse oximetry tests, representing approximately $10 million dollars in savings without a loss of screening efficacy [12].

A major drawback to a staged single-extremity initial oximetry testing is the need for reeducation and recreation of the multiple, already existent, excellent educational programs in place in many states. CDC and AHA policy makers may decide that such effort may not be worth the benefit. Certainly, for those states that have not yet established a pulse oximetry screening program, using the most efficient approach would be beneficial.

5. Conclusions

The Tennessee single extremity algorithm can more efficiently detect infants with CCHD and should be considered by new screening programs.

Author Contributions: William Walsh Conceived of the single extremity pulse oximetry algorithm, organized the State of Tennessee to use it, created the TIPQC task force and reviewed all the collected data and wrote this report. Jean A. Ballweg Detected and reviewed missed cases, provided feedback to the state CCHD detection committee and reviewed and edited this article.

Abbreviations

AAP	Academy of Pediatrics
AHA	American Heart Association
CHD	Congenital heart disease
CCHD	Critical congenital heart disease
CI	Confidence interval
CoA	Coarctation of the aorta
TIPQC	Tennessee Initiative for Perinatal Quality Care
TN	Tennessee

References

1. Wren, C.; Reinhardt, Z.; Khawaja, K. Twenty-year trends in diagnosis of life-threatening neonatal cardiovascular malformations. *Arch. Dis. Child.* **2008**, *93*, F33–F35. [CrossRef] [PubMed]
2. Oster, M.E.; Aucott, S.W.; Gildewell, J.; Hackell, J.; Kohilas, L.; Martin, G.R.; Phillippi, J.; Pinto, N.M.; Saarinen, A.; Sontag, M.; et al. Lessons Learned From Newborn Screening for Critical Congenital Heart Defects. *Pediatrics* **2016**, *137*, e20154573. [CrossRef] [PubMed]

3. Riede, F.T.; Worner, C.; Dahnert, I.; Mockel, A.; Kostelka, M.; Schneider, P. Effectiveness of neonatal pulse oximetry screening for detection of critical congenital heart disease in daily clinical routine—Results from a prospective multicenter study. *Eur. J. Pediatr.* **2010**, *169*, 975–981. [CrossRef] [PubMed]

4. De-Wahl Granelli, A.; Wennergren, M.; Sandberg, K.; Mellander, M.; Bejum, C.; Inganas, L.; Eriksson, M.; Segerdahl, N.; Ågren, A.; Ekman-Joelsson, B.-M.; et al. Impact of pulse oximetry screening on the detection of duct dependent congenital heart disease: A Swedish prospective screening study in 39,821 newborns. *BMJ* **2009**, *338*, a3037. [CrossRef] [PubMed]

5. Ewer, A.K.; Middleton, L.J.; Furmston, A.T.; Bhoyar, A.; Daniels, J.P.; Thangaratinam, S.; Deeks, J.J.; Khan, K.S.; PulseOx Study Group. Pulse oximetry screening for congenital heart defects in newborn infants (PulseOx): A test accuracy study. *Lancet* **2011**, *378*, 785–794. [CrossRef]

6. Thangaratinam, S.; Daniels, J.; Ewer, A.K.; Zamora, J.; Khan, K.S. Accuracy of pulse oximetry in screening for congenital heart disease in asymptomatic newborns: A systematic review. *Arch. Dis. Child.* **2007**, *92*, F176–F180. [CrossRef] [PubMed]

7. Kemper, A.R.; Mahle, W.T.; Martin, G.R.; Cooley, W.C.; Kumar, P.; Morrow, W.R.; Kelm, K.; Pearson, G.D.; Glidewell, J.; Grosse, S.D.; et al. Strategies for Implementing Screening for Critical Congenital Heart Disease. *Pediatrics* **2011**, *128*, e1259–e1267. [CrossRef] [PubMed]

8. Ailes, E.C.; Gilboa, S.M.; Honein, M.A.; Oster, M.E. Estimated Number of Infants Detected and Missed by Critical Congenital Heart Defect Screening. *Pediatrics* **2015**, *135*, 1001–1012. [CrossRef] [PubMed]

9. Liske, M.R.; Greeley, C.S.; Law, D.J.; Reich, J.D.; Morrow, W.R.; Baldwin, H.S.; Graham, T.P.; Strauss, A.W.; Kavanaugh-McHugh, A.L.; Walsh, W.F. Report of the Tennessee Task Force on Screening Newborn Infants for Critical Congenital Heart Disease. *Pediatrics* **2006**, *118*, 1250–1256. [CrossRef] [PubMed]

10. Mouledoux, J.H.; Walsh, W.F. Evaluating the Diagnostic Gap: Statewide Incidence of Undiagnosed Critical Congenital Heart Disease before Newborn Screening with Pulse Oximetry. *Pediatr. Cardiol.* **2013**, *34*, 1680–1686. [CrossRef] [PubMed]

11. Ewer, A.K.; Furnston, A.T.; Middleton, L.J.; Deeks, J.J.; Daniels, J.P.; Pattison, H.M.; Powell, R.; Roberts, T.E.; Barton, P.; Auguste, P.; et al. Pulse oximetry as a screening test for congenital heart defects in newborn infants: A test accuracy study with evaluation of acceptability and cost-effectiveness. *Health Technol. Assess.* **2012**, *16*, 1–184.

12. Peterson, C.; Grosse, S.D.; Oster, M.E.; Olney, R.S.; Cassell, C.H. Cost-effectiveness of routine screening for critical congenital heart disease in US newborns. *Pediatrics* **2013**, *132*, e595–e603. [CrossRef] [PubMed]

13. Thangaratinam, S.; Brown, K.; Zamora, J.; Khan, K.S.; Ewer, A.K. Pulse oximetry screening for critical congenital heart defects in asymptomatic newborn babies: A systematic review and meta-analysis. *Lancet* **2012**, *379*, 2459–2464. [CrossRef]

14. Granelli, A.W.; Ostman-Smith, I. Noninvasive peripheral perfusion index as a possible tool for screening for critical left heart obstruction. *Acta Paediatr.* **2007**, *96*, 1455–1459. [CrossRef] [PubMed]

4

Newborn Screening for CF across the Globe—*Where is it Worthwhile?*

Virginie Scotet [1,*]**, Hector Gutierrez** [2] **and Philip M. Farrell** [3]

[1]   Inserm, University of Brest, EFS, UMR 1078, GGB, F-29200 Brest, France
[2]   Department of Pediatrics, University of Alabama at Birmingham, Birmingham, AL 35233, USA; hgutierrez@peds.uab.edu
[3]   Departments of Pediatrics and Population Health Sciences, University of Wisconsin School of Medicine and Public Health, Madison, WI 53705, USA; pmfarrell@wisc.edu
*   Correspondence: virginie.scotet@inserm.fr;

Abstract: Newborn screening (NBS) for cystic fibrosis (CF) has been performed in many countries for as long as four decades and has transformed the routine method for diagnosing this genetic disease and improved the quality and quantity of life for people with this potentially fatal disorder. Each region has typically undertaken CF NBS after analysis of the advantages, costs, and challenges, particularly regarding the relationship of benefits to risks. The very fact that all regions that began screening for CF have continued their programs implies that public health and clinical leaders consider early diagnosis through screening to be *worthwhile*. Currently, many regions where CF NBS has not yet been introduced are considering options and in some situations negotiating with healthcare authorities as policy and economic factors are being debated. To consider the assigned question (*where is it worthwhile?*), we have completed a worldwide analysis of data and factors that should be considered when CF NBS is being contemplated. This article describes the lessons learned from the journey toward universal screening wherever CF is prevalent and an analytical framework for application in those undecided regions. In fact, the lessons learned provide insights about what is necessary to make CF NBS *worthwhile*.

Keywords: cystic fibrosis; newborn screening; incidence; malnutrition; cost; health policy

1. Introduction

To appreciate what makes cystic fibrosis (CF) newborn screening (NBS) *worthwhile*, if not essential, it is helpful to review briefly certain historical aspects and thereby supplement the overall history described herein by Travert [1]. In particular, the perspective that follows focuses on the lessons learned about what is needed to ensure that early diagnosis through screening is indeed *worthwhile* for individuals and targeted populations. According to the Cambridge English Dictionary, *worthwhile* means "useful, important, or good enough to be a suitable reward for the money or time spent." Currently, the majority of countries in Europe and those elsewhere populated by inhabitants with European ancestry are screening newborns for CF, as shown in Figure 1. Each of these regions faced and overcame many challenges such as those listed in Table 1. Often, the combination of laboratory difficulties and complicated but necessarily efficient follow-up systems proved daunting. It may be assumed that all these regions consider CF NBS *worthwhile*. Of course, CF NBS will not prove *worthwhile* unless sustained financial support can be anticipated and all of the essential elements shown in Figure 2 are well organized and maintained. Experience has shown that the NBS system of early diagnosis and treatment requires that every step in the process be performed with assured high quality.

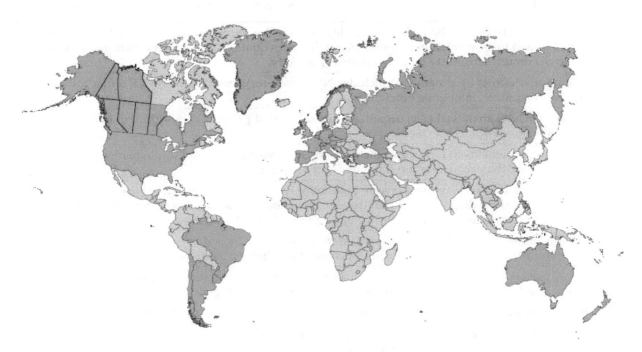

Figure 1. Worldwide implementation of cystic fibrosis newborn screening as of 2020.

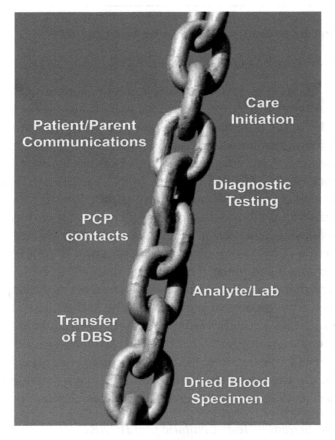

Figure 2. The sequence of processes and procedures linked together like a chain in the system of early diagnosis via newborn screening, reminding us that "a chain is only as strong as its weakest link." Abbreviations include PCP—primary care provider; DBS—dried blood specimen.

Table 1. Essential elements to ensure that cystic fibrosis newborn screening is *worthwhile*.

1	A system must be established and functioning well for the universal collection of dried blood spot specimens and their analysis in a central laboratory with quality assurance mechanisms in place and a goal to maximum sensitivity with acceptable specificity.
2	Collaborative efforts by a team that includes NBS laboratory leadership and CF center follow-up clinicians organized to operate efficiently.
3	Effective CF NBS analytical tests organized as a sequential protocol (algorithm) to maximize sensitivity and optimize specificity.
4	Quality improvements in laboratory methods must be planned for and implemented as technologies advance rather than accepting the *status quo* and resisting change.
5	Expeditious follow-up care must ensure that not only will high-quality sweat testing be provided promptly to confirm diagnoses but that the nutritional benefits are achieved immediately by a team of dedicated, experienced caregivers with gastrointestinal/nutritional expertise.
6	A cohort follow-up system must be ensured for patients diagnosed as neonates to segregate them from older patients and avoid exposure to virulent respiratory pathogens.
7	To ensure a favorable benefit: risk relationship, preventive management of potential psychosocial harms must be given priority by a skilled, dedicated follow-up team.
8	The incidence of CF must be high enough to warrant CF care centers in the NBS region.
9	The NBS system must be organized as a highly efficient operation that avoids preventable delays and ensures consistently diagnostic timeliness.
10	CF NBS guidelines should be known and adhered to throughout the sequence of integrated processes.

2. Requirements That Must Be Met for CF NBS to Be *Worthwhile*

2.1. Feasibility of Screening Newborns for CF

The requirements that must be addressed to implement and maintain a successful NBS program for CF are listed in Table 1. Although attempts to achieve early diagnosis of CF through meconium tests were organized during the 1970s [2], NBS first became feasible on a population scale in 1979 when dried blood spots were analyzed for immunoreactive trypsinogen (IRT) in New Zealand by Crossley et al. [3]. Through retrospective assessment, they found that high IRT levels revealed a significant risk for CF. The utility and convenience of dried blood spots in NBS had, of course, been obvious since their application in 1963 to phenylketonuria [4], and many public health laboratories worldwide were already screening for hereditary metabolic disorders and congenital endocrinopathies. Thus, the first requirement for the *worthwhile* implementation of CF NBS is to have a system in place and functioning well for the universal collection of dried blood spot specimens and their analysis in a central laboratory with quality assurance mechanisms in place. The seminal research in New Zealand was only possible because the NBS laboratory there collaborated closely with the University of Auckland Paediatrics Department across the street. The lesson learned there has been demonstrated repeatedly, namely that to be *worthwhile*, CF NBS must be a collaborative effort with a dedicated team that addresses every component of the sequence shown in Figure 2. For those few engaged in CF NBS using meconium tests in the 1970s, the report of Crossley et al. [3] had an immediate, profound influence, stimulating research around the world. On the other hand, the availability of a screening test alone is insufficient to justify its implementation as Wilson and Jungner [5] emphasized five decades ago.

2.2. The Need for an Excellent Screening Test: Limitations of IRT/IRT

The breakthrough discovery in New Zealand was followed by important studies in New South Wales in Australia [6], Colorado [7], and France [8]. Leaders in each of these regions recognized the potential benefits of early diagnosis ranging from epidemiologic and clinical research opportunities to care enhancement and improvement in the organization of healthcare delivery. Much skepticism remained, however, because of concerns about the IRT test per se, whether or not significant clinical benefits actually occurred, and how much adverse impact was being imposed on parents of screened neonates, i.e., the degree of psychosocial harm. In retrospect, the major concern that limited CF NBS acceptance, and thus a third lesson learned, concerns the IRT/IRT screening strategy—a method with relatively low sensitivity that requires a second, confirming blood specimen at approximately two weeks of age. Consequently, this first phase of experience with dried blood spot screening led to a realization that more research was needed on all aspects of CF NBS and the IRT method of screening needed to be improved. In fact, a decade after the report from New Zealand there was worldwide debate among health policy decision-makers whether or not CF NBS was *worthwhile* and even doubt among organizations like the U.S. Cystic Fibrosis Foundation—expressed emphatically when it sponsored a negative but influential commentary [9]. Consequently, CF NBS implementation was slow in North America and Europe, and one country (France) even discontinued their national IRT-based program.

2.3. The Value of the IRT/DNA Screening Test When CFTR Mutations Are Known

The view that IRT/IRT was not sufficiently sensitive with practical cutoff values coupled to the discovery of the *CFTR* gene in 1989 [10] and its principal disease-causing variant, p.Phe508del (F508del), led almost immediately to a search for a better screening algorithm in some regions. Others, however, continued IRT/IRT and either tolerated, or did not recognize, its relatively low sensitivity of 75–80% [11]. In retrospect, the discovery that about 90% of Europeans and Europe-derived CF populations have at least one p.Phe508del variant greatly facilitated the development of the first DNA-based NBS test, the IRT/DNA(p.Phe508del) method [12]. Soon thereafter, the DNA tier was expanded to a *CFTR* multimutation panel and a sensitivity of >95% was achieved routinely [13]. In addition, the quality of screening improved significantly by allowing test completion on the initial dried blood spot specimen, thus improving timeliness, and by providing valuable information on *CFTR* mutations. It was quickly learned with IRT/DNA(*CFTR*) that the vast majority of CF cases can be presumptively (genetically) diagnosed within a week of birth from the initial blood specimen and valuable genetic data obtained to predict pancreatic functional status.

The lesson learned from these experiences is clear: although initiating CF NBS with the IRT biomarker alone is much better than no screening for CF, regions should plan from the outset on improving their laboratory methods, ideally with a DNA-based second-tier method as *CFTR* population data emerge and enable transformation to a better, DNA-based algorithm that can make CF NBS more *worthwhile*. Another alternative is to use pancreatitis-associated protein (PAP) as an adjunct but a variety of issues limit its effectiveness [14]. The motivation for including PAP as a secondary biomarker in the screening strategy was to limit the incidental findings inherent to the use of DNA analysis such as the detection of carriers and the recognition of equivocal clinical phenotypes [14]. With any algorithm, tracking and evaluating data annually is an essential component of monitoring screening outcome measures such as sensitivity, specificity, positive predictive value, age of diagnosis to ensure that timeliness is achieved and disease incidence.

2.4. The Challenge of Evaluating and Achieving Benefits That Outweigh Risks

No NBS test has been subjected to more skepticism or scrutiny than CF screening even when the unique value of the IRT/DNA screening became evident. The rationale illustrated in Figure 3 has been considered so intuitive for other genetic conditions that implementation with little or no clinical evidence is typical for most screening tests and cost-effectiveness is generally not assessed. In retrospect, the debates in the CF community that raged over whether or not actual benefits occur and, if so, the benefit: risk relationship seems surprising when the potentially fatal salt loss in sweat and protein-energy malnutrition are well known to have plagued children with CF for decades [15]. Thus, the proof was demanded for the efficacy of CF NBS. However, the very short pre-symptomatic phase of CF, illustrated in Figure 3, was not appreciated until studies of infants diagnosed through NBS were published and revealed that malnutrition may occur within days and lung disease within weeks [15].

Eventually, convincing results from organized trials in Wales [16], Wisconsin [17], and elsewhere were published and confirmed, along with other supportive data on benefits [18]. The Wisconsin study, a randomized clinical trial assessing 650,341 infants during nine years of enrollment demonstrated short- and long-term nutritional benefits with early, aggressive care management [19,20] and less lung disease in those responding well to better nutrition [21].

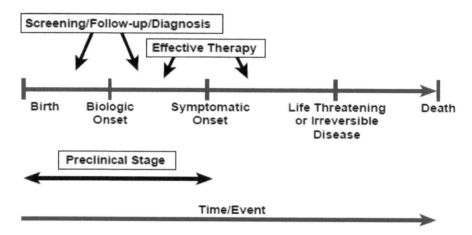

Figure 3. The rationale for early diagnosis via newborn screening by applying the principle inherent in the preventive medicine strategy to detect disease before its symptomatic onset.

In retrospect, it is much easier to evaluate nutritional outcomes after NBS than the course of lung disease, particularly in children, because of the numerous variables influencing the respiratory system as illustrated in Figure 4, including environmental factors such as respiratory pathogen exposures that are difficult to quantitate. The lesson learned from this experience is that for CF NBS to be *worthwhile*, expeditious follow-up care must ensure that not only will high-quality sweat testing be provided promptly to confirm diagnoses but that the nutritional benefits are achieved immediately by a team of dedicated, experienced caregivers with gastrointestinal/nutritional expertise. Thus, regional data tracking methods should assess multiple indices of nutritional status and monitor growth velocity carefully during the first two years of life. If growth failure occurs, comprehensive assessments and more aggressive nutritional interventions are essential, but more research is needed on supplements such as essential fatty acids.

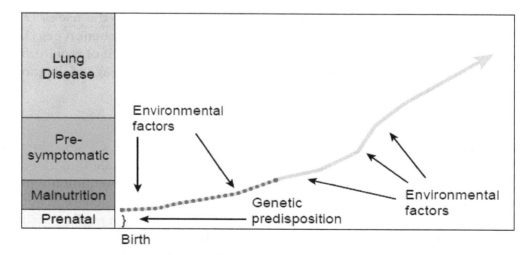

Figure 4. The many intrinsic and extrinsic variables (risk factors) that influence the course of cystic fibrosis and have much more impact on lung disease over a longer time period than those that affect nutritional status. The numerous environmental factors include exposures to smoke, virulent respiratory bacterial pathogens such as mucoid *Pseudomonas aeruginosa*, respiratory virus epidemics, etc.

Management of the respiratory complications of CF after NBS is more challenging with conventional therapies. Early diagnosis provides the opportunity to initiate some prophylactic measures, monitor for signs and symptoms of lung disease, and intervene quickly. A lesson learned in the Wisconsin trial is that infants must be segregated from older patients to avoid exposure to virulent respiratory pathogens [22]. Although cohorting non-infected patients was not the standard practice during the 20th century, this preventive strategy is essential to make CF NBS *worthwhile* [23,24]. Thus, regions contemplating the initiation of a screening program need to organize a segregated follow-up system for patients diagnosed as neonates. In addition, if/when more CFTR modulator therapy options become approved for infants with the p.Phe508del variant and routine organ preservation a routine reality, all regions will need to ensure the availability of these expensive therapies. In addition, access to care and avoidance of disparities needs to be assured.

With regard to the risks of CF NBS, many investigations worldwide have focused on potential psychosocial harms [25,26], especially in false-positive families, but it should be recognized that these risks accompany every screening test whether infants or older individuals are being screened. However, some have argued that CF NBS deserves more attention than that given to other conditions, and certainly there have been more studies on the potential risks. Recognizing the importance of the benefit: risk relationship, the Wisconsin team conducted their trial as a comprehensive longitudinal project that assessed adverse outcome potential through a variety of psychosocial studies and interviews [27,28]. The advantages and challenges of genetic counseling were also investigated and generally shown to be beneficial [29]. In summary, the lesson learned is that psychosocial harms may indeed occur, primarily due to misunderstanding of test results and their implications, but that investment by the follow-up team in proactive, excellent communication efforts can prevent and/or alleviate this risk which applies particularly to families experiencing false-positive tests. The importance of such tactics is underscored when a baby is identified as having CRMS/CFSPID (cystic fibrosis transmembrane conductance regulator-related metabolic syndrome/cystic fibrosis screen positive, inconclusive diagnosis) [30]. This condition is considered a "byproduct" of CF NBS with the IRT tier and often presents a diagnostic dilemma. In these cases, and whenever, CF is diagnosed, genetic counseling is essential and should be an integral part of the follow-up efforts [29].

3. Criteria to Implement Screening

3.1. European CF Society Guidelines

The European Cystic Fibrosis Society (ECFS) has published best practice guidelines for CF NBS [31] that are applicable to the question *Where is it worthwhile?* These deal with population characteristics such as the incidence of CF in a given region, the health and social support resources that are "minimally acceptable for newborn screening to be a valid undertaking," the quality of dried blood samples, acceptable levels of sensitivity and specificity, and the importance of timeliness. Table 2 summarizes the ECFS recommendations.

We respectfully disagree with the view that an incidence of at least 1:7000 hould guide decisions about whether or not to screen. In fact, many genetic disorders included in standard NBS panels have a much lower incidence without any challenge to their validity [32]. Many of the hereditary metabolic disorders in NBS panels have incidences of 1:200,000–3,000,000, as David et al. [32] emphasize. In addition, with CF NBS underway for extensive periods, the incidence of CF may decrease significantly [33] and even in previously high incidence regions become less than 1:7000. Certainly, these regions should not discontinue their programs. In view of the wide range of CF incidence data in countries with sufficient CF prevalence to warrant CF care centers and the reduction potential of prenatal and neonatal screening, we are reluctant to specify an incidence criterion; however, based on the typical panel of hereditary metabolic diseases in current screening programs of the western world, greater than 1:25,000 would be reasonable. It should be emphasized that the criteria established by Wilson and Jungner in 1968 [5] for the implementation of a screening program in the general population did not include the concept of a minimal incidence.

Table 2. European Cystic Fibrosis Society (ECFS) best practice guidelines: the 2018 revision [31].

1	Population characteristics that validate screening newborn infants for CF."Health authorities need to balance the benefit/risk ratio of screening newborns for CF in their population. If the incidence of CF is <1/7000 births, careful evaluation is required as to whether NBS is valid. The protocol must be shown to cause the minimum negative impact possible on the population. Other factors in making the decision on whether to implement screening should include available healthcare resources and the ability to provide a clear pathway to treatment."
2	Health and social resources that are minimally acceptable for NBS to be a valid undertaking."Infants identified with CF through a NBS program should have prompt access to specialist CF care that achieves ECFS standards. A NBS program may be a mechanism to better organize CF services, through the direct referral of infants for specialist CF care. Countries with limited resources should consider a pilot study to assess the validity of NBS and the adequacy of referral services for newly diagnosed infants in their population."
3	Acceptable number of repeat tests required for inadequate dried blood samples for every 1000 infants screened."The number of requests for repeat dried blood samples should be monitored and should be 0.5%. More than 20 repeats for every 1000 infants, is unacceptable (2%)."
4	Acceptable number of false-positive NBS results (infants referred for clinical assessment and sweat testing)."Programmes should aim for a minimum positive predictive value of 0.3 (PPV is the number of infants with a true positive NBS test divided by the total number of positive NBS tests)."
5	Acceptable number of false-negative NBS results. These are infants with a negative NBS test that are subsequently diagnosed with CF (a delayed diagnosis)."Programmes should aim for a minimum sensitivity of 95%."
6	Maximum acceptable delay between a sweat test being undertaken and the result given to the family. "The sweat test should be analyzed immediately and the result reported to the family on the same day."
7	Maximum acceptable age of an infant on the day they are first reviewed by a specialist CF team following a diagnosis of CF after NBS."The majority of infants with a confirmed diagnosis after NBS should be seen by a specialist CF team by 35 days and no later than 58 days after birth."
8	Minimum acceptable information for families of an infant recognized to be a carrier of a CF-causing mutation after NBS.Families should receive a verbal report of the result. They should also receive written information to refer to. Information should also be sent to the family Primary Care Physician. The information should be clear that the infant does not have CF; the baby is a healthy carrier; future pregnancies for this couple are not free of risk of CF and the parents may opt for genetic counseling, and there are implications that could affect reproductive decision making for extended family members and the infant when they are of childbearing age.

The ECFS recommendation that "programmes should aim for a minimum sensitivity of 95%" is appropriate but unattainable in regions using IRT/IRT or some other combination of biomarkers. Such regions are often limited by inadequate knowledge of the *CFTR* mutations prevalent in their population, but as that information is gained transformation to a more sensitive screening test can be accomplished.

The issue of follow-up efficiency was also addressed in the ECFS guidelines. First, it is stated that a sweat test result should be completed and the result reported to the family on the same day—an ideal practice but unfortunately not always routinely done. With regard to timeliness, the guidelines recommend 35–58 days after birth for the "maximum acceptable age of an infant on the day they are first reviewed by a special CF team following a diagnosis of CF after NBS." This recommendation was influenced by practical considerations in various European countries, but undoubtedly infants with CF are susceptible to potentially fatal salt loss in sweat prior to the 35–58-day interval, especially in hot climates and with breastfeeding. In addition, CF infants certainly can develop biochemically severe nutritional abnormalities within 2–4 weeks of birth and even suffer the onset of lung disease within 1–2 months. In addition, the recent data suggesting that organ preservation can be achieved with early CFTR modulator therapy [34] argues for diagnosis as soon after birth as possible. Consequently, a more efficient plan promulgated by some organizations recommends diagnosis as early as 2 weeks of age and definitely by 4 weeks of age. To be *worthwhile*, therefore, regions should organize their CF NBS programs to be highly efficient and avoid any preventable delays.

3.2. Clinical and Laboratory Standards Institute, the Association of Public Health Laboratories, the Centers for Disease Control and Prevention, and the Cystic Fibrosis Foundation

In the United States, the group of organizations listed above has worked collaboratively in the area of CF NBS to ensure expeditious nationwide implementation and ongoing attention to quality improvement. The CLSI recently published new guidelines [35] to revise the recommendations of 2011 focusing on the six aspects of CF NBS listed below as the responsible Document Development Committee identified the key areas of quality improvement.

(1) Reassessed IRT cutoff value guidelines and discussed the use of a floating rather than fixed cutoff value. The floating cutoff strategy using the 95th or 96th percentile helps overcome the seasonal and kit-related variations in IRT [11]. The recommendations included: "Recent data have shown that the traditional IRT cutoff values in the IRT/IRT algorithm were too high to minimize false-negative screening results and the 95th to 97th percentile (approximately 60 ng/mL) should be used." As expanded genetic analyses and next-generation sequencing are becoming less expensive, some CF NBS programs are operating with a lower fixed IRT (for example 40 ng/mL), thus allowing more samples for genetic testing to reduce false-negative screening results.

(2) Revised recommendations regarding *CFTR* variant panels based on the most current information including new biotechnologies such as next-generation sequencing, pointing out that "Guidelines published in 2001 and revised in 2004 include recommendations for screening with a *CFTR* variant panel of 23 disease-causing variants with a prevalence of at least 0.1% in the CF population. Although this recommended panel provides a high CF detection rate... additional variants may need to be added for improved CF detection in other ethnic groups. Many NBS programs use larger *CFTR* variant panels..."

(3) Assessed using PAP for detecting babies at risk for CF but did not make a recommendation.

(4) Discussed communications strategies related to the detecting of CF heterozygote babies and providing genetic counseling.

(5) Reviewed emerging issues related to using genetic and genomic sequencing in NBS.

(6) Described the existing CF NBS algorithms, while commenting on the advantages and disadvantages of each protocol.

The U.S. CF Foundation organized a recent diagnosis consensus with international input to (1) clarify the criteria that need to be met for diagnosis via either NBS or after signs/symptoms; (2) emphasize the importance of efficient follow-up of positive screening tests; (3) describe how to apply and communicate genetic data; (4) harmonize the definition of CRMS and CFSPID [36]. These guidelines recommend that sweat testing be performed as soon as possible after 10 days of age, ideally by 28 days of age. They also point out that treatment should not be delayed when sweat testing is unsuccessful. The Association of Public Health Laboratories, through its NewSTEPS program, has also emphasized timeliness. Lastly, the Centers for Disease Control and Prevention has established an invaluable quality assurance monitoring program for worldwide assistance *gratis* and a molecular assessment program, which conducts site visits to U.S. NBS laboratories that carry out molecular testing.

For CF NBS to be *worthwhile*, all the guidelines and recommendations summarized above should be well known to the leaders of screening regions and those that wish to implement programs. In the past, too many regions initiated CF NBS programs without taking advantage of the readily available resources and experience of established programs.

4. Incidence of CF around the World and Screening Protocols Being Employed

Figures 5 and 6 provide data on the estimated incidence of CF in many regions. Through a complete registration of cases directly at birth, the implementation of CF NBS has allowed a more accurate determination of the incidence of CF and better monitoring of its time trends. Before the implementation of NBS, the incidence estimation was mainly based on epidemiological studies that generally suffered from ascertainment bias due to under-diagnosis and/or under-reporting of cases. However, with NBS data, care must be taken when interpreting incidence data, as variations may occur depending on the patients included in the calculations (e.g., false-negatives, patients with meconium ileus, patients with CFSPID). In order to have consistent data, it is important to ensure that the calculations are based on the same population. The incidence data may also be biased by a short observation period in some studies.

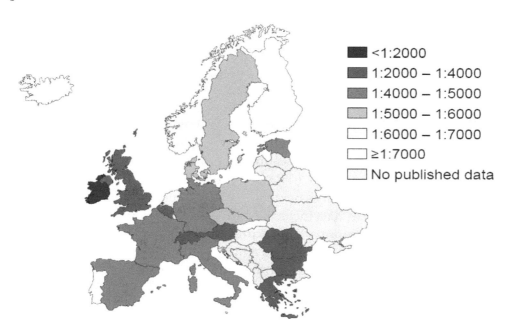

Figure 5. Incidence of cystic fibrosis in Europe.

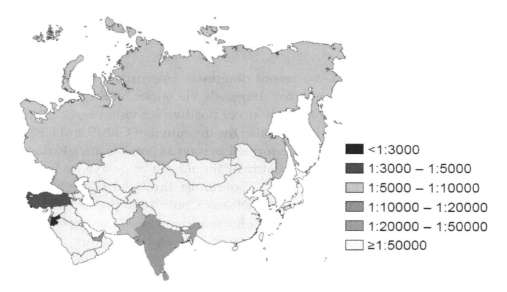

Figure 6. Incidence of cystic fibrosis in Asia.

4.1. Europe

The incidence of CF has long been estimated at 1:2500 in the European population [37]. In 2007, a review of CF NBS programs revealed that the incidence was on average 1:3500 [38] and it appears still lower nowadays. Beyond Ireland which has the highest incidence of CF in Europe (1:1353) [39], the incidence ranges from 1:2800 in the UK [38] to 1:10,000 in Russia [40] (Figure 5). It is 1:2850 in Belgium [41], about 1:4500 in France [42], Germany [14], Italy [38,43,44], and Spain (where large regional variations are observed) [45], while it oscillates between 1:5200 and 1:6500 in Central Europe (Czech Republic [32], Denmark [46], Netherlands [47], Poland [48], Slovakia [49], and Sweden [50]). The incidence appears lower than 1:7000 in three European countries (Portugal [51], Norway [52], and Russia [40]) as well as in various regions of Spain [45]. In countries without NBS, the incidence ranges from 1:2000 (Romania [53]) to 1:25,000 (Finland [54]).

The implementation of CF NBS across Europe has gradually spread, with a faster pace during the past decade. From the update performed by Barben et al. in 2016 [55] and the data acquired since, CF NBS has been implemented in 22 European countries to date (Figure 7). Nineteen countries have a national program and three have regional programs (which cover the whole country for Spain). The number of countries with a national NBS program has gradually increased over the past years, from 2 in 2007 (France and Austria) to 19 to date. Twenty-four countries have no NBS program but nine are considering or planning to implement screening protocols. The screening protocols, however, are varied and all national programs have a distinct algorithm. As illustrated in Figure 7, most programs use DNA analysis as a second-tier test, while five (Austria, Portugal, Russia, Slovakia, and Turkey) still rely exclusively on biochemical tests. The expansion of CF NBS across Europe has been successful and reveals that this screening is considered *worthwhile*.

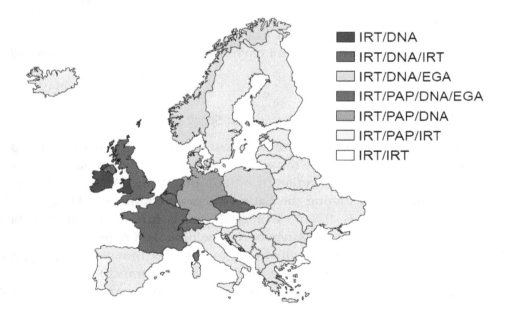

Figure 7. Protocols used in newborn screening for cystic fibrosis in Europe in 2020. Abbreviations include IRT—immunoreactive trypsinogen; EGA—expanded or extended gene analysis; PAP—pancreatitis-associated protein.

4.2. Australasia

The incidence of CF is well defined in Australasia as CF NBS has been in place for a very long time in this part of Oceania. The incidence is approximately 1:3000. It has been estimated as 1:2821 in New South Wales [56], 1:3139 in Victoria [57], and 1:3180 in New Zealand [58]. Newborn screening for CF has been performed for almost 40 years (1981) in New Zealand—which was the first country to implement a national program (1981) and for almost 20 years in all states within Australia where CF

NBS was first introduced in New South Wales during 1981 [56]. Currently, all states use a DNA-based NBS program. The very long experience of Australasia in CF NBS confirms the view that is this screening is deemed *worthwhile* in that part of the world.

4.3. United States of America

The incidence of CF for the entire population is approximately 1:4000, but ethnicity-related variations occur and have a regional impact [59]. In the white population, about 1 in 3000 babies are at risk for CF. Although limited data have been collected and analyzed on "minority" populations, it appears that the incidence and Hispanic infants are about 1:6000 and in African-Americans at least 1:10,000. Disparities in the age of diagnosis and ascertainment of CF cases may occur in these "minority" populations, so more data are needed. It has become increasingly clear that *CFTR* panels need to be expanded to reduce disparities, but NBS labs in the U.S. are notoriously slow to change methodologies as evidenced by a 10-year delay in all states transforming from IRT/IRT to IRT/DNA or IRT/IRT/DNA protocols after unequivocal evidence was published [11]. However, during the current year, all states are using DNA-based CF NBS and all consider their programs *worthwhile*.

4.4. Canada

The incidence of CF has been well defined during the past decade in Canada as all 10 provinces implemented CF NBS from 2007, beginning with Alberta, to 2017 when Québec implemented their excellent program based on clinical outcomes. In general, the Canadian population is more Euro-American than in other American countries. Therefore, it is not surprising that the incidence of CF is higher—averaging about 1:3300 [60]. Moreover, Québec in its first two years of CF NBS identified a 1:2300 incidence. The relatively high prevalence of CF throughout Canada and the excellent CF care centers providing follow-up and early treatment have certainly made CF NBS *worthwhile* there using DNA-based protocols.

4.5. Latin America—Mexico (North America), Central, and South America

The Latin American population is one of the most diverse in the world, due to a variety of ancestries, ethnicities, and races that have mixed for centuries. The dominant racial groups in the region are Caucasians, European-Amerindian (mestizo), Black, and Amerindian. The proportion of each group varies significantly among the Latin American countries [61]. Given this complex composition, the incidence of CF is difficult to foretell and is further complicated because many countries lack established clinical programs, newborn screening, and registries.

The racial distribution of CF cases, as illustrated by the 2017 Brazilian Registry, highlights the diversity of CF in Latin America. Of 5128 cases, 68% are white (branca), 25% are mestizo (parda), and 6% are black (preta). There are just a small number of cases of Asian (amarela) and Amerindian (indigena) descent.

Of 29,887 patients reported by the U.S. Cystic Fibrosis Foundation Patient Registry 2017 Annual Data Report, 8.7% are Hispanics. Extrapolating the current prevalence of CF in the US Hispanic population to Latin America, one could expect about 30,000 people with CF in the region. It should be pointed out that most of the Hispanics in the U.S. come from Mexico and Central America, which has a lower proportion of people of European descent that countries like Argentina, Uruguay, Chile, and Brazil [62]. Thus, the above prevalence might underestimate the number of people with CF.

Currently, reliable data on the incidence of CF in Latin America is lacking, in part, due to limited diagnostic accuracy. There is no neonatal screening in most of the countries, and genetic panels have a low diagnostic yield because they do not reflect the ethnic admixture of the population [63].

4.5.1. Argentina

Although Argentina approved legislation for mandatory administration of neonatal screening for CF in 1994, it has never reached meaningful national coverage (15%–20%). A recent report from the Grupo Registro Nacional de Fibrosis Quistica (National CF Registry Taskforce), verified that the neonatal screening in 2012 had coverage of 28.8%. The CF National Consensus of 2008 reported that between 1995 and 2005, CF incidence was 1:6131, after screening almost 1 million infants. There is no defined protocol for its performance. The most commonly used is IRT/IRT. The Autonomous City of Buenos Aires (CABA) started its neonatal screening in 2002, using the IRT/IRT algorithm. From 2002–2014, the incidence was 1:7444 (49/364,782; V. Rodriguez, personal communication). In 2015, Buenos Aires modified the algorithm to IRT/PAP.

4.5.2. Brazil

Brazil has developed the most robust CF care structure, similar to the OECD countries, including a CF center network, sophisticated registry, and neonatal screening. Adoption of the neonatal screening (IRT/IRT) has gained prominence in diagnosing new cases, from 32% in 2009 to 61% in 2017. The reported incidence varies among different states, higher in the South Region (Santa Catarina: 1:6500; Paraná: 1:9000), lower in others (Minas Gerais: 1:11,000), (V. Rodriguez, personal communication).

4.5.3. Chile

Studies from the mid-1990s reported an incidence of 1:4000 (Rios, 1994). More recent data from two pilot studies on neonatal screening puts the incidence between 1:8000 and 1:10,000 (2015–2017; ML Boza, personal communication). Chile anticipates starting national CF neonatal screening in 2020, using the IRT/PAP protocol.

4.5.4. Mexico

There is no accurate data on incidence. In 2016, the Secretaria de Salud (Ministry of Health) reported 350 new cases of CF per year. Averaging 2.3 million births per year over the last decade, Mexico could have an incidence of approximately 1:6700. Others have reported a lower rate (1:8500; 2002, Jose Luis Lezana, personal communication). Neonatal screening for CF was added to the national program in 2015. The screening method currently used is IRT/IRT. As it has been the norm in the Latin American countries, the use of mutation panels has low yields (A 34-mutation panel had a sensitivity of <75%; Orozco, 2000).

4.5.5. Uruguay

Uruguay implemented neonatal screening in 2010. Initially using the IRT/IRT protocol, but changing to IRT/PAP in 2012. Analysis from years 2010– 2016 totaling 322,727 screened babies, 39 confirmed diagnoses, puts the incidence in 1:8300 (C Pinchack, personal communication).

4.5.6. Other Latin American Countries

In 2019 Colombia and Peru approved the addition of CF screening into their national newborn screenings. We have no information on the protocols used. Also, the incidence in these countries has not been established. Costa Rica has had CF neonatal screening for several years but has not reached full coverage. Seven cases on average per year suggest an incidence of 1:15,000 (J. Gutierrez, personal communication). An ongoing pilot study puts the rate in 1:10,000.

4.5.7. Is CF Neonatal Screening *Worthwhile* in Latin American Countries?

With an expected high number of cases and the late age in diagnosis that presently occurs, the use of neonatal screening should be a cost-effective tool to help to identify patients at a younger age, therefore improving survival.

4.6. Asia

Although the incidence of CF in Asia has long been unknown, the existence of CF in that continent is now well established. The incidence is greatly variable and appears much higher in the Middle East than in East Asia (Figure 6). Cases of CF have been reported in many Arab countries and in some of them (where consanguinity is common), the incidence appears close to that observed in populations of European descent. It has thus been estimated to 1:2560 in Jordan [64] or to 1:5800 in Bahrain [65], while it is about 1:16,000 in the United Arab Emirates [66] and in Israel, where the incidence has dropped significantly following implementation of population carrier screening program [67]. The incidence of CF is lower in South Asian populations. It has been estimated between 1:10,000 and 1:100,000 in the Indian population [68–71] and to 1:90,000 in an Oriental population living in Hawaii [72]. The incidence is very low in Japan (1:350,000) [73] as well as in China where less than 30 cases have been reported over the two last decades [74]. Thus, CF NBS would not seem *worthwhile* in those countries.

Beyond variability in carrier frequency, the wide range observed in incidence may be in part explained by under-diagnosis and under-reporting of cases [75,76]. The incidence of CF in Asia may therefore be under-estimated. Despite the low incidence of CF in that continent, the number of CF patients must be high in some countries due to the large population size (such as India).

In Arab countries, the major challenges are to improve the diagnosis and the detection of mutations before irreversible organ damage has developed and to promote the constitution of national registries [75,76], which will help to improve CF management and health policy planning. To the best of our knowledge, no CF NBS program is implemented to date in the Arab world, but CF NBS is promoted by the annual meeting for NBS in the Middle East and North Africa. The sole country that was considering implementing an NBS program during 2020 is Israel.

In view of the high incidence of CF in some Arab countries and the genomic revolution that is underway in those countries (through the Saudi, Qatar, and Emirati genome projects), CF NBS should be *worthwhile* in the regions where CF is well managed. NBS programs would have to take into account the genetic specificities of that population (limited mutation spectrum, lower prevalence of p.Phe508del mutation, mutations found only in that population [76]) but also the high consanguinity rate.

5. Summary

Newborn screening for CF has been performed in many countries for as long as four decades and has transformed the routine method for diagnosing this genetic disease and improved the quality and quantity of life for people with this potentially fatal disorder. Each region has typically undertaken CF NBS after analysis of the advantages, costs, and challenges, particularly regarding the relationship of benefits to risks. The very fact that all regions that began screening for CF have continued their programs implies that public health and clinical leaders consider early diagnosis through screening to be *worthwhile*. In this article, after summarizing the considerations that led the majority of North American and European countries to implement CF NBS programs successfully, we analyze countries that are or should be planning to screen newborns for this relatively common genetic disorder. From this analysis, we suggest the criteria listed in Table 3. Recent, dramatic advances in therapies offer great promise for all patients diagnosed early and especially children diagnosed before pathology quickly develops irreversibly.

Table 3. Suggested criteria for cystic fibrosis newborn screening.

Incidence of CF: greater than 1:25,000
Aim at minimum sensitivity of 95%
IRT/DNA—unless unavailable or not feasible
Diagnosis including sweat chloride within 4 weeks of age
Assessment program for tests, including plans for monitoring and updating
Availability of a complete specialist CF team

Author Contributions: All authors participated in conceptualization, writing the original draft, and devoting efforts to review and editing work. V.S. was responsible for submitting the manuscript and reviewing/correcting the proofs. All authors have read and agreed to the published version of the manuscript.

Acknowledgments: The authors thank Robert Gordon of the Department of Pediatrics at the University of Wisconsin School of Medicine and Public Health for his superb computer graphics efforts to create the illustrations published herein. They also thank Jürg Barben, Kevin Southern, and Anne Munck for providing updated data on newborn screening for cystic fibrosis in Europe.

References

1. Travert, G.; Heeley, M.; Heeley, A. History of newborn screening for CF—The Early Years. *Int. J. Neonatal Screen.* **2020**, *6*, 8. [CrossRef]
2. Bruns, W.T.; Connell, T.R.; Lacey, J.A.; Whisler, K.E. Test strip meconium screening for cystic fibrosis. *Am. J. Dis. Child.* **1977**, *131*, 71–73. [CrossRef] [PubMed]
3. Crossley, J.R.; Elliott, R.B.; Smith, P.A. Dried-blood spot screening for cystic fibrosis in the newborn. *Lancet* **1979**, *1*, 472–474. [CrossRef]
4. Guthrie, R.; Susi, A. A Simple Phenylalanine Method for Detecting Phenylketonuria in Large Populations of Newborn Infants. *Pediatrics* **1963**, *32*, 338–343.
5. Wilson, J.M.G.; Jungner, Y.G. *Principles and Practice of Screening for Disease*; WHO: Geneva, Switzerland, 1968; Available online: http://www.who.int/bulletin/volumes/86/4/07-050112BP.pdf (accessed on 1 March 2020).
6. Wilcken, B.; Brown, A.R.; Urwin, R.; Brown, D.A. Cystic fibrosis screening by dried blood spot trypsin assay: Results in 75,000 newborn infants. *J. Pediatr.* **1983**, *102*, 383–387. [CrossRef]
7. Reardon, M.C.; Hammond, K.B.; Accurso, F.J.; Fisher, C.D.; McCabe, E.R.; Cotton, E.K.; Bowman, C.M. Nutritional deficits exist before 2 months of age in some infants with cystic fibrosis identified by screening test. *J. Pediatr.* **1984**, *105*, 271–274. [CrossRef]
8. Travert, G.; Duhamel, J.F. Systematic neonatal screening for mucoviscidosis using an immunoreactive trypsin blood assay. Evaluation of 80,000 tests. *Arch. Fr. Pediatr.* **1983**, *40*, 295–298.
9. Cystic Fibrosis Foundation, Ad Hoc Committee Task Force on Neonatal Screening. Neonatal screening for cystic fibrosis: Position paper. *Pediatrics* **1983**, *72*, 741–745.
10. Kerem, B.; Rommens, J.M.; Buchanan, J.A.; Markiewicz, D.; Cox, T.K.; Chakravarti, A.; Buchwald, M.; Tsui, L.C. Identification of the cystic fibrosis gene: Genetic analysis. *Science* **1989**, *245*, 1073–1080. [CrossRef]
11. Kloosterboer, M.; Hoffman, G.; Rock, M.; Gershan, W.; Laxova, A.; Li, Z.; Farrell, P.M. Clarification of laboratory and clinical variables that influence cystic fibrosis newborn screening with initial analysis of immunoreactive trypsinogen. *Pediatrics* **2009**, *123*, e338–e346. [CrossRef]
12. Gregg, R.G.; Wilfond, B.S.; Farrell, P.M.; Laxova, A.; Hassemer, D.; Mischler, E.H. Application of DNA analysis in a population-screening program for neonatal diagnosis of cystic fibrosis (CF): Comparison of screening protocols. *Am. J. Hum. Genet.* **1993**, *52*, 616–626.
13. Comeau, A.M.; Parad, R.B.; Dorkin, H.L.; Dovey, M.; Gerstle, R.; Haver, K.; Lapey, A.; O'Sullivan, B.P.; Waltz, D.A.; Zwerdling, R.G.; et al. Population-based newborn screening for genetic disorders when multiple mutation DNA testing is incorporated: A cystic fibrosis newborn screening model demonstrating increased sensitivity but more carrier detections. *Pediatrics* **2004**, *113*, 1573–1581. [CrossRef]

14. Sommerburg, O.; Hammermann, J.; Lindner, M.; Stahl, M.; Muckenthaler, M.; Kohlmueller, D.; Happich, M.; Kulozik, A.E.; Stopsack, M.; Gahr, M.; et al. Five years of experience with biochemical cystic fibrosis newborn screening based on IRT/PAP in Germany. *Pediatr. Pulmonol.* **2015**, *50*, 655–664. [CrossRef]

15. Accurso, F.J.; Sontag, M.K.; Wagener, J.S. Complications associated with symptomatic diagnosis in infants with cystic fibrosis. *J. Pediatr.* **2005**, *147*, S37–S41. [CrossRef]

16. Chatfield, S.; Owen, G.; Ryley, H.C.; Williams, J.; Alfaham, M.; Goodchild, M.C.; Weller, P. Neonatal screening for cystic fibrosis in Wales and the West Midlands: Clinical assessment after five years of screening. *Arch. Dis. Child.* **1991**, *66*, 29–33. [CrossRef]

17. Farrell, P.M.; Kosorok, M.R.; Laxova, A.; Shen, G.; Koscik, R.E.; Bruns, W.T.; Splaingard, M.; Mischler, E.H. Nutritional benefits of neonatal screening for cystic fibrosis. Wisconsin Cystic Fibrosis Neonatal Screening Study Group. *N. Engl. J. Med.* **1997**, *337*, 963–969. [CrossRef]

18. Balfour-Lynn, I.M. Newborn screening for cystic fibrosis: Evidence for benefit. *Arch. Dis. Child.* **2008**, *93*, 7–10. [CrossRef]

19. Farrell, P.M.; Kosorok, M.R.; Rock, M.J.; Laxova, A.; Zeng, L.; Lai, H.C.; Hoffman, G.; Laessig, R.H.; Splaingard, M.L. Early diagnosis of cystic fibrosis through neonatal screening prevents severe malnutrition and improves long-term growth. Wisconsin Cystic Fibrosis Neonatal Screening Study Group. *Pediatrics* **2001**, *107*, 1–13. [CrossRef]

20. Farrell, P.M.; Lai, H.J.; Li, Z.; Kosorok, M.R.; Laxova, A.; Green, C.G.; Collins, J.; Hoffman, G.; Laessig, R.; Rock, M.J.; et al. Evidence on improved outcomes with early diagnosis of cystic fibrosis through neonatal screening: Enough is enough! *J. Pediatr.* **2005**, *147*, S30–S36. [CrossRef]

21. Sanders, D.B.; Zhang, Z.; Farrell, P.M.; Lai, H.J.; Wisconsin, C.F.N.S.G. Early life growth patterns persist for 12 years and impact pulmonary outcomes in cystic fibrosis. *J. Cyst. Fibros.* **2018**, *17*, 528–535. [CrossRef]

22. Kosorok, M.R.; Jalaluddin, M.; Farrell, P.M.; Shen, G.; Colby, C.E.; Laxova, A.; Rock, M.J.; Splaingard, M. Comprehensive analysis of risk factors for acquisition of Pseudomonas aeruginosa in young children with cystic fibrosis. *Pediatr. Pulmonol.* **1998**, *26*, 81–88. [CrossRef]

23. Rosenfeld, M.; Emerson, J.; McNamara, S.; Thompson, V.; Ramsey, B.W.; Morgan, W.; Gibson, R.L.; Group, E.S. Risk factors for age at initial Pseudomonas acquisition in the cystic fibrosis epic observational cohort. *J. Cyst. Fibros.* **2012**, *11*, 446–453. [CrossRef]

24. Baussano, I.; Tardivo, I.; Bellezza-Fontana, R.; Forneris, M.P.; Lezo, A.; Anfossi, L.; Castello, M.; Aleksandar, V.; Bignamini, E. Neonatal screening for cystic fibrosis does not affect time to first infection with Pseudomonas aeruginosa. *Pediatrics* **2006**, *118*, 888–895. [CrossRef]

25. Tluczek, A.; Orland, K.M.; Cavanagh, L. Psychosocial consequences of false-positive newborn screens for cystic fibrosis. *Qual. Health Res.* **2011**, *21*, 174–186. [CrossRef]

26. Johnson, F.; Southern, K.W.; Ulph, F. Psychological impact on parents of an inconclusive diagnosis following newborn bloodspot screening for cystic fibrosis: A qualitative study. *Int. J. Neonatal Screen.* **2019**, *5*, 23. [CrossRef]

27. Tluczek, A.; Clark, R.; McKechnie, A.C.; Brown, R.L. Factors affecting parent-child relationships one year after positive newborn screening for cystic fibrosis or congenital hypothyroidism. *J. Dev. Behav. Pediatr.* **2015**, *36*, 24–34. [CrossRef]

28. Tluczek, A.; Laxova, A.; Grieve, A.; Heun, A.; Brown, R.L.; Rock, M.J.; Gershan, W.M.; Farrell, P.M. Long-term follow-up of cystic fibrosis newborn screening: Psychosocial functioning of adolescents and young adults. *J. Cyst. Fibros.* **2014**, *13*, 227–234. [CrossRef]

29. Ciske, D.J.; Haavisto, A.; Laxova, A.; Rock, L.Z.; Farrell, P.M. Genetic counseling and neonatal screening for cystic fibrosis: An assessment of the communication process. *Pediatrics* **2001**, *107*, 699–705. [CrossRef]

30. Munck, A.; Mayell, S.J.; Winters, V.; Shawcross, A.; Derichs, N.; Parad, R.; Barben, J.; Southern, K.W.; ECFS Neonatal Screening Working Group. Cystic Fibrosis Screen Positive, Inconclusive Diagnosis (CFSPID): A new designation and management recommendations for infants with an inconclusive diagnosis following newborn screening. *J. Cyst. Fibros.* **2015**, *14*, 706–713. [CrossRef]

31. Castellani, C.; Duff, A.J.A.; Bell, S.C.; Heijerman, H.G.M.; Munck, A.; Ratjen, F.; Sermet-Gaudelus, I.; Southern, K.W.; Barben, J.; Flume, P.A.; et al. ECFS best practice guidelines: The 2018 revision. *J. Cyst. Fibros.* **2018**, *17*, 153–178. [CrossRef]

32. David, J.; Chrastina, P.; Peskova, K.; Kozich, V.; Friedecky, D.; Adam, T.; Hlidkova, E.; Vinohradska, H.; Novotna, D.; Hedelova, M.; et al. Epidemiology of rare diseases detected by newborn screening in the Czech Republic. *Cent. Eur. J. Public Health* **2019**, *27*, 153–159. [CrossRef]

33. Scotet, V.; Dugueperoux, I.; Saliou, P.; Rault, G.; Roussey, M.; Audrezet, M.P.; Ferec, C. Evidence for decline in the incidence of cystic fibrosis: A 35-year observational study in Brittany, France. *Orphanet J. Rare Dis.* **2012**, *7*, 14. [CrossRef]

34. De Boeck, K. Cystic fibrosis in the year 2020: A disease with a new face. *Acta Paediatr.* **2020**. [CrossRef]

35. CLSI. *Newborn Screening for Cystic Fibrosis*, 2nd ed.; CLSI Guideline NBS05; CLSI: Wayne, PA, USA, 2019.

36. Ren, C.L.; Borowitz, D.S.; Gonska, T.; Howenstine, M.S.; Levy, H.; Massie, J.; Milla, C.; Munck, A.; Southern, K.W. Cystic Fibrosis Transmembrane Conductance Regulator-Related Metabolic Syndrome and Cystic Fibrosis Screen Positive, Inconclusive Diagnosis. *J. Pediatr.* **2017**, *181S*, S45–S51. [CrossRef]

37. Romeo, G.; Devoto, M.; Galietta, L.J. Why is the cystic fibrosis gene so frequent? *Hum. Genet.* **1989**, *84*, 1–5. [CrossRef]

38. Southern, K.W.; Munck, A.; Pollitt, R.; Travert, G.; Zanolla, L.; Dankert-Roelse, J.; Castellani, C.; ECFS CF Neonatal Screening Working Group. A survey of newborn screening for cystic fibrosis in Europe. *J. Cyst. Fibros.* **2007**, *6*, 57–65. [CrossRef]

39. Farrell, P.; Joffe, S.; Foley, L.; Canny, G.J.; Mayne, P.; Rosenberg, M. Diagnosis of cystic fibrosis in the Republic of Ireland: Epidemiology and costs. *Ir. Med. J.* **2007**, *100*, 557–560.

40. Newsletter ECFS Neonatal Screening Working Group. January 2014. Available online: https://www.ecfs.eu/sites/default/files/general-content-files/working-groups/NSWG_newsletter06Jan14.pdf (accessed on 1 March 2020).

41. Lucotte, G.; Hazout, S.; De Braekeleer, M. Complete map of cystic fibrosis mutation DF508 frequencies in Western Europe and correlation between mutation frequencies and incidence of disease. *Hum. Biol.* **1995**, *67*, 797–803.

42. Audrezet, M.P.; Munck, A.; Scotet, V.; Claustres, M.; Roussey, M.; Delmas, D.; Ferec, C.; Desgeorges, M. Comprehensive *CFTR* gene analysis of the French cystic fibrosis screened newborn cohort: Implications for diagnosis, genetic counseling, and mutation-specific therapy. *Genet. Med.* **2015**, *17*, 108–116. [CrossRef]

43. Castellani, C.; Picci, L.; Tridello, G.; Casati, E.; Tamanini, A.; Bartoloni, L.; Scarpa, M.; Assael, B.M.; Veneto, C.F.L.N. Cystic fibrosis carrier screening effects on birth prevalence and newborn screening. *Genet. Med.* **2016**, *18*, 145–151. [CrossRef]

44. Terlizzi, V.; Mergni, G.; Buzzetti, R.; Centrone, C.; Zavataro, L.; Braggion, C. Cystic fibrosis screen positive inconclusive diagnosis (CFSPID): Experience in Tuscany, Italy. *J. Cyst. Fibros.* **2019**, *18*, 484–490. [CrossRef]

45. Bauca, J.M.; Morell-Garcia, D.; Vila, M.; Perez, G.; Heine-Suner, D.; Figuerola, J. Assessing the improvements in the newborn screening strategy for cystic fibrosis in the Balearic Islands. *Clin. Biochem.* **2015**, *48*, 419–424. [CrossRef]

46. Skov, M.; Baekvad-Hansen, M.; Hougaard, D.M.; Skogstrand, K.; Lund, A.M.; Pressler, T.; Olesen, H.V.; Duno, M. Cystic fibrosis newborn screening in Denmark: Experience from the first 2 years. *Pediatr. Pulmonol.* **2020**, *55*, 549–555. [CrossRef]

47. Dankert-Roelse, J.E.; Bouva, M.J.; Jakobs, B.S.; Janssens, H.M.; de Winter-de Groot, K.M.; Schonbeck, Y.; Gille, J.J.P.; Gulmans, V.A.M.; Verschoof-Puite, R.K.; Schielen, P.; et al. Newborn blood spot screening for cystic fibrosis with a four-step screening strategy in the Netherlands. *J. Cyst. Fibros.* **2019**, *18*, 54–63. [CrossRef]

48. Sobczynska-Tomaszewska, A.; Oltarzewski, M.; Czerska, K.; Wertheim-Tysarowska, K.; Sands, D.; Walkowiak, J.; Bal, J.; Mazurczak, T.; NBS CF Working Group. Newborn screening for cystic fibrosis: Polish 4 years' experience with CFTR sequencing strategy. *Eur. J. Hum. Genet.* **2013**, *21*, 391–396. [CrossRef]

49. Soltysova, A.; Tothova Tarova, E.; Ficek, A.; Baldovic, M.; Polakova, H.; Kayserova, H.; Kadasi, L. Comprehensive genetic study of cystic fibrosis in Slovak patients in 25 years of genetic diagnostics. *Clin. Respir. J.* **2018**, *12*, 1197–1206. [CrossRef]

50. Lannefors, L.; Lindgren, A. Demographic transition of the Swedish cystic fibrosis community–results of modern care. *Respir. Med.* **2002**, *96*, 681–685. [CrossRef]

51. Marcao, A.; Barreto, C.; Pereira, L.; Guedes Vaz, L.; Cavaco, J.; Casimiro, A.; Felix, M.; Reis Silva, T.; Barbosa, T.; Freitas, C.; et al. Cystic fibrosis newborn screening in Portugal: PAP value in populations with stringent rules for genetic studies. *Int. J. Neonatal Screen.* **2018**, *4*, 22. [CrossRef]

52. Lundman, E.; Gaup, H.J.; Bakkeheim, E.; Olafsdottir, E.J.; Rootwelt, T.; Storrosten, O.T.; Pettersen, R.D. Implementation of newborn screening for cystic fibrosis in Norway. Results from the first three years. *J. Cyst. Fibros.* **2016**, *15*, 318–324. [CrossRef]

53. Popa, I.; Pop, L.; Popa, Z.; Schwarz, M.J.; Hambleton, G.; Malone, G.M.; Haworth, A.; Super, M. Cystic fibrosis mutations in Romania. *Eur. J. Pediatr.* **1997**, *156*, 212–213. [CrossRef]

54. Kere, J.; Estivill, X.; Chillon, M.; Morral, N.; Nunes, V.; Norio, R.; Savilahti, E.; de la Chapelle, A. Cystic fibrosis in a low-incidence population: Two major mutations in Finland. *Hum. Genet.* **1994**, *93*, 162–166. [CrossRef]

55. Barben, J.; Castellani, C.; Dankert-Roelse, J.; Gartner, S.; Kashirskaya, N.; Linnane, B.; Mayell, S.; Munck, A.; Sands, D.; Sommerburg, O.; et al. The expansion and performance of national newborn screening programmes for cystic fibrosis in Europe. *J. Cyst. Fibros.* **2017**, *16*, 207–213. [CrossRef]

56. Wilcken, B.; Wiley, V.; Sherry, G.; Bayliss, U. Neonatal screening for cystic fibrosis: A comparison of two strategies for case detection in 1.2 million babies. *J. Pediatr.* **1995**, *127*, 965–970. [CrossRef]

57. Massie, R.J.; Curnow, L.; Glazner, J.; Armstrong, D.S.; Francis, I. Lessons learned from 20 years of newborn screening for cystic fibrosis. *Med. J. Aust.* **2012**, *196*, 67–70. [CrossRef]

58. Wesley, A.W.; Stewart, A.W. Cystic fibrosis in New Zealand: Incidence and mortality. *N. Z. Med. J.* **1985**, *98*, 321–323.

59. Kosorok, M.R.; Wei, W.H.; Farrell, P.M. The incidence of cystic fibrosis. *Stat. Med.* **1996**, *15*, 449–462. [CrossRef]

60. Lilley, M.; Christian, S.; Hume, S.; Scott, P.; Montgomery, M.; Semple, L.; Zuberbuhler, P.; Tabak, J.; Bamforth, F.; Somerville, M.J. Newborn screening for cystic fibrosis in Alberta: Two years of experience. *Paediatr. Child Health* **2010**, *15*, 590–594. [CrossRef]

61. Eyheramendy, S.; Martinez, F.I.; Manevy, F.; Vial, C.; Repetto, G.M. Genetic structure characterization of Chileans reflects historical immigration patterns. *Nat. Commun.* **2015**, *6*, 6472. [CrossRef]

62. Lay-Son, G.; Puga, A.; Astudillo, P.; Repetto, G.M.; Collaborative Group of the Chilean National Cystic Fibrosis Program. Cystic fibrosis in Chilean patients: Analysis of 36 common CFTR gene mutations. *J. Cyst. Fibros.* **2011**, *10*, 66–70. [CrossRef]

63. Silva Filho, L.V.; Castanos, C.; Ruiz, H.H. Cystic fibrosis in Latin America-Improving the awareness. *J. Cyst. Fibros.* **2016**, *15*, 791–793. [CrossRef]

64. Nazer, H.M. Early diagnosis of cystic fibrosis in Jordanian children. *J. Trop. Pediatr.* **1992**, *38*, 113–115. [CrossRef]

65. Al-Mahroos, F. Cystic fibrosis in Bahrain incidence, phenotype, and outcome. *J. Trop. Pediatr.* **1998**, *44*, 35–39. [CrossRef]

66. Frossard, P.M.; Lestringant, G.; Girodon, E.; Goossens, M.; Dawson, K.P. Determination of the prevalence of cystic fibrosis in the United Arab Emirates by genetic carrier screening. *Clin. Genet.* **1999**, *55*, 496–497. [CrossRef]

67. Stafler, P.; Mei-Zahav, M.; Wilschanski, M.; Mussaffi, H.; Efrati, O.; Lavie, M.; Shoseyov, D.; Cohen-Cymberknoh, M.; Gur, M.; Bentur, L.; et al. The impact of a national population carrier screening program on cystic fibrosis birth rate and age at diagnosis: Implications for newborn screening. *J. Cyst. Fibros.* **2016**, *15*, 460–466. [CrossRef]

68. Goodchild, M.C.; Insley, J.; Rushton, D.I.; Gaze, H. Cystic fibrosis in 3 Pakistani children. *Arch. Dis. Child.* **1974**, *49*, 739–741. [CrossRef]

69. Powers, C.A.; Potter, E.M.; Wessel, H.U.; Lloyd-Still, J.D. Cystic fibrosis in Asian Indians. *Arch. Pediatr. Adolesc. Med.* **1996**, *150*, 554–555. [CrossRef]

70. Kapoor, V.; Shastri, S.S.; Kabra, M.; Kabra, S.K.; Ramachandran, V.; Arora, S.; Balakrishnan, P.; Deorari, A.K.; Paul, V.K. Carrier frequency of F508del mutation of cystic fibrosis in Indian population. *J. Cyst. Fibros.* **2006**, *5*, 43–46. [CrossRef]

71. Kabra, S.K.; Kabra, M.; Lodha, R.; Shastri, S. Cystic fibrosis in India. *Pediatr. Pulmonol.* **2007**, *42*, 1087–1094. [CrossRef]

72. Wright, S.W.; Morton, N.E. Genetic studies on cystic fibrosis in Hawaii. *Am. J. Hum. Genet.* **1968**, *20*, 157–169.

73. Yamashiro, Y.; Shimizu, T.; Oguchi, S.; Shioya, T.; Nagata, S.; Ohtsuka, Y. The estimated incidence of cystic fibrosis in Japan. *J. Pediatr. Gastroenterol. Nutr.* **1997**, *24*, 544–547. [CrossRef]

74. Liu, Y.; Wang, L.; Tian, X.; Xu, K.F.; Xu, W.; Li, X.; Yue, C.; Zhang, P.; Xiao, Y.; Zhang, X. Characterization of gene mutations and phenotypes of cystic fibrosis in Chinese patients. *Respirology* **2015**, *20*, 312–318. [CrossRef]

75. Singh, M.; Rebordosa, C.; Bernholz, J.; Sharma, N. Epidemiology and genetics of cystic fibrosis in Asia: In preparation for the next-generation treatments. *Respirology* **2015**, *20*, 1172–1181. [CrossRef]

76. Al-Sadeq, D.; Abunada, T.; Dalloul, R.; Fahad, S.; Taleb, S.; Aljassim, K.; Al Hamed, F.A.; Zayed, H. Spectrum of mutations of cystic fibrosis in the 22 Arab countries: A systematic review. *Respirology* **2019**, *24*, 127–136. [CrossRef]

5

Thalassemias

Michael Angastiniotis [1,*] **and Stephan Lobitz** [2]

[1]   Thalassemia International Federation, Strovolos 2083, Nicosia, Cyprus
[2]   Department of Pediatric Oncology/Hematology, Kinderkrankenhaus Amsterdamer Straße, 50735 Cologne, Germany; LobitzS@Kliniken-Koeln.de
*   Correspondence: michael.angastiniotis@thalassaemia.org.cy;

Abstract: Thalassemia syndromes are among the most serious and common genetic conditions. They are indigenous in a wide but specific geographical area. However, through migration they are spreading across regions not previously affected. Thalassemias are caused by mutations in the α (*HBA1/HBA2*) and β globin (*HBB*) genes and are usually inherited in an autosomal recessive manner. The corresponding proteins form the adult hemoglobin molecule (HbA) which is a heterotetramer of two α and two β globin chains. Thalassemia-causing mutations lead to an imbalanced globin chain production and consecutively to impaired erythropoiesis. The severity of the disease is largely determined by the degree of chain imbalance. In the worst case, survival is dependent on regular blood transfusions, which in turn cause transfusional iron overload and secondary multi-organ damage due to iron toxicity. A vigorous monitoring and treatment regime is required, even for the milder syndromes. Thalassemias are a major public health issue in many populations which many health authorities fail to address. Even though comprehensive care has resulted in long-term survival and good quality of life, poor access to essential components of management results in complications which increase the cost of treatment and lead to poor outcomes. These requirements are not recognized by measures such as the Global Burden of Disease project, which ranks thalassemia very low in terms of disability-adjusted life years (DALYs), and fails to consider that it ranks highly in the one to four-year-old age group, making it an important contributor to under-5 mortality. Thalassemia does not fulfil the criteria to be accepted as a target disease for neonatal screening. Nevertheless, depending on the screening methodology, severe cases of thalassemia will be detected in most neonatal screening programs for sickle cell disease. This is very valuable because: (1) it helps to prepare the affected families for having a sick child and (2) it is an important measure of secondary prevention.

Keywords: thalassemia; burden of disease; newborn screening; hemoglobinopathies

1. Introduction

The hereditary disorders of the hemoglobin molecule are among the commonest of clinically serious genetic conditions [1]. They are of two general types: those in which a mutation interferes with the amount of protein produced (thalassemias), and those that result in a structural change of the hemoglobin molecule, leading to the production of a variant protein (hemoglobinopathies).

In this article we will review the pathophysiology and the clinical and public health consequences of thalassemias. These include two categories, the α- and β-thalassemias, according to which the globin chain of the hemoglobin molecule is inadequately produced. The clinically most serious conditions are the β-thalassemias in the homozygous state, while the α-thalassemia homozygotes are usually lethal in utero.

The numbers of affected patients are not known. Very few countries maintain a patient registry and in many others, children die from the more severe transfusion-dependent syndromes before they are even diagnosed. Rough estimates of expected global annual births are around

60,000 [1]. The distribution of the thalassemia genes stretches from the Mediterranean basin and Sub-Saharan Africa through the Middle East to the Far East including South China and the Pacific Islands. In northern regions, these genes are rare in the indigenous populations, but population movements, both for economic reasons and due topolitical instability, are contributing to a changing epidemiology [2,3]. The necessity for lifelong treatment, the prevention of serious complications through regular monitoring, and premature deaths in many patients make these disorders a significant health burden requiring public health planning and policy making [4]. This is a process which countries with few resources are often unable to follow. Even in the well-resourced countries of the West, the rarity of the condition does not always allow for expertise to develop, and optimum care is also lacking here.

2. Pathophysiology of Thalassemias

In the physiological state, the hemoglobin molecule is a heterotetramer consisting of two α and two non-α globin chains, each carrying a heme molecule with a central iron. In this state, the oxygen-carrying capacity of the molecule is maximal. The non-α globin chains can be β chains which coupled with α chains form adult hemoglobin (HbA), while α chains and δ chains form a minor fraction of adult hemoglobin (HbA$_2$). Finally, α and γ chains form the fetal hemoglobin (HbF). The production of the globin chains is regulated by the α globin cluster on chromosome 16 with the two α globin genes *HBA1* and *HBA2*, and the β globin cluster on chromosome 11 with the genes for the γ, δ, and β globin chains. The physiological situation is characterized by a balanced production of the α and the non-α globin chains that ensures a reciprocal pairing into the normal tetramers. In the thalassemias, this equilibrium is disrupted by the defective production of one of the globin chains. Any reduced production of one of the globin chains within the developing red cell will cause an accumulation of the normally produced chain that can no longer find the equivalent amount of its heterologous partner to assemble to the normal heterotetramer. If α globin chains are not produced in adequate amounts there will be an accumulation of β globin chains (α-thalassemia); if β globin chains are inadequately produced then α globin chains will accumulate (β-thalassemia). These observations were made possible by the introduction of methods to separate and quantify these globin chains [5,6]. These studies enabled the understanding of the pathophysiology of these conditions as being the result of the chain imbalance [7].

The excess unpaired and insoluble α globin chains in β-thalassemia cause apoptosis of red cell precursors, resulting in ineffective erythropoiesis. The excess non-α globin chains in α-thalassemia assemble as γ_4 tetramers (Hb Bart's) in intrauterine life and β_4 tetramers (HbH) after birth. Both of these abnormal homotetramers are poor carriers of oxygen (too high affinity for oxygen). The excess chains have further devastating effects on the function of erythrocytes and their ability to deliver oxygen [8,9].

- The production of hemoglobin starts in the proerythroblast and increases during erythroid maturation through the basophilic, polychromatophilic and orthochromatic phases of red cell maturation. In erythroblasts, the excess α globin chains in β-thalassemia precipitate at the cell membrane and cause oxidative membrane damage and premature cell death by apoptosis. This happens within the erythropoietic tissue and so results in ineffective erythropoiesis [10].
- Some of the immature red cells pass into the circulation. Because of their membrane defect, they are fragile and prone to hemolysis. They also exhibit an altered deformability and are trapped by the spleen where they are destroyed by macrophages. This leads to an enlargement of the spleen which can become massive, leading to the development of functional hypersplenism with removal of platelets and white cells as well as red cells.
- Ineffective erythropoiesis, removal of abnormal cells by the spleen, and hemolysis all contribute to an anemia of variable severity.

The response to anemia is twofold:

- The kidneys increase secretion of erythropoietin (EPO). EPO is a cytokine that targets red cell precursors in response to the oxygen requirement of tissues. EPO secretion results in an increased red cell production, but because of the defect of erythroblast maturation this will make the ineffective erythropoiesis worse. This is a vicious cycle that results in expansion of hematopoietic tissue within the bone marrow and the destruction of bone architecture, thus contributing to bone disease and fragility. In some patients, extramedullary hematopoietic masses develop within the liver, the spleen, and the reticuloendothelial system.

- Hepcidin is a regulator of iron absorption [11] and produced by liver cells. It regulates the expression of ferroportin, a protein which directly facilitates enterocytic iron absorption in the gut. Independently of the cause, in severe anemia, hepcidin production is suppressed which results in increased iron absorption [12]. This contributes to iron overload, especially in patients who are not regularly transfused.

The degree of anemia is variable and depends on the mutation or combination of mutations in each individual patient. There are about 200 known mutations on the β gene cluster. Some mutations do not allow any β globin chain production. These are known as β^0 mutations while other mutations allow some β globin chain production and are referred to as β^+ and β^{++} mutations, respectively [13]. Likewise, in α-thalassemia more than 100 varieties have been described [14]. The degree of anemia and the severity of the clinical effect can be modified by other mitigating factors. The most common of these is the co-inheritance of factors that reduce globin chain imbalance such as when α-thalassemia is co-inherited in β-thalassemia homozygotes, resulting in a milder β-thalassemia syndrome.

The treatment of severe anemia is blood transfusion. In the serious transfusion dependent forms, regular transfusions from early childhood lead to severe iron overload. In the physiological state 1–2 mg of iron are absorbed from food sources daily and the same amount is excreted fecally. Increased gastrointestinal absorption of iron in thalassemia aggravates transfusional iron burden and results in the excess iron being taken up by proteins produced in the liver, including transferrin and ferritin. Protein bound iron is stored mainly in the liver and is not toxic. However, since each unit of transfused blood contains 100–200 mg of iron (0.47 mg/mL), in regularly transfused patients, the capacity of these proteins to bind iron is saturated soon and non-transferrin bound iron (NTBI) is released into the plasma [15,16]. This free iron, particularly a species known as labile plasma iron (LPI), generates reactive-oxygen species resulting in organelle damage and cell death, especially of hepatocytes, cardiomyocytes and the cells of endocrine glands [17]. Vital organ function is disturbed in this way, leading to serious complications which may be lethal. This necessitates the daily consumption of iron chelating agents to prevent complications and ensure survival. The degree to which these effects of iron overload occur is related to transfusion dependency. In non-transfusion dependent forms of thalassemia (NTDT), such as β-thalassemia intermedia and α-thalassemia, there is also iron overload secondary to increased absorption from the gut. However, this develops at a much slower rate than in transfusion-dependent thalassemia (TDT) [18]. Complications in these NTDT appear later in life, mostly in the second and third decades (the clinical effects of NTDT are summarized below).

3. Clinical Considerations

According to the causative genetic defect, the thalassemia syndromes are usually classified as β- or α-thalassemias. Here, in Table 1, we attempt to use a classification according to clinical severity, which may include several genetic types in one category.

Table 1. Thalassemia groupings according to clinical severity.

α-Thalassemia hydrops fetalis	Leads to death in utero in most cases
Transfusion-dependent (β) thalassemia	Leads to death in early infancy unless treated
Non transfusion-dependent thalassemia	Occasional blood transfusions required (may become transfusion-dependent in later life)
Thalassemia minor	Mostly heterozygotes for thalassemia genes (carriers), but may include some homozygotes/compound heterozygotes for very mild β-thalassemia mutations and HbE

Alpha thalassemia hydrops fetalis is caused by deletion or inactivation of all four α globin alleles. The result is that excess gamma globin chains form tetramers (γ_4 = Hb Bart's) in uterine life, which because of their high oxygen affinity cannot effectively deliver oxygen to tissues. This leads to severe hypoxia [19]. Intrauterine anemia leads to heart failure although the underlying mechanisms are still to be fully understood [20]. There are signs of pronounced fetal edema, hepatosplenomegaly and hydramnios. Maternal pre-eclampsia and the need for caesarean section endanger mother's health and life. These possible outcomes have made it a rule that prenatal diagnosis is offered to at-risk pregnancies with termination of pregnancy before maternal health is affected. However, intra-uterine blood transfusions have led some pregnancies to a successful outcome and the babies to survive as transfusion dependent patients [21]. The molecular defects that can cause hydrops include deletional mutations found in the Mediterranean countries like $-^{MED}/-^{MED}$, but more commonly in Asia like $-^{SEA}/-^{SEA}$; in addition, in South East Asia severe non-deletional mutations are more common, and so hydrops is more commonly encountered in that region. Some of these non-deletional mutations correspond to a mixed defect in which the thalassemic determinant is associated with an unstable abnormal hemoglobin. Examples are Constant Spring (common), Quong Sze, Suan Dok, Pakse, and Adana (rare) hemoglobin [22].

TDTs are the most serious clinical entities which become clinically apparent in infancy and result from β^0 or severe β^+ homozygosity. Triplication or quadruplication of α genes aggravate β-thalassemia and can even transform a classically asymptomatic β-thalassemia heterozygosity into a clinically relevant condition.

The hallmark of TDT is a steadily progressive anemia which makes the child transfusion-dependent from the first few months of life. The onset of clinical symptoms coincides with the fetal to adult hemoglobin switch in which HbF production decreases and is normally replaced by the production of HbA. However, because of the thalassemic defect, the switch is either abolished (β^0/β^0 homozygosity) or the production of HbA is grossly insufficient to compensate for the HbF decrease (β^0/β^+ or severe β^+/β^+). The continuous fall of the hemoglobin level and all the consequences described above lead to the need for repeated blood transfusions. The therapeutic aim is to keep a level of hemoglobin that will not only ensure good oxygenation, but also reduce the stimulus for EPO secretion and thus reduce endogenous erythropoiesis [23]. Keeping the pre-transfusion hemoglobin above 9–10 g/dL achieves this aim and allows for physical development with reduced or no bony changes and deformities. Regular lifelong transfusions have several possible adverse effects which include immunological reactions and transmission of infectious agents of which the hepatitis C virus is currently the most common. In many countries, inadequate supplies of donors result in low hemoglobin levels, with the consequences of anemia described before. The most important side effect, however, is the accumulation of iron, the pathophysiological consequences of which have been described above. The life endangering effects of iron toxicity necessitate close monitoring and quantification of the iron load in the tissues and removal of the iron by iron chelating agents [24]. The thalassemia patient is therefore subjected to a series of tests aiming at prevention or at least early recognition of tissue toxicity.

Regular monitoring of regularly transfused patients includes

- Regular blood tests: hematology, biochemistry and serology
- Imaging: MRI (to measure heart and liver iron load), abdominal ultrasound, bone density
- Echocardiography to assess cardiac function and pulmonary hypertension
- Ophthalmological examinations and audiometry
- Organ biopsies as required (largely replaced by MRI)

On a global level, effective iron chelation is hampered by:

- Poor availability of drugs in many countries and catastrophic out of pocket expenses [25].
- Patient non-adherence to prescribed treatment [26]. In many clinics, non-adherence is regarded as a major cause of treatment failure. This is not surprising since chelation treatment is a daily routine, and any short or long interruption leads to the exposure of cells to free iron radicals with consecutive tissue damage. Various interventions have been suggested to reduce this phenomenon mainly relying on psychosocial support and the patient partaking in management decisions which concern them. Understanding patient concerns is still an open subject [27,28] and effective interventions are still a problem in everyday life of thalassemia clinics across the world.
- Inexperience and inadequate adherence of physicians to evidence based guidelines. This is a phenomenon which is not well documented in scientific publications but is a common experience where rare conditions are concerned [29]. Due to the rarity of the condition in many localities, thalassemia suffers from all the weaknesses reported by EURORDIS and other rare disease organizations, such as delayed diagnosis and recognizing life-threatening complications too late [30].

The long survival experienced by the latest birth cohorts of patients with the most severe thalassemia syndromes, mainly treated in centers of expertise, is due toa combination of safe and effective blood transfusion, adequate iron chelation and early recognition of complications with effective interventions by a multidisciplinary team of experts. The excellent outcomes in terms of survival and quality of life were not achieved by the introduction of new additional therapies [31], but by adherence to evidence-based guidelines. New treatments are expected in the near future [32] which will probably further improve quality of life. Curative treatments, apart from haemopoietic stem cell transplantation (HSCT) which has long been available [33], are also in the pipeline, utilizing genetic therapies.

Milder, non-transfusion dependent forms (NTDT), which can survive without regular blood transfusions may require occasional transfusions during intercurrent illnesses or pregnancies. However, regular transfusions may be required in later life due tocomplications. NTDT syndromes are caused by mild β^{++} mutations (allowing some β globin chain production) and/or the co-inheritance of mitigating factors such as α-thalassemia or persistence of fetal hemoglobin which reduce the globin chain imbalance. Another mechanism is the co-inheritance of another hemoglobin variant, the most common being HbE which is commonly encountered in South East Asia [34]. HbE is a "thalassemic variant", i.e., a hemoglobin variant that is produced insufficiently and thus promotes anemia.

Since erythropoietic tissue expansion is not suppressed early in life by transfusions, its effects on bone marrow expansion and extramedullary erythropoiesis continues and so damage to bone structure, leading to deformities and relatively early onset of osteopenia/osteoporosis and pressure from hematopoietic masses, characterize this syndrome. Chronic anemia and ineffective erythropoiesis persist despite a relatively steady hemoglobin level with the result of increasing iron absorption from the gut through hepcidin suppression. This causes iron toxicity mainly to the liver while the heart remains relatively free of iron-related damage [35–37]. Iron overload with the increased circulation of NTBI leads to hepatocyte damage which progresses to fibrosis, presumably due tolonger duration of exposure [38] and to hepatocellular carcinoma, which is more frequent in NTDT. Erythropoietic expansion as evidenced by the respective markers like soluble transferrin receptors (sTfR), increased nucleated red cells (NRBCs) and growth differentiation factor 15 (GDF-15) [39], will also contribute to splenomegaly leading many clinicians to recommend splenectomy. The pathophysiological effects of splenectomy and hypercoagulability are more often encountered in NTDT compared to TDT and so stroke, pulmonary hypertension and vascular disease are more frequent in NTDT compared to regularly transfused patients. It is because of these complications that splenectomy is avoided and that regular transfusions are initiated in NTDT patients when complications arise such as symptomatic extramedullary hematopoietic masses, pulmonary hypertension, thrombotic events, and leg ulcers [40]. Interestingly, causative factors of NTDT are variable, including mostly β-thalassemia intermedia and HbE/β-thalassemia but also HbH disease (which belongs to the α-thalassemia group). There are differences in both the biomarkers of iron metabolism and erythropoiesis as well as in the clinical manifestations among the various causative factors [39]. For instance, HbH disease in the Mediterranean has the mildest effects but can be severe in South East Asia. Similarly, for unknown reasons, HbE/β-thalassemia presentation varies from relatively moderate to very severe.

4. Management of the Thalassemia Syndromes: The Global Perspective

It is not possible here to go over the details of all treatment modalities and their possible effectiveness or side effects. The impression in many high prevalence areas is that providing adequate supplies of 'clean' blood and a choice of iron chelating agents is the basis of managing these syndromes effectively. This is particularly true if the thalassemia population consists of children. From adolescence and even earlier, a monitoring schedule should be in place, aiming to recognize early complications which should be dealt with. Centers, mainly in the economically developed world, which are able to fully follow internationally accepted guidelines [41] are serving a minority of the global community of patients [1,3,4]. Such privileged patients are now surviving to their fifties with a good quality of life. Even in locations with few resources, essential components of care cannot be ignored or put aside because of "other priorities". The reason is that any reductions will increase the chance of complications and so increase the cost of care and/or result in premature death. This is a waste of resources that is often not recognized. The burden of disease, in the case of congenital disorders, cannot be simply assessed by the numbers of patients affected. In the reports of the Global Burden of Disease (GBD), thalassemia was ranked 68th in 2010 in terms of DALYs, yet it ranked 24th when the one-to-four-year age group was considered, indicating its important contribution to under-5 mortality [42]. It is doubtful whether this ranking is based on accurate data since many children in countries with high prevalence of thalassemia and with less privileged populations may die without even a diagnosis. National policies are usually formulated by public health officials who have no clinical experience and use DALYs and GBD data to rank their country's priorities. The hemoglobin disorders are therefore not regarded as a priority. Late-onset diseases such as cardiovascular disorders and diabetes are given high ranking and are prioritized, even by WHO in its non-communicable disease (NCD) program, leaving congenital and hereditary disorders with no plan either for patient survival or even for prevention. The results are disastrous, and early death often makes the problem invisible [4]. Any improvements in thalassemia management will benefit health services for many needs in the community:

- Adequacy of blood supplies—Regularly transfused patients require more blood than the general population and so blood collection drives, donor education, and good practices in donor management are organized. These efforts which aim to have adequate supplies will benefit the whole community and patients who require blood transfusion circumstantially for whatever reason will also benefit
- Safe blood—Regularly transfused patients are at higher risk from contaminated blood from both bacteria and viruses, and in some locations malaria is also a threat. Having strict screening procedures to screen donors will make blood safer for all the community.

- Reactions to blood transfusion are more common in regularly transfused patients, especially alloimmunization. Having procedures and technology for leukodepletion and extended antigen typing (including molecular typing) in place, will help many patients in the community (N.B., regularly transfused patients are not only those with hemoglobin disorders but include other congenital anemias, myelodysplasias, and bleeding disorders).

- Having availability of quality medication, so that effectiveness and safety of drugs is guaranteed, is a universal requirement. As generic drugs are increasingly becoming available and affordable, their quality should be more strictly controlled. This will help all patients, especially those with life-long dependency due tochronic disease.

- Centers of expertise are healthcare facilities where standards of care for chronic and rare diseases can be guaranteed. Coordinated multidisciplinary teams have been shown to improve patient outcomes where multi-organ disorders are concerned [43]. Centers of expertise can support other centers with fewer patients and less experience in an organized and officially recognized networking system. This is a universal recommendation supported by a system of accreditation of centers. This concept has been recognized by the European Commission through projects like EURORDIS and ENERCA which has resulted in criteria for centers of expertise [44,45] and the creation of European Reference Networks (ERNs) for rare diseases including rare anemias. The Thalassemia International Federation (TIF) is now developing disease-specific standards aiming at the accreditation of centers as a means for quality improvement.

- Following evidence-based guidelines is another universal recommendation.

  - Universal health coverage will ensure that families are not bankrupted by the demands of a chronic lifelong condition. Out of pocket expenses are the major reason why in some countries optimum care is not accessible for all patients—with all the known consequences. "Health is a human right. No one should get sick and die just because they are poor, or because they cannot access the health services they need" (Dr. Tedros Adhanom Ghebreyesus, Director General WHO, World Health Day 2018 Advocacy Toolkit; 7th April 2018; https://www.who.int/campaigns/world-health-day/2018/World-Health-Day-2018-Policy-Advocacy-Toolkit-Final.pdf?ua=1; last access: 20 March 2019)

5. Prevention and Screening

Prevention programs have reduced the birth prevalence of thalassemia in some countries and possibly saved resources for patient care. Such programs require planning and investment in order to include public awareness, screening to identify carriers, genetic counselling aiming to assist couples in making informed choices, and finally making available solutions such as prenatal diagnosis [46]. There are considerable differences in the attitude of people towards screening as well as for prenatal diagnosis and termination of pregnancy. Cultural, religious, ethical, and legal considerations must be considered in each country, but also, in this era of increasing population mix, different attitudes within communities in any country have to be considered in planning services [47]. Even though prevention has been shown to be cost-effective [48] very few countries have adopted nationally planned programs.

Neonatal screening to identify thalassemia syndromes early is not of great benefit especially in high prevalence areas where full prevention programs are in effect, since the clinical manifestations and transfusion dependency appear early in life. Where neonatal screening for sickle cell disease is established, some thalassemia homozygote cases and hemoglobin variants can be identified using the same laboratory techniques (mainly high-pressure liquid chromatography [48] and/or capillary electrophoresis and even isoelectric focusing). However, in many countries' patients are not identified and/or there is no patient registry on a national level and so the numbers are not known. In these situations, neonatal screening (when universal) can be useful in collecting more accurate data than surveys which often include small cohorts of a population:

- Hemoglobin variants can be accurately identified and so result in the well-known benefits of screening for sickle cell disease and epidemiological data on other variants can be obtained.
- Epidemiology of α-thalassemia can also be obtained through the detection of Hb Bart's [49].
- Thalassemia major can be identified in neonatal blood by using a cut off value of 1.5% HbA [50,51].

These tests are useful for secondary prevention and epidemiological studies, especially if supplemented by molecular studies. Other forms of technology such as tandem mass spectrometry may even be sensitive enough to identify β-thalassemia heterozygotes [52].

6. Conclusions

The thalassemia syndromes are hereditary disorders with a complex pathophysiology and serious multi-organ involvement. Current treatment may lead to long survival and a good quality of life. This includes benefitting from a full education, marriage, and parenthood, as well as contributing to the society as ordinary citizens do. In contrast, for the majority of patients, access to quality and holistic care is not possible. For these patients, thalassemia is a tragic disease with life-threatening complications which imply death in adolescence or early adulthood and result in a life of disability. Even in well-organized and well-resourced health services the provision of adequate supplies of safe blood and iron chelation are thought to meet patient needs, often ignoring the role of endocrine, cardiac, and liver monitoring by specialized teams which can deal with emerging vital organ dysfunction. The need for at least one expert reference center supporting secondary centers within each country in an organized network must be part of a policy directed and supported at the central level. This is in accordance with the concept of European Reference Networks (ERNs) for rare disorders; thalassemia falls into this category of disease in most countries.

Emerging new therapies, such as genetic interventions aiming to reduce globin chain imbalance, are likely to benefit those able to afford current management modalities leaving the "silent majority" to struggle with what basic treatments that they can afford. The solution is for health authorities to meet their obligations to those born with these conditions and persuade society and economists that investment in their health is meeting an obligation to human rights.

In this picture the question is whether neonatal screening programs can effectively contribute to achieve the desired outcomes. In areas where effective pre-conceptual or premarital prevention programs are fully applied, few cases will be picked up postnatally. In such a setting, new-born affected infants are often in families which have been informed and have chosen to give birth to an affected child. Even where there is no prevention policy, infants generally present clinically at a very young age and require immediate intervention due tosevere anemia. To develop a policy solely for the early detection of thalassemia does not seem necessary. However, where there is a program for the detection of sickle cell disease, some thalassemia syndromes and most variants may be identified. This can be beneficial for secondary prevention but also in some settings for the early detection of new cases.

Author Contributions: Conceptualization, M.A.; Writing—Original Draft Preparation, M.A.; Writing—Review & Editing, M.A., S.L.

References

1. Modell, B.; Darlison, M. Global epidemiology of haemoglobin disorders and derived service indicators. *Bull. World Health Organ.* **2008**, *86*, 480–487. [CrossRef]
2. Angastiniotis, M.; Vives Corrons, J.L.; Soteriades, E.S.; Eleftheriou, A. The impact of migrations on the health services of Europe: The example of haemoglobin disorders. *Sci. World J.* **2013**, *2013*, 727905. [CrossRef] [PubMed]
3. Weatherall, D.J. The inherited diseases of haemoglobin are an emerging global health burden. *Blood* **2010**, *115*, 4331–4333. [CrossRef] [PubMed]

4. Weatherall, D.J. The challenge of haemoglobinopathies in poor resource countries. *Br. J. Haematol.* **2011**, *154*, 736–744. [CrossRef] [PubMed]

5. Clegg, J.B.; Naughton, M.A.; Weatherall, D.J. An improved method for the characterisation of human haemoglobin mutants: Identification of alpha-2-beta-95 GLU haemoglobin N (Baltimore). *Nature* **1965**, *207*, 944. [CrossRef]

6. Weatherall, D.J.; Clegg, J.B.; Naughton, M.A. Globin synthesis in thalassaemia: An in vitro study. *Nature* **1965**, *208*, 1061–1065. [CrossRef] [PubMed]

7. Nathan, D.G.; Gunn, R.B. Thalassemia: The consequence of unbalanced haemoglobin synthesis. *Am. J. Med.* **1966**, *41*, 815–830. [CrossRef]

8. Nathan, D.G.; Strossel, T.B.; Gunn, R.B.; Zarkowsky, H.S.; Laforet, M.T. Influence of haemoglobin precipitation on erythrocyte metabolism in alpha and beta thalassaemia. *J. Clin. Investig.* **1969**, *48*, 33–41. [CrossRef] [PubMed]

9. Nienhuis, A.W.; Nathan, D.G. Pathophysiology and clinical manifestations of the β-thalassemias. *Cod. Spring Harb. Perspect. Med.* **2012**, *2*, a011726. [CrossRef]

10. Rivella, S. Ineffective erythropoiesis and thalassemias. *Curr. Opin. Hematol.* **2009**, *16*, 187–194. [CrossRef]

11. Ganz, T. Hepcidin, a key regulator of iron metabolism and mediator of anemia of inflammation. *Blood* **2003**, *102*, 783–788. [CrossRef]

12. Papanikolaou, G.; Tzilianos, M.; Christakis, J.I.; Bagdanos, D.; Tsimirika, K.; MacFarlane, J.; Goldberg, Y.P.; Sakellaropoulos, N.; Ganz, T.; Nemeth, E. Hepcidin in iron overload disorders. *Blood* **2005**, *105*, 4103–4105. [CrossRef]

13. Higgs, D.R.; Engel, J.D.; Stamatoyannopoulos, G. Thalassaemia. *Lancet* **2012**, *379*, 373–383. [CrossRef]

14. Piel, F.; Weatherall, D.J. The alpha thalassaemias. *N. Engl. J. Med.* **2014**, *371*, 1908–1916. [CrossRef]

15. Porter, J.B. Practical management of iron overload. *Br. J. Haematol.* **2001**, *115*, 239–252. [CrossRef]

16. Porter, J.B.; Garbowski, M. The pathophysiology of transfusion iron overload. *Hematol. Oncol. Clin. N. Am.* **2014**, *28*, 683. [CrossRef]

17. Fibach, E.; Rachmilevitz, E. The role of anti-oxidants and iron chelators in the treatment of oxidative stress in thalassaemia. *Ann. N. Y. Acad. Sci.* **2010**, *1202*, 10–16. [CrossRef]

18. Taher, A.; Weatherall, D.J.; Cappellini, M.D. Thalassaemia. *Lancet* **2018**, *391*, 115–167. [CrossRef]

19. Origa, R.; Moi, P. Alpha thalassaemia. In *GeneReviews®[Internet]*; Adam, M.P., Ardinger, H.H., Pagon, R.A., Wallace, S.E., Bean, L.J.H., Stephens, K., Amemiya, A., Eds.; University of Washington, Seattle: Seattle, WA, USA, 2005.

20. Jatavan, P.; Chattipakorn, N.; Tongsong, T. Fetal haemoglobin Bart's hydrops fetalis: Pathophysiology, prenatal diagnosis and possibility of intrauterine treatment. *J. Mater. Fetal. Neonatal. Med.* **2018**, *31*, 946–957. [CrossRef]

21. Songdej, D.; Babbs, C.; Higgs, D.R.; BHFS Consortium. An international registry of survivors with haemoglobin Bart's hydrops fetalis syndrome. *Blood* **2017**, *129*, 1251–1259. [CrossRef]

22. Farashi, S.; Harteveld, C.L. Molecular basis of α-thalassaemia. *Blood Cells Mol. Dis.* **2018**, *70*, 43–53. [CrossRef] [PubMed]

23. Cazzola, M.; De Stefano, P.; Ponchio, L.; Locatelli, F.; Beguin, Y.; Dessi, C.; Barella, S.; Cao, A.; Galanello, R. Relationship between transfusion regimen and suppression of erythropoiesis in beta-thalassaemia major. *Br. J. Haematol.* **1995**, *89*, 473–478. [CrossRef] [PubMed]

24. Porter, J.B.; Garbowski, M.W. Interaction of transfusion and iron chelation in thalassaemia. *Hematol. Oncol. Clin. N. Am.* **2018**, *32*, 247–259. [CrossRef]

25. Hisam, A.; Sadiq Khan, N.; Tariq, N.A.; Irfan, H.; Arif, B.; Noor, M. Perceived stress and monetary burden among thalassaemia patients and their caregivers. *Pak. J. Med. Sci.* **2018**, *34*, 901–906. [CrossRef]

26. Fortin, P.M.; Fisher, S.A.; Madgwick, K.V.; Trivella, M.; Hopewell, S.; Doree, C.; Estcourt, L.J. Strategies to increase adherence to iron chelation therapy in people with sickle cell disease or thalassaemia. *Cochrane Database Syst. Rev.* **2018**. [CrossRef] [PubMed]

27. Trachtenberg, F.L.; Mednick, L.; Kwiatkowski, J.L.; Neufeld, E.J.; Haines, D.; Pakbaz, Z.; Thompson, A.A.; Quinn, C.T.; Grady, R.; Sobota, A.; et al. Beliefs about chelation among thalassemia patients. *Health Qual. Life Outcomes* **2012**, *10*, 148. [CrossRef] [PubMed]

28. Vosper, J.; Evangeli, M.; Porter, J.B.; Shah, F. Psychological factors associated with episodic chelation adherence in thalassaemia. *Hemoglobin* **2018**, *42*, 30–36. [CrossRef] [PubMed]

29.   Budych, K.; Helms, T.M.; Schultz, C. How do patients with rare diseases experience the medical encounter? Exploring role behaviour and the impact on patient physician interaction. *Health Policy* **2012**, *105*, 154–164. [CrossRef]

30.   EURORDIS. Rare Disease: Understanding the Public Health Policy. 2005. Available online: www.eurordis.org (accessed on 20 March 2019).

31.   Taher, A.T.; Cappellini, M.D. How I manage medical complications of beta thalassemia in adults. *Blood* **2018**, *132*, 1781–1791. [CrossRef] [PubMed]

32.   Cappellini, M.D.; Porter, J.B.; Viprakasit, V.; Taher, A.T. A paradigm shift on beta thalassaemia treatment: How will we manage this old disease with new therapies? *Blood Rev.* **2018**, *32*, 300–311. [CrossRef]

33.   Shenoy, S.; Angelucci, E.; Arnold, S.D.; Baker, K.S.; Bhatia, M.; Bresters, D.; Dietz, A.C.; De La Fuente, J.; Duncan, C.; Gaziev, J.; et al. Current Results and Future Research Priorities in Late Effects after Hematopoietic Stem Cell Transplantation for Children with Sickle Cell Disease and Thalassemia: A Consensus Statement from the Second Pediatric Blood and Marrow Transplant Consortium International Conference on Late Effects after Pediatric Hematopoietic Stem Cell Transplantation. *Biol. Blood Marrow. Transplant.* **2017**, *23*, 552–561. [PubMed]

34.   Sleiman, J.; Tarhini, A.; Bou-Fakhredin, R.; Saliba, A.N.; Cappellini, M.D.; Taher, A.T. Non-Transfusion-Dependent Thalassemia: An Update on Complications and Management. *Int. J. Mol. Sci.* **2018**, *19*, 182. [CrossRef] [PubMed]

35.   Bou-Fakhredin, R.; Bazarbachi, A.H.; Chaya, B.; Sleiman, J.; Cappellini, M.D.; Taher, A.T. Iron Overload and Chelation Therapy in Non-Transfusion Dependent Thalassemia. *Int. J. Mol. Sci.* **2017**, *18*, 2778. [CrossRef] [PubMed]

36.   Mavrogeni, S.; Gotsis, E.; Ladis, V.; Berdousis, E.; Verganelakis, D.; Toulas, P.; Cokkinos, D.V. Magnetic resonance evaluation of liver and myocardial iron deposition in thalassemia intermedia and b-thalassemia major. *Int. J. Cardiovasc. Imaging* **2008**, *24*, 849–854. [CrossRef] [PubMed]

37.   Origa, R.; Barella, S.; Argiolas, G.M.; Bina, P.; Agus, A.; Galanello, R. No evidence of cardiac iron in 20 never- or minimally-transfused patients with thalassemia intermedia. *Haematologica* **2008**, *93*, 1095–1096. [CrossRef]

38.   Olynyk, J.K.; St Pierre, T.G.; Britton, R.S.; Brunt, E.M.; Bacon, B.R. Duration of hepatic iron exposure increases the risk of significant fibrosis in hereditary hemochromatosis: A new role for magnetic resonance imaging. *Am. J. Gastroenterol.* **2005**, *100*, 837–841. [CrossRef]

39.   Porter, J.B.; Cappellini, M.D.; Kattamis, A.; Viprakasit, V.; Mussalam, K.M.; Zhu, Z.; Taher, A.T. Iron overload across the spectrum of non-transfusion dependent thalassaemias: Role of erythropoiesis, splenectomy and transfusions. *Br. J. Haematol.* **2017**, *176*, 288–299. [CrossRef] [PubMed]

40.   Taher, A.; Vichinsky, E.; Mussalam, K.M.; Cappellini, M.D.; Viprakasit, V. *Guidelines for the Management of Non-Transfusion Dependent Thalassaemia (NTDT)*, 2nd ed.; Thalassaemia International Federation: Nicosia, Cyprus, 2017.

41.   Cappellini, M.D.; Cohen, A.; Porter, J.; Taher, A.; Viprakasit, V. *Guidelines for the Management of Transfusion Dependent Thalassaemia (TDT)*, 3rd ed.; Thalassaemia International Federation: Nicosia, Cyprus, 2014.

42.   Piel, F. The present and future Global Burden of the inherited disorders of haemoglobin. *Hematol. Oncol. Clin. N. Am.* **2016**, *30*, 327–341. [CrossRef]

43.   Kattamis, C.; Sofocleous, C.; Ladis, V.; Kattamis, A. Athens University thalassemia expertise unit: Evolution, structure, perspectives and patients' expectations. *Georgian Med. News* **2013**, *222*, 94–98.

44.   Vives-Corrons, J.L.; Manu Pereira, M.M.; Romeo-Casabona, C.; Ncolas, P.; Gulbis, B.; Eleftheriou, A.; Angastiniotis, M.; Aguilar-Martinez, P.; Bianchi, P.; Van Wijk, R.; et al. Recommendations for centres of expertise in rare anaemias. The ENERCA White book. *Thalass. Rep.* **2014**, *4*, 4878.

45.   EUCERD Recommendations for Centres of Expertise for Rare Diseases 2013. Available online: www.eucerd. eu (accessed on 20 March 2019).

46.   Angastiniotis, M.; Eleftheriou, A.; Galanello, R.; Harteveld, C.L.; Petrou, M.; Traeger-Synodinos, J.; Giordano, P.; Jauniaux, E.; Modell, B.; Serour, G.; et al. *Prevention of Thalassaemias and Other Haemoglobin Disorders: Volume 1: Principles [Internet]*, 2nd ed.; Thalassaemia International Federation: Nicosia, Cyprus, 2013.

47.   Cousens, N.E.; Gaff, C.L.; Metcalf, S.A.; Delatycki, M.B. Carrier screening for beta thalassaemia: A review of international practice. *Eur. J. Hum. Genet.* **2010**, *18*, 1077–1083. [CrossRef]

48. Koren, A.; Profeta, L.; Zalman, L.; Palmor, H.; Levin, C.; Zamir, R.B.; Shalev, S.; Blondheim, O. Prevention of β-thalassemia in Northern Israel—A Cost-Benefit Analysis. *Med. J. Hematol. Infect. Dis.* **2014**, *6*, e2014012. [CrossRef]

49. Allaf, B.; Patin, F.; Elion, J.; Couque, N. New approaches to accurate interpretation of sickle cell disease newborn screening by applying multiple of median cut offs and ratios. *Pediatr. Blood Cancer* **2018**, *65*, e27230. [CrossRef]

50. Rugless, M.J.; Fisher, C.A.; Stephens, A.D.; Amos, R.J.; Mohammed, T.; Old, J.M. Hb Bart's in cord blood: An accurate indicator of alpha-thalassemia. *Hemoglobin* **2006**, *30*, 57–62. [CrossRef]

51. Streely, A.; Latinovic, R.; Henthorn, J.; Daniel, Y.; Dormandy, E.; Darbyshire, P.; Mantio, D.; Fraser, L.; Farrar, L.; Will, A.; et al. Newborn blood spots results: Predictive value of screen positive test for thalassaemia major. *J. Med. Screen* **2013**, *20*, 183–187. [CrossRef]

52. Yu, C.; Huang, S.; Wang, M.; Zhang, J.; Liu, H.; Yuan, Z.; Wang, X.; He, X.; Wang, J.; Zou, L. A novel tandem mass spectrometry method for first line screening of mainly beta-thalassaemia from dried blood spots. *J. Proteom.* **2017**, *154*, 78–84. [CrossRef]

6

Pancreatitis-Associated Protein in Neonatal Screening for Cystic Fibrosis: Strengths and Weaknesses

Olaf Sommerburg [1,2,*] **and Jutta Hammermann** [3]

[1] Division of Pediatric Pulmonology & Allergy and Cystic Fibrosis Center, Department of Pediatrics III, University of Heidelberg, Im Neuenheimer Feld 430, D-69120 Heidelberg, Germany

[2] Translational Lung Research Center Heidelberg (TLRC), Member of the German Center for Lung Research (DZL), Im Neuenheimer Feld 350, D-69120 Heidelberg, Germany

[3] Pediatric Department, University Hospital of Dresden, Fetscherstr. 74, D-01307 Dresden, Germany; Jutta.Hammermann@uniklinikum-dresden.de

[*] Correspondence: olaf.sommerburg@med.uni-heidelberg.de

Abstract: There are currently four countries and one local region in Europe that use PAP in their newborn screening programme. The first country to employ PAP at a national level was the Netherlands, which started using IRT/PAP/DNA/EGA in 2011. Germany followed in 2016 with a slightly different IRT/PAP/DNA strategy. Portugal also started in 2016, but with an IRT/PAP/IRT programme, and in 2017, Austria changed its IRT/IRT protocol to an IRT/PAP/IRT program. In 2018, Catalonia started to use an IRT/PAP/IRT/DNA strategy. The strengths of PAP are the avoidance of carrier detection and a lower detection rate of CFSPID. PAP seems to have advantages in detecting CF in ethnically-diverse populations, as it is a biochemical approach to screening, which looks for pancreatic injury. Compared to an IRT/IRT protocol, an IRT/PAP protocol leads to earlier diagnoses. While PAP can be assessed with the same screening card as the first IRT, the second IRT in an IRT/IRT protocol requires a second heel prick around the 21st day of the patient's life. However, IRT/PAP has two main weaknesses. First, an IRT/PAP protocol seems to have a lower sensitivity compared to a well-functioning IRT/DNA protocol, and second, IRT/PAP that is performed as a purely biochemical protocol has a very low positive predictive value. However, if the advantages of PAP are to be exploited, a combination of IRT/PAP with genetic screening or a second IRT as a third tier could be an alternative for a sufficiently performing CF-NBS protocol.

Keywords: cystic fibrosis; newborn screening; biochemical screening; pancreatitis associated protein; immunoreactive trypsinogen

1. Introduction

Cystic Fibrosis Newborn screening (CF NBS) is widely accepted, but there is no universal screening strategy [1]. All programs start with a measurement of immunoreactive trypsinogen (IRT) in dried blood spots. As the second tier, a repeat measurement of the IRT concentration can be performed at the age of 2–3 weeks, but in the most common CF NBS protocols, IRT measurement as the first tier are combined with the search for population-specific *CFTR* mutations, which provides good sensitivity and specificity [2]. However, the use of *CFTR* mutation analysis is also associated with a few unsolved problems. For example, the detection of healthy carriers and of infants in whom the diagnosis of CF is inconclusive (CFSPID) is not the goal of CF NBS. Furthermore, with increasing migration in the world and the mixing of different ethnic groups, especially in big cities, there is a tendency in countries with genetic CF NBS to increase the number of *CFTR* mutations tested to ensure sufficient sensitivity. This leads to a further increase in the number of carriers and CFSPID. However, this makes information and counselling for families with children with CF, carriers, or CFSPID in these countries increasingly challenging [3,4]. In addition, in countries where informed consent for CF NBS is required, genetic CF NBS can significantly complicate the parental education and consent process.

In 1994, a French group suggested pancreatitis associated protein (PAP) as candidate for a marker for screening CF [5]. PAP is a secretory protein which is not measurable in blood under normal conditions, but which can be detected in high quantities in the context of pancreatic injury [6]. Two pilot studies showed that almost all IRT-negative newborns and most IRT-positive newborns without cystic fibrosis had normal PAP, while PAP was increased in newborns with CF [5,7]. Yet, the increase in PAP observed in newborns is not strictly CF-specific. If the measurement of PAP were used for CF NBS alone, it would have a similarly low specificity as the use of IRT alone. In the first French pilot studies, however, it was found that newborns with CF always had both an increased IRT and an increased PAP; in a further study, it was concluded that both parameters should be evaluated. The aim of this feasibility study was to compare the sensitivity and specificity of the combined measurement of IRT and PAP in the same neonatal population with the screening strategy (IRT/DNA/IRT) used in France at that time [8]. In this study, 204,748 newborns were included; the results published in 2005 showed that the performance of the IRT/PAP strategy was not inferior to that of the IRT/DNA/IRT strategy applied in parallel [8].

2. The Evolution of the PAP Kit

It is important to mention right at the beginning that the PAP kit has undergone several changes and improvements since it first appeared. For the data of the first publications on the use of PAP in CF NBS obtained from 1994 to 2003, an ELISA kit using a polyclonal antibody for antigen capture and detection was used [5,8,9]. When Sarles et al. published their lauded paper on the IRT/PAP protocol including recommended cut-offs in 2005 [8], the manufacturer (Dynabio, Marseille, France) had already changed the ELISA kit used for this evaluation, and the original kit, to which the recommendations referred, was no longer available. At that time, a new kit, called "MucoPAP", was available, which uses monoclonal antibodies to capture and detect antigens. Unfortunately, there were no new recommendations for the cut-off values for this MucoPAP kit to serve as guidelines. Thus, pilot studies that were later conducted in other European countries and which are described below used the cut-off values that were actually set with the previously-marketed kit. The new cut-off recommendations for the MucoPAP kit with the monoclonal antibody were published by Sarles et al., but not before 2014 [10]. In the meantime, however, results from other European pilot studies had been published [11–13]. Some had used different cut-off values in their protocols or had used different safety net strategies to ensure sufficient sensitivity [11,12,14]. During the pilot study in the Netherlands, which will be discussed below [12], the researchers realized that the dilution factor recommended in the product description of the manufacturer of the MucoPAP kit for calculating the measured values after comparison with the reference standard was incorrect. After contact with Dynabio, this was officially corrected, but this meant that the originally recommended cut-off values had to be corrected by a factor of 1.67. To avoid further confusion for the reader, we will mention from now on in this review only the values with the corrected dilution factors, but we will add the noncorrected values in parenthesis, if these values were used in the respective original articles (e.g., in [8,11,13]).

From 2013 onwards, a further version of the PAP-ELISA, the MucoPAP-F-Kit, was available from DynaBio, which uses an alternative readout system. With this kit, the antigen–antibody complexes are detected by a streptavidin–europium conjugate, which serves as fluorescence enhancement solution. This makes it possible to detect highly fluorescent chelates that emit at 620 nm when excited at 337 nm. Compared to measurements with the MucoPAP kit with photometric detection, the MucoPAP-F kit seems to be much more stable and has a higher reproducibility. It is important to note that the cut-off values of PAP measurements with MucoPAP and MucoPAP-F are not directly comparable.

In 2016, Dynabio launched a new version of its PAP kit with photometric detection, the "MucoPAP II". The company claimed that this test had a much better intraspot reproducibility of ranges and controls compared to the previous MucoPAP kit, but the calculations from the new ranges were ~1.5 times lower than with the old kit. As a result, the PAP cut-off values had to be changed again, as done for the Austrian CF NBS in 2017.

Unfortunately, the different PAP cut-off values published over the years have meant that publications on the performance of PAP-based CF-NBS protocols are very difficult to compare.

3. Description of Selected European Pilot Studies

In 2005, Sarles et al. published their study, which demonstrated the feasibility of using PAP in conjunction with IRT [8]. While IRT and PAP were measured in parallel during the study, after an evaluation, the authors proposed a protocol in which IRT is used as the first tier and PAP as the second, which is only performed in case of increased IRT. In this respect, the so-called IRT/PAP protocol was very similar to the IRT/IRT and IRT/DNA protocols known before. In the protocol proposed by Sarles et al., a fixed IRT cut-off value of 50 µg/L was used to ensure sufficient sensitivity. For PAP, two IRT-dependent cut-off values were proposed to reduce the number of newborns with CFSPID and improve the positive predictive value (PPV): If IRT was measured between 50.0–99.9 µg/L, a PAP cut-off value of 3.0 (before correction of the dilution factor 1.8) µg/L should have been applied; if IRT was > 100 µg/L, a PAP cut-off of 1.67 (before correction of the dilution factor 1.0) µg/L should have been used [8] (Figure 1A). This protocol was the starting point for all changes that were later made in other CF NBS protocols based on PAP.

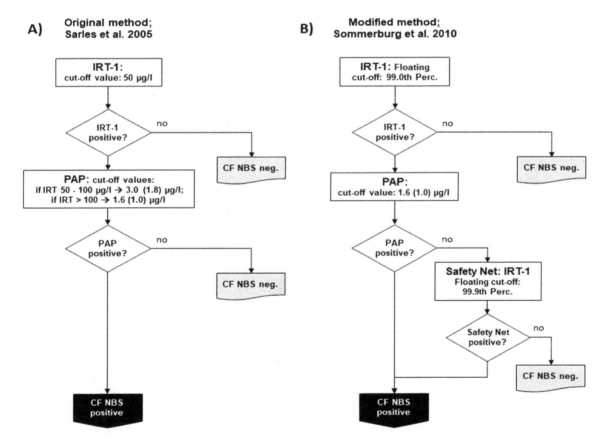

Figure 1. Schemes of the two main variants of the pure biochemical IRT/PAP protocol: (**A**) IRT/PAP protocol published by Sarles et al. 2005 [8] and (**B**) the IRT/PAP-SN protocol with IRT-dependent safety net modified by Sommerburg et al. [11]. Values in parenthesis show the PAP cut-off values as given before correction of the dilution factor by the manufacturer (see explanation in the main Text).

After the publication of this study in 2005, many specialists involved in CF NBS were interested in PAP as a new biochemical parameter and as an alternative to genetic CF screening. Although IRT/DNA protocols became the gold standard for CF NBS in terms of sensitivity and PPV, they had the disadvantages described above. However, if IRT/PAP is used as a pure biochemical protocol, the detection of healthy carriers can be completely avoided. This was the reason why studies were started in several countries around the world in the following years to verify the results of the French study and to adapt the method to local requirements. Unfortunately, not all the results of these studies were published. To the best of our knowledge, data are currently available only from France [10], Germany [11,15], The Netherlands [12,16], Czech Republic [13] and Portugal [17].

In 2008, new pilot studies started in the Netherlands and Germany. In the study in the Netherlands, samples from 145,499 newborns were measured using the slightly modified IRT/PAP protocol proposed by Sarles et al. [8], and the results were compared with those of an IRT/DNA/EGA protocol [12]. In the modified IRT/PAP protocol, the IRT cut-off used was set at 60 instead of 50 μg/L. Furthermore, the photometric measurement of the commercially available MucoPAP kit (Dynabio, Marseille, France) was replaced by a flouroimmunoassay using a Streptavidin-Europium tracer for the detection of PAP in a manner that is similar to that later introduced in the MucoPAP-F kit. The two IRT dependent PAP cut-offs were performed as follows: a positive result for PAP was defined if IRT was ≥ 100 μg/L and PAP was ≥ 1.6 μg/L or IRT was ≥ 60 μg/L and PAP was ≥ 3.0 μg/L. In the IRT/DNA protocol, the *CFTR* gene was sequenced (extended gene analysis, EGA) if, in an initial search with a panel of 35 *CFTR* mutations, none or only one *CFTR* mutation was found. In a post hoc analysis, a combination of both strategies (IRT/PAP/DNA(35)/EGA) was shown to be the best compromise for the requirements of the CF NBS program in the Netherlands.

In Germany, separate pilot studies were started in 2008 in two NBS centres (Dresden and Heidelberg) and continued until the start of the nationwide CF NBS programme in 2016. However, it should be mentioned that preliminary IRT/PAP trials had already been carried out in the CF NBS centre Dresden since 2005. The IRT/PAP protocol there was performed as originally described by Sarles et al. [8,14], but, as in the Netherlands, the ELISA MucoPAP kit (Dynabio, Marseille, France) was used for PAP quantification, and the photometric detection was replaced by fluorometric measurements [14]. Every year, 18,000 newborns are examined in Dresden and 110,000 in Heidelberg. In Heidelberg, however, less than half of the hospitals that send Guthrie cards to the NBS centre participated in the CF NBS pilot study. The IRT/PAP strategy in Heidelberg has been modified by applying a floating cut-off for IRT using the 99.0th percentile, which is often used in other CF NBS protocols. For PAP, the Heidelberg protocol relied only on one PAP cut-off using the lower PAP cut-off of the two IRT-dependent PAP cut-offs of the original protocol by Sarles et al. [8], which was defined at ≥ 1.67 μg/L (before correction of the dilution factor ≥ 1.0 μg/L) (Figure 1B). In both Dresden and Heidelberg, a safety net strategy was applied from the first year of the study due to ongoing discussions about the possibility of low sensitivity when using PAP. According to this, CF NBS was positive when the IRT ≥ was 99.9 percentile, regardless of the PAP value, which was measured as 2nd tier test. From 2008 until 2016 in Heidelberg, but not in Dresden, a genetic CF NBS protocol searching for the four most common *CFTR* mutations in Germany (IRT/DNA (4)) was run in parallel as a reference.

In 2009, another pilot study was started in the Czech Republic (Prague). In this prospective study 106,522 newborns from Bohemia, the western region of the Czech Republic, were examined to compare the IRT/PAP protocol, as originally published by Sarles et al. [8], with an IRT/DNA/IRT protocol that had been started two years earlier. While for the IRT/PAP protocol the same IRT and PAP cut-offs values were used as originally published, for the IRT/DNA/IRT protocol, the initial IRT was rated positive when the value was ≥ 65 μg/L. The initial DNA test included 32 CFTR mutations, while from July 2010, it contained 50 CFTR mutations, which represented 90.8% and 92.8% of all CFTR mutations of Czech CF patients, respectively. The results of these two protocols were compared and used to simulate an IRT/PAP/DNA(50) protocol, whose performance was then compared to that of the IRT/PAP and IRT/DNA(50)/IRT protocol.

Some of the questions concerning the PAP-based CF NBS protocols could only be answered through cooperation and combinations of study results, as done with those from Heidelberg, Dresden, and Prague. This was the only way to answer questions about the initial IRT cut-off value, the PAP cut-off values, the need for an IRT-dependent safety net, and the performance of a CF NBS strategy using the product of the IRT and PAP values [14,18].

Another PAP-based CF NBS study with 255,000 newborns started in Portugal at the end of 2013 [17]. To the best of our knowledge, this study was the first to test an IRT/PAP/IRT strategy. The cut-off value of the initial IRT was first set at 50 µg/L, but was increased to 65 µg/L after only four months. The second IRT measurement as a third stage strategy was either performed when the initial IRT ≥ was 150 µg/L (SN strategy), the PAP ≥ was 0.5 and the IRT was between 100 and 150 µg/L, or the PAP was ≥ 1.6 µg/L. For PAP analysis, the MucoPAP-F kit (Dynabio, Marseille, France) was used.

4. Findings from the Pilot Studies

4.1. IRT/PAP Protocols Detect Less Healthy Carriers

The obvious advantage of an IRT/PAP strategy is the complete avoidance of the detection of healthy carriers of *CFTR* mutations by using the pure biochemical parameters IRT and PAP. Interestingly, however, the published results from the Netherlands, Heidelberg (Germany), and the Czech Republic also showed that only 10–20% of newborns who tested positive in IRT/PAP were healthy carriers [11–13]. This shows that the heterozygous presence of a *CFTR* mutation alone does not lead to an increased PAP value in the majority of cases, which, in turn, excludes a direct dependence on the presence of certain *CFTR* mutations. This fact may seem unimportant at first glance, but it is of considerable relevance when the decision has to be made in countries with very heterogeneous ethnic populations about whether a genetic or a biochemical CF NBS should be used. While an increased number of *CFTR* mutations in the panel of an IRT/DNA protocol inevitably also increases the number of healthy carriers, a significantly lower detection rate of carriers can be achieved by adding a PAP test prior to the search for *CFTR* mutations. In the pilot study in the Netherlands, the reduction of carriers by the IRT/PAP/DNA(35)/EGA strategy was 88% in comparison to the IRT/DNA (35)/EGA strategy [12].

4.2. IRT/PAP Protocols Detect Less CFSPID

The notion that PAP-based CF NBS protocols detect less CFSPID was primarily based on the fact that the first IRT/PAP protocol by Sarles et al., with its two IRT-dependent PAP cut-off levels, was designed in a way that the majority of CFSPID patients are not detected [8]. The reason for using this design was based on the assumption that in the IRT range from 50.0 to 99.9 µg/L, lower PAP values could reflect mild CF phenotypes that are not the goal of CF NBS. As expected, those IRT/PAP protocols showed also in the following pilot studies a significantly lower detection rate of newborns with CFSPID [12,13]. However, so far, there is no evidence that the PAP concentration generally correlates with the severity of CF disease. This fact is also supported by data from the other pilot studies showing higher PAP concentrations in CFSPID or patients with *CFTR* mutations leading to pancreatic sufficiency and low PAP concentrations in some patients with *CFTR* mutations leading to pancreatic insufficiency and a severe CF phenotype (e.g., [18]). When the pilot study on the IRT/PAP strategy was started in Heidelberg in 2008, it was decided that only a single PAP cut-off level of ≥ 1.67 µg/L (before correction of the dilution factor 1.0 µg/L) [11] should be used. Nevertheless, even with this protocol, a significantly lower detection rate for newborns with CFSPID was found. While only 1.6% of the children positively screened by the IRT/PAP protocol with subsequent detection of 2 *CFTR* mutations were newborns with CFSPID, the rate with the IRT/DNA [4] protocol run in parallel was 7.3% [18]. These results indicate that a CF NBS with PAP alone can reduce the detection of CFSPID.

4.3. IRT/PAP Protocols May Show Lower Sensitivity than IRT/DNA Protocols

The published pilot studies by Sarles et al. showed that the IRT/PAP strategy had the same—if not better—sensitivity than the IRT/DNA(20/30)/IRT protocol conducted in parallel [8,10]. However, these results could not really be confirmed in any of the other pilot studies (e.g., [12,13,15]). However, it turned out that there may be a variety of reasons for possible reductions of the sensitivity of an

IRT/PAP protocol. Several of these drawbacks were addressed in the pilot studies, and it became clear that some of them could be overcome by minor protocol changes. Nevertheless, most of the sensitivity improvements proposed below are at the expense of the PPV, another important quality criterion of CF-NBS protocols.

1. *The use of an IRT-dependent safety net:* When the pilot studies were started in the Germany, the general concern was that the PAP strategy had a worse sensitivity than a well-performing genetic CF NBS. Similar to the IRT/DNA protocols with a restricted mutation panel, an IRT-dependent safety net was added six months after starting the pilot studies. Therefore, CF NBS is considered positive if the initial IRT is above the 99.9th percentile, regardless of the PAP result. When the results of the pilot study conducted in Prague (Czech Republic) were published in 2012, the IRT/PAP strategy showed a very low sensitivity of only 76% [13]. After a re-evaluation for a joint, posthoc analysis of the raw data from Prague, Dresden and Heidelberg, it was found that the sensitivity of the Prague PAP-based CF NBS would have been 89.5% if the colleagues there had used the original IRT/PAP protocol but with the IRT-dependent safety net, as was done in the German centres [18]. Furthermore, a recently published paper on the Dutch CF NBS shows that out of eight CF patients not detected in the IRT/PAP part of the IRT/PAP/DNA(35)/EGA strategy, five would probably have been found if such an IRT-dependent safety net had been used [16].

2. *Renouncing the two IRT-dependent PAP cut-off values:* As mentioned, the reason to use the two IRT-dependent PAP cut-offs was based on the assumption that such a protocol would avoid the detection of CFSPID. In addition, IRT/PAP protocols with two IRT-dependent PAP cut-off values were proposed to detect less healthy newborns as false positives compared to protocols with only one PAP cut-off value. However, the results of the aforementioned joint posthoc analysis of the data from Prague, Dresden, and Heidelberg suggest that IRT/PAP protocols with two IRT-dependent PAP cut-off values may have limited sensitivity compared to those with only one PAP cut-off value. In a joint simulation of raw data from Prague and Heidelberg, it was found that by using two PAP cut-off values, four newborns with two mutations in the *CFTR* gene would have been missed, but would have been detected by the protocol with one PAP cut-off. Only one out of these four newborns carried a *CFTR* mutation with varying clinical consequence and had a normal sweat chloride. The other three newborns were diagnosed with classical CF with pancreatic insufficiency. Two out of these three CF patients suffered from MI and would have been diagnosed clinically. However, the third CF patient would have been missed by all IRT/PAP protocols relying on two IRT-dependent PAP cut-offs [18]. It can be argued whether one has to consider three missed patients with CF or only one, since two out of these three presented with MI.

3. Anyway, the fact that newborns carrying two CF-causing mutations were not detected due to the IRT/PAP protocol with two PAP cut-offs raises the question of whether such a protocol can achieve sufficient sensitivity. It is interesting to note that if the colleagues in Prague had used the same IRT/PAP protocol as that used in Heidelberg, not only with the IRT dependent safety net, but also with only one PAP cut-off value, the sensitivity would have been 94.7%. Also, in a recently published work on the aforementioned Dutch CF NBS program, it was shown that if only one PAP cut-off value had been used, one CF patient out of the eight CF patients not found would still have been detected. With the five CF patients that would have been found by the safety Net, six of the eight CF patients would have been found [16].

4. *Lowering of PAP cut-off values:* Due to the fact that all the pilot studies mentioned above were started with a MucoPAP kit whose PAP cut-off values had not yet been sufficiently evaluated, the most obvious solution for sensitivity problems would have been to simply adjust the PAP cut-off values downwards. Actually, this was also done later by Sarles et al. and reported in a publication in 2014 [10]. However, significantly lowered PAP cut-off values were not only found there, but were seen in recent years also in other PAP-based protocols (e.g., [17]). Yet, it is precisely this approach that significantly increases the number of false-positive newborns detected.

5. *Using both biochemical markers, IRT and PAP, at the same time:* In all current PAP-based CF-NBS protocols, IRT and PAP are used sequentially. However, the simultaneous use of both biomarkers instead of two steps, e.g., by using the product of IRT and PAP, has the potential to make the screening strategy significantly more sensitive than in the IRT/PAP protocols currently in use. Despite the simultaneous use of both parameters, IRT can still be used as a first-tier-parameter that triggers the PAP measurement if it is above a certain cut-off value. Such an approach was demonstrated by the Dresden group in a posthoc analysis using raw data from the pilot studies of the two German CF NBS centres, i.e., Dresden and Heidelberg [14]. The data from Heidelberg showed the highest sensitivity with the IRTxPAP product (98.3%), in contrast to the revised strategy of Sarles et al. published in 2014 (94.9%), and also in contrast to the Heidelberg IRT/PAP-SN protocol (96.6%).

6. *Time-dependent sampling of the dried blood for neonatal screening:* There is unpublished local experience from Australia, still acknowledged by a number of CF NBS specialists, that the use of PAP is not sensitive enough if the dried blood sample for NBS is taken from the infant before the age of 48 h. As a reason for this, it was assumed that the PAP blood levels in infants with cystic fibrosis increase over time. According to our experience, this could be true, but not only in CF infants. In Germany, the collection of the dried blood sample is usually carried out between the 36th and 72nd hour of life, but for special reasons, we sometimes see early or late sampling. If we group all available PAP values of the infants studied in recent years into 12-h intervals, we see a trend of an increase in the 25th, 50th, and 75th percentiles from 24 h to 72 h (personal communication O. Sommerburg). However, when we focused on CF patients not found in our IRT/PAP protocol, we could not confirm that these CF patients were missed because the time of collection of the dry blood sample was before the 48th hour of life. In this regard, after more than 10 years of PAP-based CF NBS, we consider it to be proven that PAP screening with samples collected between 36 and 48 h of life is feasible. Yet, if the majority of infants in a country are screened for NBS before the 36th hour of life, we might imagine that PAP blood levels might still be too low. In this case, we would recommend a comprehensive pilot study to test the feasibility of a PAP-based CF NBS also under these conditions.

4.4. Pure Biochemical IRT/PAP Protocols Show a Relatively Low Positive Predictive Value

The reason why no current PAP-based CF-NBS screening program uses a purely biochemical IRT/PAP strategy has to do with the associated low PPV. In various publications from the pilot studies mentioned above, the PPV was stated to be 7.8–15.3% [12–15]. Furthermore, it is remarkable that almost all of the aforementioned interventions to improve the sensitivity of the PAP step in an IRT/PAP strategy lead to a further reduction of the PPV. However, it should be noted that the disadvantage of a higher false positive rate is compensated for by the expected higher sensitivity. Of note, also a DNA-based protocol, especially with a limited *CFTR* mutation panel, does not guarantee that the required PPV of 30% is reached, as seen with the IRT/DNA protocol run in parallel in the CF-NBS centre Heidelberg (15.3%) and in the French study published 2014 (27.1%) [10,15] (Table 1). However, the combination of a PAP-based two-tier protocol with a third step test such as a search for *CFTR* mutations or a second IRT will maintain the higher sensitivity but eliminate the disadvantage of the lower PPV. This is the reason why all CF NBS protocols currently in use are based on PAP three- or even four-tier strategies. In DNA-based CF-NBS strategies today, extended gene analysis is often used as the 3rd step after the 2nd step was performed with a limited CFTR mutation panel. This strategy also improves both the sensitivity and the PPV of the protocol. However, it does detect significantly more newborns with CFSPID, which is not really desirable. In this respect, a well-performing IRT/PAP/DNA protocol would be superior to a genetic protocol, as described above.

Table 1. Performance indicators sensitivity (%), positive predictive value (PPV, (%)) and CF/CFSPID ratio of a number of representative genetic and PAP-based CF-NBS protocols of different countries and regions compared to the ECFS standard. The numbers in parentheses within the protocol name reflect the CFTR mutations in the panel used.

2nd Tier Test	Reference	Protocol	Region/Country	n Screened	Prevalence of CF	Sensitivity (%) w/o MI	PPV (%)
	ECFS standard [19]					≥95	≥30
IRT	Calvin et al. 2012 [20]	IRT/IRT	East Anglia (UK)	582,966	1:2286	93.8	67.3
DNA	Calvin et al. 2012 [20]	IRT/DNA(29)/IRT	East Anglia (UK)	147,764	1:2111	90.2	85.9
	Sommerburg et al. 2015 [15]	IRT/DNA(4)+SN	Southwest Germany	252,020	1:4582	95.1	15.3
	Kharrazi et al. 2015 [21]	IRT/DNA(28–40)/EGA	California	2,573,293	1:6899	92	34
	Sontag et al. 2016 [22]	IRT/IRT/DNA(41–48)	Colorado, Wyoming, Texas	1,520,079	1:5548	96.2	19.7
	Lundman et al. 2016 [23]	IRT/DNA/EGA	Norway	181,859	1:8660	95	43
	Skov et al. [24]	IRT/DNA(1)/EGA	Denmark	126,338	1:4866	91.7	84.6
PAP	Sommerburg et al. 2015 [15]	IRT/PAP+SN	Southwest Germany and East-Saxony (Germany)	328,176	1:4860	96.0	8.8
	Weidler et al. [14]	IRTxPAP	Southwest Germany and East-Saxony (Germany)	410,111	1:5258	97.4	8.2
	Marcao et al. 2018 [17]	IRT/PAP/IRT	Portugal	255,000	1:7500	94.4	41.3
	Dankert-Roelse et al. 2019 [16]	IRT/PAP/DNA(35)/EGA	The Netherlands	819,879	1:6029	90	63

4.5. Current PAP-Based CF Screening Protocols in Use

Today, PAP-based CF NS protocols may achieve sufficient performance. One strength of a PAP-based CF NBS is the possibility to use it in multiethnic populations where an appropriate genetic screening is either not possible or is too cost-intensive. Table 1 gives an overview of the performance of PAP-based protocols compared to selected purely biochemical IRT/IRT- or genetic CF NBS protocols. There are currently five European countries where a CF NBS strategy based on PAP is used either in a national or regional setting.

The Netherlands: The first country to use PAP at nationwide level after a pilot study [12] was the Netherlands, which started its national screening program with an IRT/PAP/DNA(35)/EGA protocol in 2011 [16] (Figure 2A). The program started using the commercially-available MucoPAP kit (Dynabio, Marseille, France), but, as mentioned above, the photometric measurement was replaced by a flouroimmunoassay during the pilot study. Until 2016, the IRT/PAP part of the protocol was performed as proposed by Sarles et al. [8], except for the increased IRT cut-off values (now 60 µg/L). However, after the last evaluation published in 2019 [16], the IRT/PAP part of the screening protocol was changed in two points. Firstly, the lower of the two PAP cut-off values was reduced, and secondly, a safety net was introduced for the PAP step, which is based on the 99.9th IRT percentile, as in the protocol according to Sommerburg et al. [11,18]. It may be expected that this variant of the CF-NBS protocol will now have a very high sensitivity and a very good PPV. So far, however, there are no newly-published data on this.

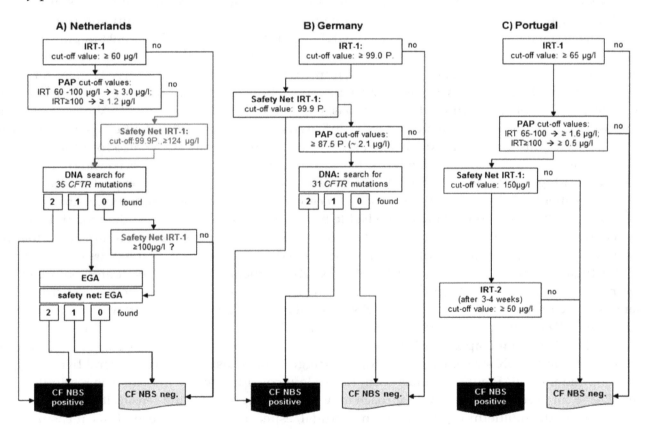

Figure 2. Simplified schemes of three selected PAP-based CF NBS protocols currently used: (**A**) The Netherlands: IRT/PAP/DNA(35)/EGA protocol including last modifications from 2016, (**B**) Germany: IRT/PAP-SN/DNA(31) protocol, (**C**) Portugal: IRT/PAP-SN/IRT protocol.

To the best of our knowledge, after the MucoPAP-F became commercially available, it was used for this program. However, it should be noted that in the Netherlands, the two IRT-dependent PAP cut-offs as proposed by Sarles (IRT ≥ 100 µg/L: PAP cut-off ≥ 1.6 µg/L and IRT 60–100 µg/L: PAP cut-off ≥ 3.0 µg/L) were maintained, although it has been recognised that the fluorometric read-out of

MucoPAP is higher than that with photometric detection. Nevertheless, this is not a disadvantage for the overall performance. In the genetic part of the protocol, an initial screen will be performed with 35 *CFTR* mutations. Following a different procedure in the past, there is, today, a very comprehensive genetic approach (Figure 2A). All samples showing only 1 *CFTR* mutation and those without mutation but with an IRT > 100 (safety net) receive a very high level extensive gene analysis. Nevertheless, the overall sensitivity of the protocol in the evaluated five years is only 90%, which does not meet the criteria of the ECFS standards of care [19]. The reason for this is clearly the IRT/PAP part and not the DNA (35)/EGA part of the protocol. As shown by Dankert-Roelse et al. 2019 [16] (given also in Table 1), seven CF patients were missed by a low IRT and eight by a low PAP. While problems with a low IRT are difficult to circumvent, the majority of CF patients missed by PAP, as described above, might have been found if a protocol like the one according to Sommerburg et al. [11,18] or Weidler et al. [14] had been used.

In Germany, a PAP-based protocol with a DNA analysis as third tier is also used (Figure 2B). The IRT/PAP-SN part follows the recommendations of Sommerburg et al. 2014, and contains a floating IRT cut-off at the 99.0th percentile and only one PAP cut-off value. Originally, the lower PAP cut-off value (1.6 µg/L) according to Sarles et al. 2005 was used; however, the recommendation is now to apply the 87.5th PAP percentile calculated from PAP values of a nonpreselected population of newborns [25].

After the introduction of the new MucoPAP-F-Kit, the PAP cut-off value, e.g., at the CF NBS centre Heidelberg, is 2.1 µg/L.

If a sample is PAP positive, a search for the 31 most common disease-causing *CFTR* mutations detected by the German national register will be done. If one or two CFTR mutations are found, the sample is rated CF NBS positive. Also, the IRT-dependent safety net (IRT ≥ 99.9th percentile) is used. While samples whose IRT is between 99.0 and 99.9th percentile will be tested for PAP and DNA, samples with an IRT ≥ 99.9th percentile will be immediately rated CF NBS positive [25]. As a reason for this decision, the authorities argued that CF patients whose CFTR mutations were not included in the panel should not be discriminated on the basis of their origin. The expected PPV was calculated in a post hoc analysis and was expected to be 20%, which would not meet the European standards of care [19,26]. This kind of IRT-dependent safety net remains questionable also for other reasons. For example, there is currently no modern CF NBS protocol in which a sample is considered positive after an ultra-high IRT alone. Furthermore, it was shown that, as previously expected, only about 25% of CF patients diagnosed with this protocol received a search for *CFTR* mutations during the CF NBS protocol [26]. Based on data from the Heidelberg IRT/PAP+SN pilot study, the sensitivity of the protocol was estimated to be 96% in the post hoc analysis mentioned above [26]. A complete evaluation of the CF NBS protocol used in Germany is now scheduled to be conducted after 3 years of application.

Portugal started in 2016 with an IRT/PAP-SN/IRT protocol which was evaluated before in the aforementioned pilot study (Figure 2C) [17]. To the best of our knowledge, there are currently no changes in the protocol. The IRT cut-off level was set at 65 µg/L. PAP is measured with the Muco PAP F kit. The PAP cut-off values are IRT dependent: If the IRT value is between 65 and 100 µg/L, a PAP cut-off value of ≥ 1.6 µg/L applies, with an IRT value of ≥ 100 µg/L a PAP cut-off value of ≥ 0.5 applies. Furthermore, an IRT SN strategy (≥150 µg/L) also triggers the measurement of a second IRT (50 µg/L). In our opinion, the PAP cut-off values seem rather low considering the fluorimetric readout of the MucoPAP-F kit used. However, this approach may be advantageous for the sensitivity of the protocol with regard to the multiethnic population in Portugal, especially since the second IRT measurement in IRT/PAP positive neonates will achieve a PPV as required by the European standards. In the pilot study the sensitivity was 94.4% and the PPV 41.03% [17].

In 2017, Austria changed from an IRT/IRT to an IRT/PAP-SN/IRT protocol. PAP measurement is done with the MucoPAP II kit. For the initial IRT, a cut-off value of 65 ng/L was set. The PAP measurement is based on Sarles et al. with two IRT-dependent PAP cut-off values [8,10] that were adapted to the conditions of MucoPAP II: If IRT is between 65 and 100 µg/L, a PAP cut-off value of ≥ 2.5 µg/L applies, if IRT is ≥ 100 µg/L, a PAP cut-off value of ≥ 1.33 µg/L is valid. In addition an

IRT-dependent SN (IRT ≥ 130 µg/L) is used. Both an increased PAP and an ultra-high IRT (SN) trigger the second IRT (sampled after 3–4 weeks of age, cut-off value 50 µg/L) [27].

In 2018, Catalonia started using an IRT/PAP-SN/IRT/DNA strategy. PAP measurement is done with the MucoPAP-F kit. The initial IRT cut-off value was set at 50 ng/L. For the second tier, two IRT-dependent PAP cut-off values [8,10] are used, but with other cut-off values, as published elsewhere: If IRT is between 50 and 80 µg/L, a PAP cut-off value of ≥ 1.95 µg/L is used, if IRT is ≥ 80 µg/L, a PAP cut-off value of ≥ 1.0 µg/L applies. An IRT dependent SN with an IRT cut-off value of ≥ 130 µg/L was also implemented in Catalonia. Both an increased PAP and an ultra-high IRT (SN) trigger the second IRT (sampled after 21–30 days of life, IRT cut-off value 35 µg/L). If the second IRT is positive, a comprehensive genetic analysis is performed [28].

Of the PAP-based CF NBS protocols currently used in a national or regional screening programme, only the Netherlands has so far provided performance data of sufficient quality [16]. It is obvious that the data from the other programmes must also be evaluated without delay and the results published. PAP-based protocols definitely have advantages in multiethnic populations, and help to detect less carriers and CFSPID. While the problem of a too low PPV caused by purely biochemical IRT/PAP protocols is probably no longer relevant, as currently, only protocols with at least three tiers are in use, the problem of sufficient sensitivity remains of high relevance.

References

1. Castellani, C.; Southern, K.W.; Brownlee, K.; Roelse, J.D.; Duff, A.; Farrell, M.; Mehta, A.; Munck, A.; Pollitt, R.; Sermet-Gaudelus, I.; et al. European best practice guidelines for cystic fibrosis neonatal screening. *J. Cyst. Fibros.* **2009**, *8*, 153–173. [CrossRef] [PubMed]
2. Wilcken, B.M.; Wiley, V. Newborn screening methods for cystic fibrosis. *Paediatr. Respir. Rev.* **2003**, *4*, 272–277. [CrossRef]
3. Munck, A.; Delmas, M.; Audrézet, M.-P.; Lemonnier, L.; Cheillan, D.; Roussey, M. Optimization of the French cystic fibrosis newborn screening programme by a centralized tracking process. *J. Med Screen.* **2017**, *25*, 6–12. [CrossRef] [PubMed]
4. Terlizzi, V.; Mergni, G.; Buzzetti, R.; Centrone, C.; Zavataro, L.; Braggion, C. Cystic fibrosis screen positive inconclusive diagnosis (CFSPID): Experience in Tuscany, Italy. *J. Cyst. Fibros.* **2019**, *18*, 484–490. [CrossRef] [PubMed]
5. Iovanna, J.L.; Férec, C.; Sarles, J.; Dagorn, J.C. The pancreatitis-associated protein (PAP). A new candidate for neonatal screening of cystic fibrosis. *Comptes Rendus de l'Académie des Sciences Series III Sciences de la Vie* **1994**, *317*, 561–564.
6. Iovanna, J.L.; Keim, V.; Nordback, I.; Montalto, G.; Camarena, J.; Letoublon, C.; Levy, P.; Berthézène, P.; Dagorn, J.-C. Serum levels of pancreatitis-associated protein as indicators of the course of acute pancreatitis. *Gastroenterology* **1994**, *106*, 728–734. [CrossRef]
7. Sarles, J.; Barthellemy, S.; Férec, C.; Iovanna, J.; Roussey, M.; Farriaux, J.-P.; Toutain, A.; Berthelot, J.; Maurin, N.; Codet, J.-P.; et al. Blood concentrations of pancreatitis associated protein in neonates: Relevance to neonatal screening for cystic fibrosis. *Arch. Dis. Child. Fetal Neonatal Ed.* **1999**, *80*, F118–F122. [CrossRef] [PubMed]
8. Sarles, J.; Berthézène, P.; Le Louarn, C.; Somma, C.; Perini, J.-M.; Catheline, M.; Mirallié, S.; Luzet, K.; Roussey, M.; Farriaux, J.-P.; et al. Combining Immunoreactive Trypsinogen and Pancreatitis-Associated Protein Assays, a Method of Newborn Screening for Cystic Fibrosis that Avoids DNA Analysis. *J. Pediatr.* **2005**, *147*, 302–305. [CrossRef] [PubMed]
9. Barthellemy, S.; Maurin, N.; Roussey, M.; Férec, C.; Murolo, S.; Berthézène, P.; Iovanna, J.L.; Dagorn, J.C.; Sarles, J. Evaluation of 47,213 infants in neonatal screening for cystic fibrosis, using pancreatitis-associated protein and immunoreactive trypsinogen assays. *Arch. Pédiatrie* **2001**, *8*, 275–281. [CrossRef]

10. Sarles, J.; Giorgi, R.; Berthézène, P.; Munck, A.; Cheillan, D.; Dagorn, J.-C.; Roussey, M. Neonatal screening for cystic fibrosis: Comparing the performances of IRT/DNA and IRT/PAP. *J. Cyst. Fibros.* **2014**, *13*, 384–390. [CrossRef] [PubMed]

11. Sommerburg, O.; Lindner, M.; Muckenthaler, M.; Kohlmueller, D.; Leible, S.; Feneberg, R.; Kulozik, A.E.; Mall, M.A.; Hoffmann, G.F. Initial evaluation of a biochemical cystic fibrosis newborn screening by sequential analysis of immunoreactive trypsinogen and pancreatitis-associated protein (IRT/PAP) as a strategy that does not involve DNA testing in a Northern European population. *J. Inherit. Metab. Dis.* **2010**, *33*, 263–271. [CrossRef] [PubMed]

12. Langen, A.M.M.V.-V.; Loeber, J.G.; Elvers, B.; Triepels, R.H.; Gille, J.J.; Van Der Ploeg, C.P.B.; Reijntjens, S.; Dompeling, E.; Dankert-Roelse, J.E. Novel strategies in newborn screening for cystic fibrosis: A prospective controlled study. *Thorax* **2012**, *67*, 289–295. [CrossRef] [PubMed]

13. Krulisova, V.; Balaščaková, M.; Skalická, V.; Piskackova, T.; Holubova, A.; Padĕrová, J.; Krenkova, P.; Dvořáková, L.; Zemkova, D.; Kracmar, P.; et al. Prospective and parallel assessments of cystic fibrosis newborn screening protocols in the Czech Republic: IRT/DNA/IRT versus IRT/PAP and IRT/PAP/DNA. *Eur. J. Nucl. Med. Mol. Imaging* **2012**, *171*, 1223–1229.

14. Weidler, S.; Stopsack, K.H.; Hammermann, J.; Sommerburg, O.; Mall, M.A.; Hoffmann, G.F.; Kohlmüller, D.; Okun, J.G.; Macek, M.; Votava, F.; et al. A product of immunoreactive trypsinogen and pancreatitis-associated protein as second-tier strategy in cystic fibrosis newborn screening. *J. Cyst. Fibros.* **2016**, *15*, 752–758. [CrossRef] [PubMed]

15. Sommerburg, O.; Hammermann, J.; Lindner, M.; Stahl, M.; Muckenthaler, M.; Kohlmueller, D.; Happich, M.; Kulozik, A.E.; Stopsack, M.; Gahr, M.; et al. Five years of experience with biochemical cystic fibrosis newborn screening based on IRT/PAP in Germany. *Pediatr. Pulmonol.* **2015**, *50*, 655–664. [CrossRef] [PubMed]

16. Dankert-Roelse, J.E.; Bouva, M.J.; Jakobs, B.S.; Janssens, H.M.; Groot, K.D.W.-D.; Schönbeck, Y.; Gille, J.J.; Gulmans, V.A.; Verschoof-Puite, R.K.; Schielen, P.; et al. Newborn blood spot screening for cystic fibrosis with a four-step screening strategy in the Netherlands. *J. Cyst. Fibros.* **2019**, *18*, 54–63. [CrossRef] [PubMed]

17. Marcão, A.; Barreto, C.; Pereira, J.B.; Vaz, L.; Cavaco, J.; Casimiro, A.; Félix, M.; Silva, T.R.; Barbosa, T.; Freitas, C.; et al. Cystic Fibrosis Newborn Screening in Portugal: PAP Value in Populations with Stringent Rules for Genetic Studies. *Int. J. Neonatal Screen.* **2018**, *4*, 22. [CrossRef]

18. Sommerburg, O.; Krulišová, V.; Hammermann, J.; Lindner, M.; Stahl, M.; Muckenthaler, M.; Kohlmueller, D.; Happich, M.; Kulozik, A.E.; Votava, F.; et al. Comparison of different IRT-PAP protocols to screen newborns for cystic fibrosis in three central European populations. *J. Cyst. Fibros.* **2014**, *13*, 15–23. [CrossRef]

19. Castellani, C.; Duff, A.; Bell, S.C.; Heijerman, H.G.; Munck, A.; Ratjen, F.; Sermet-Gaudelus, I.; Southern, K.W.; Barben, J.; A Flume, P.; et al. ECFS best practice guidelines: The 2018 revision. *J. Cyst. Fibros.* **2018**, *17*, 153–178. [CrossRef]

20. Calvin, J.; Hogg, S.L.; McShane, D.; McAuley, S.A.; Iles, R.; Ross-Russell, R.; MacLean, F.M.; Heeley, M.E.; Heeley, A.F. Thirty-years of screening for cystic fibrosis in East Anglia. *Arch. Dis. Child.* **2012**, *97*, 1043–1047. [CrossRef]

21. Kharrazi, M.; Yang, J.; Bishop, T.; Lessing, S.; Young, S.; Graham, S.; Pearl, M.; Chow, H.; Ho, T.; Currier, R.; et al. Newborn Screening for Cystic Fibrosis in California. *Pediatrics* **2015**, *136*, 1062–1072. [CrossRef] [PubMed]

22. Sontag, M.; Lee, R.; Wright, D.; Freedenberg, D.; Sagel, S.D. Improving the Sensitivity and Positive Predictive Value in a Cystic Fibrosis Newborn Screening Program Using a Repeat Immunoreactive Trypsinogen and Genetic Analysis. *J. Pediatr.* **2016**, *175*, 150–158.e1. [CrossRef] [PubMed]

23. Lundman, E.; Gaup, H.J.; Bakkeheim, E.; Olafsdottir, E.J.; Rootwelt, T.; Storrøsten, O.T.; Pettersen, R.D. Implementation of newborn screening for cystic fibrosis in Norway. Results from the first three years. *J. Cyst. Fibros.* **2016**, *15*, 318–324. [CrossRef] [PubMed]

24. Skov, M.; Baekvad-Hansen, M.; Hougaard, D.M.; Skogstrand, K.; Lund, A.M.; Pressler, T.; Olesen, H.V.; Duno, M. Cystic fibrosis newborn screening in Denmark: Experience from the first 2 years. *Pediatr. Pulmonol.* **2019**, *55*, 549–555. [CrossRef]

25. Gemeinsamer Bundesausschuss. Kinder-Richtlinie: Änderung des Beschlusses zur Neufassung—Screening auf Mukoviszidose (Zystische Fibrose)—Tragende Gründe zum Beschluss. Available online: https://www.g-ba.de/informationen/beschluesse/2316/ (accessed on 3 November 2015).

26. Sommerburg, O.; Stahl, M.; Hammermann, J.; Okun, J.G.; Kulozik, A.; Hoffmann, G.; Mall, M. Neugeborenenscreening auf Mukoviszidose in Deutschland: Vergleich des neuen Screening-Protokolls mit einem Alternativprotokoll. *Klin. Pädiatrie* **2017**, *229*, 59–66. [CrossRef] [PubMed]
27. Zeyda, M.; (Medical University of Vienna, Vienna, Austria). Personal communication, 2020.
28. Gartner, S.; (Tilburg School of Catholic Theology, Tilburg, The Netherlands). Personal communication, 2020.

7

The Changing Face of Cystic Fibrosis and its Implications for Screening

Lutz Naehrlich

Department of Pediatrics, Justus-Liebig-University Giessen, D-35392 Giessen, Germany;
lutz.naehrlich@paediat.med.uni-giessen.de;

Abstract: Early diagnosis, multidisciplinary care, and optimized and preventive treatments have changed the face of cystic fibrosis. Life expectancy has been expanded in the last decades. Formerly a pediatric disease, cystic fibrosis has reached adulthood. Mutation-specific treatments will expand treatment options and give hope for further improvement of quality of life and life expectancy. Newborn screening for CF fits perfectly into these care structures and offers the possibility of preventive treatment even before symptoms occur. Especially in countries without screening, newborn screening will fulfill that promise only with increased awareness and new care structures.

Keywords: cystic fibrosis; newborn screening; diagnosis; therapy; prognosis

1. Introduction

Cystic fibrosis (CF) is a life-shortening multisystem disease with an autosomal recessive inheritance pattern that affects nearly 100,000, mainly Caucasian, people worldwide. The disease is caused by dysfunction of the exocrine gland chloride channel protein, the cystic fibrosis transmembrane conductance regulator (*CFTR*). CF mainly involves the pancreas and the lungs, but also the upper airways, liver, intestine, skin, and reproductive organs. Improved diagnosis, a multidisciplinary team approach, and symptomatic treatment have improved the health and survival prospects of persons with CF. Early diagnosis by newborn screening (NBS) [1] and prophylactic treatment are critical components for overall success. The approval of causally directed, mutation-specific treatments creates hope for reduced morbidity and increased life expectancy in the near future. The face of CF has changed over the last decades. This has implications for CF NBS, especially in countries in which it is not yet established.

2. Changing Face of Cystic Fibrosis

2.1. Diagnosis

Since the first description of CF [2,3] in the 1930s, clinical and pathophysiological knowledge and diagnostic and therapeutic possibilities have changed and influenced each other. In the beginning, CF was diagnosed based on clinical symptoms, such as meconium ileus, exocrine pancreatic insufficiency, chronic pneumonia, or post-mortem findings of cystic fibrosis of the pancreas and the lung [2]. During a heat wave in New York in 1948, disturbances of electrolytes were detected in CF patients [4]. The increased sweat chloride concentration was described in 1953 as a characteristic finding in CF, [5] and since then has been used as a diagnostic tool. In 1959, Gibson and Cooke published a method for sweat induction by pilocarpine iontophoresis on a small body surface area [6], and it remains the diagnostic gold standard for CF even today. Measuring conductivity by Nanoduct® can facilitate the diagnosis of screening-positive newborns, but is less specific than the sweat chloride measurement [7] and not recommended as a diagnostic measurement [8].

A close observation of families with CF led to its description as an autosomal recessive genetic disorder in 1946 [9]. In 1989, the cystic fibrosis gene on the long arm of chromosome 7 was identified [10], paving the way for genetic diagnosis. To date, more than 2000 *CFTR* mutations have been described (http://www.genet.sickkids.on.ca) [11]. Functional and clinical analyses have led to the characterization of 432 variants, including 352 disease–causing variants (https://www.cftr2.org) [12] and the concept of functional mutation classes [13]. Worldwide, F508del is the major CF variant, but the prevalence varies between ethnic groups (for example, 70% in Germany and 25% in Turkey) [14]. Despite extensive *CFTR* sequencing, around 1% of *CFTR* variants have not been identified. To confirm the diagnosis in these cases, in vivo functional *CFTR* testing, such as nasal potential difference measurement and intestinal current measurement were implemented [8].

Due to the consistent clinical characterization of CF patients, the first pancreatic-sufficient CF patients were reported in the 1950s [15]. This group of patients, characterized by *CFTR* mutations with residual *CFTR* function, accounts for 10–15% of all CF patients [16]. They can present with similar severity of lung disease, but as a group have a better prognosis than others. In 1975, the first pancreatic-insufficient CF patient with a normal sweat chloride test was reported [17]. A normal sweat chloride test was reported in 3.5% of all patients in the US in 2015 [18], these patients were diagnosed based on two CF-causing mutations or pathologic CFTR functional tests. In the 1990s, the first CF diagnoses in adolescents and adults were reported [19]. The patients are mainly pancreatic sufficient but infertile due to an obstructive azoospermia and suffer from respiratory symptoms [19]. In Germany, 5% of all CF-patients are diagnosed at age 18 years or older [20]. The expanding knowledge of patients with a clinical entity associated with CFTR-dysfunction that does not fulfill the diagnostic criteria for CF widened the spectrum and led to the description of *CFTR*-related disorders [21]. International guidelines [8] have been updated regularly and reflect the expanding knowledge of the spectrum of *CFTR* dysfunction and the widely varying clinical presentation of CF.

2.2. Care

CF care today is seen as multidisciplinary, to fit the medical, psychosocial, physiotherapeutic, and nutritional needs of CF patients, prevent chronic infection and malnutrition, minimize deterioration, maintain independence, optimize quality of life, and maximize life expectancy [22].

Until the 1950s, many pediatricians took care of CF-patients, and only a few doctors, those dedicated to CF, treated more than a handful of patients. Broader experience with the spectrum of the disease and rare complications, the ability to analyze treatment options and outcome in a more systematic way, and long-term follow-up are the major advantages of CF-center care and also drive clinical research and progress. In 1958, Shwachmann and Kulczycki published their results from a large cohort of 105 patients, marking the beginning of center-based care worldwide [23]. The Cystic Fibrosis Foundation in the USA established an accredited care network in 1961 by creating centers devoted to treating CF. The number of Foundation-accredited care centers in the USA grew to more than 100 by 1978 and there are currently 130 (https://www.cff.org/About-Us/About-the-Cystic-Fibrosis-Foundation/Our-History/). In 1963, the CFF Foundation published the first guidelines for the diagnosis and treatment of CF. These achievements inspired colleagues and parents to establish a national CF foundation and CF care centers across the world and to deliver structured care, including annual checkups and regular outpatient visits [24]. The integration of clinical research reflected by the establishment of clinical trial networks in the USA, Canada, and Europe have sped up the development of clinical trials [25]. This combination of clinical research and best care practices has been cited as a model of effective and efficient healthcare delivery for other chronic diseases. A transition from pediatric to adult care began in the 1960s with the increasing number of adults with CF, but it is still a challenge globally.

2.3. Therapy

The paradigm for comprehensive and preventive treatment programs for CF was introduced by Matthews, who first suggested and funded a program in 1957 in Cleveland [26]. Accurate early diagnosis and treatment from diagnosis had a dramatic impact on survival and morbidity at this time. This paradigm has been adopted globally and is the basis of our Standards of Care today [24]. The evolution of the diagnostic and therapeutic Standards of Care for CF was based on clinical experience and controlled studies. Until the 1990s, almost all therapeutic strategies for CF were based on center experiences and comparisons with historical controls. Since then, drug development has been based mainly on randomized placebo-controlled studies. Neither strategy answers all relevant clinical questions, and both leave room for interpretation and individual treatment regimens.

The symptomatic treatment of pancreatic insufficiency, which affects 85–90% of all CF patients, started in the 1930s (in the absence of pancreatic enzyme replacement) as a low-fat, high-protein diet. Pancreatic enzyme replacement was established in the 1940s, but required high doses due to the enzymes' lack of resistance to gastric acid. After gastric-acid resistant pancreatic enzyme therapy was established in the 1980s based on a historical comparison of center data, dietary recommendations changed from a low-fat diet to a high-fat, high-calorie diet. Instead of a standard dosage regimen, individual dosage adjustment of pancreatic enzymes and fat-soluble vitamins and nutritional advice from a specialized dietician are critical to overcoming malnutrition and achieving sufficient blood vitamin levels [27].

Symptomatic mucolytic therapy today is mainly based on inhalation of DNase [28], hypertonic saline, [29] or mannitol [30] in combination with physiotherapy. High quality studies comparing the mucolytic drugs are still lacking, and the individual experiences of patients and caregivers explain the high variability of their use globally. Mucolytic therapy was shown to reduce pulmonary exacerbation frequency and to improve and stabilize lung function. Physiotherapy is an important daily prophylactic and therapeutic component of care, and is based on personalized experience and different approaches [24].

Chronic bacterial pneumonia has been a continuous challenge for CF care since the first description of CF. *Staphylococcus aureus* and *Pseudomonas aeruginosa* (PA) are the most important bugs [18]. The concept of early detection and eradication of *P. aeruginosa* was established in the 1990s in order to postpone chronic infection [31], which is defined by more than 50% of the preceding 12 months being PA culture positive [32]. Methicillin resistant *Staphylococcus aureus* and nontuberculous mycobacteria are emerging pathogens in CF [18]. Aggressive antibiotic treatment of pulmonary exacerbations is the backbone of pulmonary treatment. Lower treatment thresholds, higher dosages, and longer treatment durations compared with those typical for non-CF patients are mainly based on clinical experience. Chronic suppression therapy by inhalation of antibiotics was first described in the 1980s [33]. A placebo-controlled trial in the 1990s confirmed the concept [34]. Infection control at home and in the hospital are critical components of avoidance of both cross-infection and infection with multi-resistant bugs. These concepts have been defined in the last 10 years and contribute to the control of chronic bacterial infection in CF.

The active surveillance of CF-related complications, such as liver disease, diabetes mellitus, bone disease, and their active treatments have become important components of annual checkups and therapeutic concepts [24]. Lung transplantation has a major impact on survival. In France and Belgium, 10–13% of all CF patients have undergone lung transplantation, compared to less than 2% in most eastern European countries [16].

In the last decade, causally directed, mutation-specific treatments have been evolving. In contrast to gene therapy, [35] orally administered small molecules with systemic effects have been shown to increase CFTR function (reducing sweat chloride), lung function, body weight, and quality of life significantly. These effects depend highly on the particular drugs, which are divided into correctors and modulators, and the mutation classes. The proof of concept has been shown with Ivacaftor for patients with at least one gating mutation (3% of all CF patients in Europe) [36–38]. This treatment is licensed in the European Union (EU) for use from the age of 6 months. Ivacaftor treatment in children aged 12 to 24 months with a gating mutation support the potential of Ivacaftor to protect against progressive exocrine pancreatic dysfunction [38]. In utero treatment provided partial protection from pathologies in pancreas, intestine, and male reproductive tract in a ferret model [39]. A combination of Elexacaftor/Tezacaftor/Ivacaftor has shown comparable data in patients with at least one F508del mutation (90% of all patients in Europe) [40,41]. This drug was licensed in the USA in 2019 for patients older than 12 years of age, and the decision of the European Medical Agency is expected in 2020. Another combination, of Lumacaftor/Ivacaftor, is licensed in the EU for F508del homozygous patients (45% of all patients in Europe) for use from the age of 2 years [42], but its effect is limited compared with Elexacaftor/Tezacaftor/Ivacaftor. All these trial developments are the result of close cooperation between clinical trial networks, CF centers, and industry, and the drugs have been tested as an add-on to the standard symptomatic therapy. These developments offer great hope for parents of newborns with CF by improving quality of life and life expectancy in the near future.

2.4. Prognosis

CF was seen as a pediatric disease for many decades, affecting only a few adult patients. This has changed dramatically since the 1990s. With reduced pediatric morbidity and mortality, more pediatric patients are surviving to adulthood [43]. For example, the rate of malnutrition declined from 26% to 17% in children and adolescents and from 26% to 14% in adults in Germany from 2009 to 2018 [20,44]. The rate of chronic *Pseudomonas* infection in 16–19-year-old patients dropped from 43.9% in 2009 to 25.5% in 2018 in the UK [45]. Nearly 40% of all adults 18–29 years of age had normal lung function (FEV1%pred) of more than 80% in 2017, compared with 30% in 2008/2009 in Europe [16,46].

During the last decades, great improvements in survival were achieved. In 1980, 31.1 % of the US CF population was over the age of 18 years, compared with 54.6% in 2018. In Belgium, Denmark, Netherland, Norway, and Sweden, adults were reported to make up 60–65% of all CF patients in 2017 [16]. This comes with dramatic improvements in increasing the age of death, survival of birth cohorts, and median survival age over time [43]. For the period 2012–2016, the median age of survival was estimated to be 53.3 (95% CI: unknown) in Canada, 47.5 years (95% CI: 44.8–49.7) in Germany, 47.0 years (95% CI: 44.7–48.2) in the UK, and 42.7 years (95% CI: 41.7–43.9) in the USA [47].

These improvements have far-reaching implications in terms of care structures and resources. To fulfill the increasingly promising prognosis, access to care including dedicated multidisciplinary CF teams and a broad range of medicines is critical. Socioeconomic status (SES) is a major confounder and must be taken into account. Studies in the USA have found that medical insurance status [48] and median household income [49] are both independently associated with significant differences in survival, even within a country with a high mean gross net income. Comparing the highest SES countries with the lowest SES countries in Europe showed a significant decrease in the hazard of mortality [50].

3. Implications for Newborn Screening

Despite the continuously improving quality of life and life expectancy of patients over the last decades and promising therapeutic developments, CF is still a chronic, life-limiting disease. Early diagnosis and multidisciplinary treatment according to current standards of care are critical in avoiding early severe complications. The following are some key implications of screening that must be discussed.

The awareness of cystic fibrosis in general, but especially of the improving prognosis and treatment options, is critical for the success of NBS. The common problems of late diagnosis and underdiagnosis in some countries reflect the low awareness of CF among caregivers, parents, and health authorities. The promising prognosis has to be emphasized. Patient representatives and organizations could help to support this important public health topic by personalizing experiences and helping to create a supportive environment for families after diagnosis. CF caregivers are responsible for advocacy for CF, especially among healthcare professionals, and for providing obstetricians, surgeons, pediatricians, and general practitioners with updated information about CF in general, the spectrum of disease presentation, diagnostic and therapeutic options, and improving overall prognosis. Patient registries are important tools for collecting, reporting, and comparing international and national epidemiologic data. CF caregivers and patient organizations should jointly stand up to raise awareness (and resources) amongst health authorities, provide information about medical needs, and discuss and propose care structures for each country.

CF core diagnostic and care facilities with established multidisciplinary teams must be established and promoted in each country. Pediatric facilities should be integrated within a NBS tracking system and take an active role in providing information to local caregivers, patients, and health authorities. The confirmation of the diagnosis should be performed at the earliest stage in specialized CF centers. The results have to be discussed by a CF experienced doctor on the day the diagnosis is confirmed. Critical components of the service are a high-quality sweat chloride test to minimize the rate of sweat tests with insufficient volume and give reliable results on the day of the confirmation visit, a multidisciplinary team to counsel the parents and establish the treatment plan immediately, and strict infection control to minimize the risk of *P. aeruginosa* acquisition. Without this essential infrastructure, even the best NBS program cannot succeed [51].

High specificity of the newborn screening program reduces the recall rate, the parents' burden and stress, and the burden of CF centers. Due to the low number of CF centers in some countries, the travel distance and burden for families should not be underestimated. The genetic component of each individual NBS program is critical to achieving the goal. The selection of mutations for screening has to be adapted to the genetic and ethnic spectrum of each country/region and could be based on registry data or epidemiologic studies. The detection of mutations with varying consequences through newborn screening should be avoided as it will complicate interpretation and overextend caregivers and patients. An expanded mutation panel or genotyping should not be "abused" to substitute for robust confirmation of diagnosis. Unfortunately, commercial panel testing does not fit this need. Measuring pancreatitis associated protein in addition to immunoreactive trypsinogen might be an additional 2nd tier to reduce the use of genetic analyses [52]. Learning from international experience is the best way to build up individual NBS programs for each country. Even the best CF screening program will not detect all patients at birth, and awareness of the possibility of later diagnosis is needed anyway.

Changes in diagnostic and therapeutic dogmas are driven fundamentally by NBS. Unlike symptomatic patients who are diagnosed by confirmation of *CFTR* dysfunction, asymptomatic patients are diagnosed based on proven *CFTR* dysfunction. In contrast to symptomatic treatment, which is often well received and accepted by parents, the diagnosis and prophylactic treatment of asymptomatic children is often mistrusted and seen as a greater burden by parents. The developing mutation-specific treatments offer great hope for parents of newborns with CF. Only if healthcare providers (including primary care providers) and parents are convinced and have hope that early diagnosis and treatment offers a benefit for the patient, such as avoiding or postponing malnutrition or pulmonary and other complications, will NBS fulfill its promise.

4. Conclusions

NBS for CF should be seen as a game changer in CF care, not reduced to simply a diagnostic procedure. Its final success depends on the general awareness of the disease, the integration of NBS within well-established CF care structures, and the engagement and interaction of obstetricians, primary caregivers, pediatricians, CF centers, and health authorities.

References

1. Castellani, C.; Massie, J.; Sontag, M.; Southern, K.W. Newborn screening for cystic fibrosis. *Lancet Respir. Med.* **2016**, *4*, 653–661. [CrossRef]
2. Andersen, D.H. Cystic fibrosis of the pancreas and its relation to celiac disease: A clinical and pathological study. *Am. J. Dis. Child.* **1938**, *56*, 344–399. [CrossRef]
3. Fanconi, G.; Uehlinger, E.; Knauer, C. Das Coeliakie-syndrom bei angeborener zystischer Pankreasfibromatose und Bronchiektasien. *Wien. Med. Wchnschr* **1936**, *86*, 753–756.
4. Kessler, W.R.; Andersen, D.H. Heat prostration in fibrocystic disease of the pancreas and other conditions. *Pediatrics* **1951**, *8*, 648–656.
5. Di Sant'Agnese, P.A.; Darling, R.C.; Perera, G.A.; Shea, E. Abnormal electrolyte composition of sweat in cystic fibrosis of the pancreas; clinical significance and relationship to the disease. *Pediatrics* **1953**, *12*, 549–563.
6. Gibson, L.E.; Cooke, R.E. A test for concentration of electrolytes in sweat in cystic fibrosis of the pancreas utilizing pilocarpine by iontophoresis. *Pediatrics* **1959**, *23*, 545–549. [PubMed]
7. Rueegg, C.S.; Kuehni, C.E.; Gallati, S.; Jurca, M.; Jung, A.; Casaulta, C.; Barben, J. Comparison of two sweat test systems for the diagnosis of cystic fibrosis in newborns. *Pediatr. Pulmonol.* **2019**, *54*, 264–272. [CrossRef] [PubMed]
8. Farrell, P.M.; White, T.B.; Howenstine, M.S.; Munck, A.; Parad, R.B.; Rosenfeld, M.; Sommerburg, O.; Accurso, F.J.; Davies, J.C.; Rock, M.J.; et al. Diagnosis of Cystic Fibrosis in Screened Populations. *J. Pediatr.* **2017**, *181*, S33–S44.e2. [CrossRef] [PubMed]
9. Andersen, D.H.; Hodges, R.G. Celiac syndrome; genetics of cystic fibrosis of the pancreas, with a consideration of etiology. *Am. J. Dis. Child.* **1946**, *72*, 62–80. [CrossRef] [PubMed]
10. Kerem, B.; Rommens, J.M.; Buchanan, J.A.; Markiewicz, D.; Cox, T.K.; Chakravarti, A.; Buchwald, M.; Tsui, L.C. Identification of the cystic fibrosis gene: Genetic analysis. *Science* **1989**, *245*, 1073–1080. [CrossRef]
11. Cystic Fibrosis Mutation Database (CFTR1). Available online: http://www.genet.sickkids.on.ca (accessed on 17 May 2020).
12. Sosnay, P.R.; Siklosi, K.R.; Van Goor, F.; Kaniecki, K.; Yu, H.; Sharma, N.; Ramalho, A.S.; Amaral, M.D.; Dorfman, R.; Zielenski, J.; et al. Defining the disease liability of variants in the cystic fibrosis transmembrane conductance regulator gene. *Nat. Genet.* **2013**, *45*, 1160–1167. [CrossRef] [PubMed]
13. Boyle, M.P.; De Boeck, K. A new era in the treatment of cystic fibrosis: Correction of the underlying CFTR defect. *Lancet Respir. Med.* **2013**, *1*, 158–163. [CrossRef]
14. World Health Organization. The Molecular Genetic Epidemiology of Cystic Fibrosis. Available online: http://www.who.int/genomics/publications/reports/en/index.html (accessed on 29 June 2020).
15. Dooley, R.R.; Guilmette, F.; Leubner, H.; Patterson, P.R.; Shwachman, H.; Weil, C. Cystic fibrosis of the pancreas with varying degrees of pancreatic insufficiency. *AMA J. Dis. Child.* **1956**, *92*, 347–368. [PubMed]
16. Zolin, A.; Orenti, A.; Naehrlich, L.; van Rens, J.; Fox, A.; Krasnyk, M.; Jung, A.; Mei-Zahav, M.; Cosgriff, R.; Storms, V.; et al. *ECFSPR Annual Report 2017*; European Cystic Fibrosis Society: Karup, Denmark, 2019.
17. Sarsfield, J.K.; Davies, J.M. Negative sweat tests and cystic fibrosis. *Arch. Dis. Child.* **1975**, *50*, 463–466. [CrossRef] [PubMed]
18. Cystic Fibrosis Foundation. *Cystic Fibrosis Foundation Patient Registry—2015 Annual Data Report*; Cystic Fibrosis Foundation: Bethesda, MD, USA, 2016.
19. Gan, K.H.; Geus, W.P.; Bakker, W.; Lamers, C.B.; Heijerman, H.G. Genetic and clinical features of patients with cystic fibrosis diagnosed after the age of 16 years. *Thorax* **1995**, *50*, 1301–1304. [CrossRef]
20. Nährlich, L.; Burkhart, M.; Wosniok, J. *German Cystic Fibrosis registry—Annual Report 2018*; Mukoviszidose Institut GmbH: Bonn, Germany, 2019.
21. Bombieri, C.; Claustres, M.; De Boeck, K.; Derichs, N.; Dodge, J.; Girodon, E.; Sermet, I.; Schwarz, M.; Tzetis, M.; Wilschanski, M.; et al. Recommendations for the classification of diseases as CFTR-related disorders. *J. Cyst. Fibros.* **2011**, *10*, S86–S102. [CrossRef]
22. Smyth, A.R.; Bell, S.C.; Bojcin, S.; Bryon, M.; Duff, A.; Flume, P.; Kashirskaya, N.; Munck, A.; Ratjen, F.; Schwarzenberg, S.J.; et al. European Cystic Fibrosis Society Standards of Care: Best Practice guidelines. *J. Cyst. Fibros.* **2014**, *13*, S23–S42. [CrossRef]
23. Shwachman, H.; Kulczycki, L.L. Long-term study of one hundred five patients with cystic fibrosis; studies made over a five- to fourteen-year period. *AMA J. Dis. Child.* **1958**, *96*, 6–15. [CrossRef]

24. Castellani, C.; Duff, A.J.A.; Bell, S.C.; Heijerman, H.G.M.; Munck, A.; Ratjen, F.; Sermet-Gaudelus, I.;
     Southern, K.W.; Barben, J.; Flume, P.A.; et al. ECFS best practice guidelines: The 2018 revision. *J. Cyst. Fibros.*
     2018, *17*, 153–178. [CrossRef]
25. De Boeck, K.; Bulteel, V.; Fajac, I. Disease-specific clinical trials networks: The example of cystic fibrosis.
     Eur. J. Pediatr. **2016**, *175*, 817–824. [CrossRef]
26. Doershuk, C.F.; Matthews, L.W.; Tucker, A.S.; Nudleman, H.; Eddy, G.; Wise, M.; Spector, S. A 5year clinical
     evaluation of a therapeutic program for patients with cystic fibrosis. *J. Pediatr.* **1964**, *65*, 677–693. [CrossRef]
27. Turck, D.; Braegger, C.P.; Colombo, C.; Declercq, D.; Morton, A.; Pancheva, R.; Robberecht, E.; Stern, M.;
     Strandvik, B.; Wolfe, S.; et al. ESPEN-ESPGHAN-ECFS guidelines on nutrition care for infants, children,
     and adults with cystic fibrosis. *Clin. Nutr.* **2016**, *35*, 557–577. [CrossRef] [PubMed]
28. Yang, C.; Chilvers, M.; Montgomery, M.; Nolan, S.J. Dornase alfa for cystic fibrosis. *Cochrane Database
     Syst. Rev.* **2016**, *4*, Cd001127. [CrossRef]
29. Wark, P.; McDonald, V.M. Nebulised hypertonic saline for cystic fibrosis. *Cochrane Database Syst. Rev.* **2009**,
     15, Cd001506. [CrossRef] [PubMed]
30. Nolan, S.J.; Thornton, J.; Murray, C.S.; Dwyer, T. Inhaled mannitol for cystic fibrosis. *Cochrane Database
     Syst. Rev.* **2015**, *10*, Cd008649. [CrossRef]
31. Valerius, N.H.; Koch, C.; Hoiby, N. Prevention of chronic Pseudomonas aeruginosa colonisation in cystic
     fibrosis by early treatment. *Lancet* **1991**, *338*, 725–726. [CrossRef]
32. Lee, T.W.; Brownlee, K.G.; Conway, S.P.; Denton, M.; Littlewood, J.M. Evaluation of a new definition for
     chronic Pseudomonas aeruginosa infection in cystic fibrosis patients. *J. Cyst. Fibros.* **2003**, *2*, 29–34. [CrossRef]
33. Jensen, T.; Pedersen, S.S.; Garne, S.; Heilmann, C.; Hoiby, N.; Koch, C. Colistin inhalation therapy in cystic
     fibrosis patients with chronic Pseudomonas aeruginosa lung infection. *J. Antimicrob. Chemother.* **1987**,
     19, 831–838. [CrossRef]
34. Ramsey, B.W.; Pepe, M.S.; Quan, J.M.; Otto, K.L.; Montgomery, A.B.; Williams-Warren, J.; Vasiljev, K.M.;
     Borowitz, D.; Bowman, C.M.; Marshall, B.C.; et al. Intermittent administration of inhaled tobramycin in
     patients with cystic fibrosis. Cystic Fibrosis Inhaled Tobramycin Study Group. *N. Engl. J. Med.* **1999**,
     340, 23–30. [CrossRef]
35. Alton, E.; Armstrong, D.K.; Ashby, D.; Bayfield, K.J.; Bilton, D.; Bloomfield, E.V.; Boyd, A.C.; Brand, J.;
     Buchan, R.; Calcedo, R.; et al. Repeated nebulisation of non-viral CFTR gene therapy in patients with cystic
     fibrosis: A randomised, double-blind, placebo-controlled, phase 2b trial. *Lancet Respir. Med.* **2015**, *3*, 684–691.
     [CrossRef]
36. Ramsey, B.W.; Davies, J.; McElvaney, N.G.; Tullis, E.; Bell, S.C.; Drevinek, P.; Griese, M.; McKone, E.F.;
     Wainwright, C.E.; Konstan, M.W.; et al. A CFTR potentiator in patients with cystic fibrosis and the G551D
     mutation. *N. Engl. J. Med.* **2011**, *365*, 1663–1672. [CrossRef] [PubMed]
37. Davies, J.C.; Wainwright, C.E.; Canny, G.J.; Chilvers, M.A.; Howenstine, M.S.; Munck, A.; Mainz, J.G.;
     Rodriguez, S.; Li, H.; Yen, K.; et al. Efficacy and safety of ivacaftor in patients aged 6 to 11 years with cystic
     fibrosis with a G551D mutation. *Am. J. Respir. Crit. Care Med.* **2013**, *187*, 1219–1225. [CrossRef] [PubMed]
38. Rosenfeld, M.; Wainwright, C.E.; Higgins, M.; Wang, L.T.; McKee, C.; Campbell, D.; Tian, S.; Schneider, J.;
     Cunningham, S.; Davies, J.C. Ivacaftor treatment of cystic fibrosis in children aged 12 to <24 months and
     with a CFTR gating mutation (ARRIVAL): A phase 3 single-arm study. *Lancet Respir. Med.* **2018**, *6*, 545–553.
     [CrossRef]
39. Sun, X.; Yi, Y.; Yan, Z.; Rosen, B.H.; Liang, B.; Winter, M.C.; Evans, T.I.A.; Rotti, P.G.; Yang, Y.; Gray, J.S.; et al.
     In utero and postnatal VX-770 administration rescues multiorgan disease in a ferret model of cystic fibrosis.
     Sci. Transl. Med. **2019**, *11*, eaau7531. [CrossRef] [PubMed]
40. Heijerman, H.G.M.; McKone, E.F.; Downey, D.G.; Van Braeckel, E.; Rowe, S.M.; Tullis, E.; Mall, M.A.;
     Welter, J.J.; Ramsey, B.W.; McKee, C.M.; et al. Efficacy and safety of the elexacaftor plus tezacaftor
     plus ivacaftor combination regimen in people with cystic fibrosis homozygous for the F508del mutation:
     A double-blind, randomised, phase 3 trial. *Lancet* **2019**, *394*, 1940–1948. [CrossRef]
41. Middleton, P.G.; Mall, M.A.; Drevinek, P.; Lands, L.C.; McKone, E.F.; Polineni, D.; Ramsey, B.W.;
     Taylor-Cousar, J.L.; Tullis, E.; Vermeulen, F.; et al. Elexacaftor-Tezacaftor-Ivacaftor for Cystic Fibrosis
     with a Single Phe508del Allele. *N. Engl. J. Med.* **2019**, *381*, 1809–1819. [CrossRef]

42. Ratjen, F.; Hug, C.; Marigowda, G.; Tian, S.; Huang, X.; Stanojevic, S.; Milla, C.E.; Robinson, P.D.; Waltz, D.; Davies, J.C. Efficacy and safety of lumacaftor and ivacaftor in patients aged 6-11 years with cystic fibrosis homozygous for F508del-CFTR: A randomised, placebo-controlled phase 3 trial. *Lancet Respir. Med.* **2017**, *5*, 557–567. [CrossRef]

43. Stephenson, A.L.; Stanojevic, S.; Sykes, J.; Burgel, P.R. The changing epidemiology and demography of cystic fibrosis. *Presse Med.* **2017**, *46*, e87–e95. [CrossRef]

44. Stern, M.; Sens, B.; Wiedemann, B.; Busse, O.; Damm, G.; Wenzlaff, P. *Qualitätssicherung Mukoviszidose—Überblick über den Gesundheitszustand der Patienten in Deutschland 2009*; Hippocampus-Verlag: Bad Honnef, Germany, 2010.

45. UK Cystic Fibrosis Registry. *Annual Data Report 2018.*; Cystic Fibrosis Trust: London, UK, 2019.

46. Vivani, L.; Zolin, A.; Olesen, H. *ECFSPR Annual Report 2008–2009*; European Cystic Fibrosis Society: Karup, Denmark, 2012.

47. Naehrlich, L. Survival analyis of the German Cystic Fibrosis Registry. *J. Cyst. Fibros.* **2019**, *18*, S75. [CrossRef]

48. Schechter, M.S.; Shelton, B.J.; Margolis, P.A.; Fitzsimmons, S.C. The association of socioeconomic status with outcomes in cystic fibrosis patients in the United States. *Am. J. Respir. Crit. Care Med.* **2001**, *163*, 1331–1337. [CrossRef]

49. O'Connor, G.T.; Quinton, H.B.; Kneeland, T.; Kahn, R.; Lever, T.; Maddock, J.; Robichaud, P.; Detzer, M.; Swartz, D.R. Median household income and mortality rate in cystic fibrosis. *Pediatrics* **2003**, *111*, e333–e339. [CrossRef] [PubMed]

50. McKone, E.; Ariti, C.; Jackson, A.; Zolin, A.; Carr, S.; VanRens, J.; Colomb, V.; Lemonnier, L.; Keogh, R.; Naehrlich, L. Cystic fibrosis survival and socioeconomic status across Europe. *J. Cyst. Fibros.* **2017**, *16*, S20. [CrossRef]

51. Barreda, C.B.; Farrell, P.M.; Laxova, A.; Eickhoff, J.C.; Braun, A.T.; Coller, R.J.; Rock, M.J. Newborn screening alone insufficient to improve pulmonary outcomes for cystic fibrosis. *J. Cyst. Fibros.* **2020**. [CrossRef] [PubMed]

52. Sommerburg, O.; Krulisova, V.; Hammermann, J.; Lindner, M.; Stahl, M.; Muckenthaler, M.; Kohlmueller, D.; Happich, M.; Kulozik, A.E.; Votava, F.; et al. Comparison of different IRT-PAP protocols to screen newborns for cystic fibrosis in three central European populations. *J. Cyst. Fibros.* **2014**, *13*, 15–23. [CrossRef]

8

Barriers to the Implementation of Newborn Pulse Oximetry Screening

Martin Kluckow

Department of Neonatal Medicine, Royal North Shore Hospital and University of Sydney, Sydney, NSW 2065, Australia; martin.kluckow@sydney.edu.au;

Abstract: Pulse oximetry screening of the well newborn to assist in the diagnosis of critical congenital heart disease (CCHD) is increasingly being adopted. There are advantages to diagnosing CCHD prior to collapse, particularly if this occurs outside of the hospital setting. The current recommended approach links pulse oximetry screening with the assessment for CCHD. An alternative approach is to document the oxygen saturation as part of a routine set of vital signs in each newborn infant prior to discharge, delinking the measurement of oxygen saturation from assessment for CCHD. This approach, the way that many hospitals which contribute to the Australian New Zealand Neonatal Network (ANZNN) have introduced screening, has the potential benefits of decreasing parental anxiety and expectation, not requiring specific consent, changing the interpretation of false positives and therefore the timing of the test, and removing the pressure to perform an immediate echocardiogram if the test is positive. There are advantages of introducing a formal screening program, including the attainment of adequate funding and a universal approach, but the barriers noted above need to be dealt with and the process of acceptance by a national body as a screening test can take many years.

Keywords: pulse oximetry; neonate; congenital heart disease; screening

1. Introduction

Reviews suggest that about 30% of infants with critical congenital heart disease (CCHD) leave hospital undiagnosed and that, in cardiovascular deaths occurring within the first week of life, the malformation was not identified before death in one out of four [1,2]. Neurological outcome is related to the presentation of the disease, with infants who collapse prior to presentation having a significantly worse outcome than those that are identified prior to collapse [3]. There is therefore a need for the development of effective screening tests for CCHD. Current screening for congenital heart defects has relied on a mid-trimester ultrasound scan, which is operator-dependent and at present detects <50% of CHD and about 60% of CCHD requiring surgery in the first month of life [4,5]. In Sweden, 26% of newborns with CCHD were sent home without being diagnosed [6].

Pulse oximetry has been evaluated in multiple studies as a screening test for CCHD. A high sensitivity is clearly important where a test is used to screen for a serious but treatable disease. Ewer et al. [7] in a test accuracy study showed that pulse oximetry had a sensitivity of 58% for critical (likely to require treatment in the first month) and 29% for all major (likely to require treatment in the first year) lesions when antenatal screening was negative. A systematic review and meta-analysis by Thangaratinam et al. [8] including 13 studies and almost 230,000 babies showed the overall sensitivity of pulse oximetry for the detection of critical congenital heart defects was 76.5%. In this review, there were no significant differences in sensitivity for pulse oximetry in the foot alone versus in both foot and right hand. The specificity was 99.9%, with an overall false-positive rate of 0.14%. The equipment is readily available and does not require calibration; the monitoring is minimally invasive and familiar to most parents and staff. Despite all of these potential screening advantages, the uptake of pulse oximetry screening for CCHD has not been universal. This paper aims to identify and review the barriers to the implementation of pulse oximetry as a screening test for CCHD.

2. Australian/New Zealand Progress

The adoption of pulse oximetry for screening for critical congenital heart disease has progressed substantially around the world, led by the development and adoption of screening guidelines in North America by the American Academy of Pediatrics (AAP) in 2011 [9]. The adoption of pulse oximetry screening in Australia/New Zealand has been on a hospital-by-hospital, state-by-state basis. New Zealand has recently proposed a countrywide adoption of screening at all health care facility levels and is currently exploring the feasibility of this [10]. A recent survey of all of the Australian/New Zealand Neonatal Intensive Care Units (Unpublished 2017) concluded that 77% of all units have implemented a screening program. Three units in New Zealand were not screening pending the introduction of a National screening program. Two units in Australia had suspended their screening programs due to resourcing implications both at the primary screen and in dealing with positive test results. Most units have adopted a screening guideline similar to either the AAP-recommended one or one based on the PulseOx study [7], but with some practical differences, particularly in terms of the timing of the screen and response to a positive screen. None of the units required a mandatory echocardiogram as part of the response to a positive screen.

The approach in Australia has been driven in part by some modification of the basic tenants of pulse oximetry screening for CCHD. Whilst the focus in the USA and the UK has been on the implementation of a formal screening program for CCHD, the discussion in Australia and New Zealand has been on the use of the terminology of "Pulse oximetry screening for critical congenital heart disease" versus "Pulse oximetry screening of the well newborn", the timing of pulse oximetry screening, the interpretation and significance of false positives, and the appropriate action for babies who screen positive, all of which have been areas of controversy during the implementation of universal routine pulse oximetry screening in many countries, including the United Kingdom [11].

3. Challenges in Introducing Pulse Oximetry Screening for CCHD

3.1. Screening for CCHD or Documentation of a Vital Sign

Pulse oximetry is used routinely in the assessment of adult patients admitted to hospital. Early warning scores have been developed, inclusive of routine saturation checks, to identify patients before clinical deterioration and preventing admissions to the intensive care unit. Saturation documentation forms part of Paediatric early warning systems, such as the Cardiff and Vale Paediatric Early Warning System and the Melbourne criterion for activation of medical emergency teams [12]. In Australia, local state health authorities have implemented programs such as "Between the Flags" to recognise and respond to patients when their clinical condition starts to deteriorate, which include documenting oxygen saturation [13]. Saturation monitoring has been proposed as an adjunct to the assessment of the newborn in the delivery room and as a routine vital sign assessment [14]. It is proposed that the documentation of oxygen saturation in the newborn should be an integral part of normal vital sign documentation, equivalent in importance to pulse, respirations, heart rate, and blood pressure. Introducing pulse oximetry as part of a routine observational assessment changes the emphasis of a pulse oximetry measure from screening for CCHD (still achieved) to documentation of the fifth vital sign [15]. As a result, it has been our observation that many of the barriers to CCHD screening are minimized, including parental anxiety about the link with CCHD and subsequent refusal of the screen [16], the need to obtain consent in some programs, which can be threatening to parents necessitating an opt-out clause in some countries, including the USA [17], the concept of a false positive for CCHD when the infant has a positive pulse oximetry screen (i.e., is noted to be hypoxic) but is not diagnosed with CCHD, and finally the response to a positive screen, which does not have to be a mandated echocardiogram with all of its resource implications [18].

3.2. Linking 'Pulse Oximetry Screening' to 'Screening for CCHD'

Referring to the screening program as "Pulse oximetry screening of the well newborn" rather than a "Program to screen for critical congenital heart disease" has resulted in better acceptance of the screening program for clinicians and parents in our setting [18]. Pulse oximetry screening identifies some forms of cyanotic heart disease, but does not screen for all CCHD. Some babies with CCHD are missed using pulse oximetry screening, particularly those with obstruction of the aorta. There is a risk of false parental reassurance of absence of congenital heart diseases with the use of the term 'Pulse oximetry screening for CCHD'.

The terminology "Screening for CCHD" may raise anxiety, as it introduces the possibility of a child having a serious health condition. In a recent article by Powell et al. [16] evaluating the acceptability of pulse oximetry screening to mothers, white British and Irish mothers had the lowest rate of decline (5%), while all other minor ethnic groups had an increased likelihood of declining the screening in a research setting (up to 21% in African women). Post-hoc analysis indicated that participants of minor ethnic origin were more anxious, more depressed, less satisfied, and more stressed than the white population who participated in the study. In our opinion, replacing the terminology with "routine pulse oximetry screening" as a documentation of a vital sign undertaken on all babies born in hospital is less likely to raise unnecessary anxiety in parents. The interesting requirement for an opt-out clause in the pulse oximetry screening program in the United States [17] is likely to have resulted from similar observations of parental anxiety.

3.3. Timing of Pulse Oximetry Screening and Significance of False Positives

The AAP work group recommends that screening should not begin until after 24 h of life, or as late as possible if an earlier discharge is planned, and be completed on the second day of life. Dawson et al. [19] have defined reference data for oxygen saturation in healthy full-term infants during their first 24 h of life. The time to reach a stable saturation >95% is generally 20 min in healthy babies (range 3–90 min), so waiting for 24 h is cautious. Earlier screening can lead to more false-positive results because of the transition from fetal to neonatal circulation and the stabilization of systemic oxygen saturation levels [9]. Thangaratinam et al. [8] showed that the false-positive rate for detection of CCHD was particularly low when newborn pulse oximetry was done after 24 h from birth than when it was done before 24 h: 0.05% versus 0.50%. Consequently, many screening programs have chosen to screen after 24 h to decrease the false positives for CCHD. An alternative way of looking at this is that the infants picked up on a positive screening test are infants with low oxygen saturation, regardless of the aetiology, and that any infant with low saturation requires investigation. When the population of infants with a false positive for CCHD are reviewed in the large data sets of screening, more than 50% of them will have important pathology, including congenital pneumonia, sepsis, meconium aspiration syndrome, milder forms of congenital heart disease, and failure to transition (eg. persistent pulmonary hypertension of the newborn (PPHN), transient tachypnea of the newborn (TTN)) [7,20–22]. Although these studies were not specifically designed to assess the cohort of false positives, a false positive result suggests a 'hypoxic' baby and a baby with undiagnosed Group B streptococcal sepsis, pneumonia, or PPHN is just as likely to collapse and die as a baby with undiagnosed CCHD. If documentation of saturation is agreed to be a routine vital sign, are we delaying the documentation of saturation in our babies for the wrong reasons?

When combined with the routine anomaly scan and newborn physical examination, early (4–24 h) pulse oximetry screening adds value to existing screening procedures and is likely to be useful for the identification of cases of CCHD that would otherwise go undetected. The added value in pulse oximetry screening over and above physical examination has been quantitated in two studies. deWahl Granelli [23] showed an increase in sensitivity of CCHD detection from 63% to 83% with specificity remaining at 98%. Similarly, Zhao et al. showed increased sensitivity of CCHD detection from 77.4% to 93.2% with the addition of pulse oximetry screening to the newborn examination [24].

There is clear data to show that infants with CCHD who present collapsed will have a worse neurological outcome than those who are identified before a collapse [3]. As a significant number of infants with CCHD present in the first 24 h with early ductal closure [25], planning a screening program in the first 24 h will result in less collapsed presentations and provide an opportunity for earlier stabilization and intervention. An added benefit is that screening within the first 24 h is less likely to interfere with the discharge process, particularly in those false positive cases that require only minimal intervention, such as a period of observation. The pros and cons of early versus late screening are presented in Table 1.

Table 1. Pros and cons of screening before and after 24 h of age.

<24 h of Age	>24 h of Age
Increased detection of significant and major CHD	Increased detection of significant and major CHD
Optimal for prevention of postnatal hypoxia	Not optimal but still prevents some hypoxic events
Higher false positive rate for CCHD (0.5%)	Lower false positive rate for CCHD (0.05%)
Detection of other pathology (up to 50% of all false positives)	Detection of other pathology (up to 50% of all false positives)
Often still in hospital: doesn't disrupt discharge process	May disrupt discharge process

CHD: congenital heart disease; CCHD: critical congenital heart disease.

3.4. Response to a Positive Screen

The number of false positives for CCHD arising from the physical examination is significantly more than that from pulse oximetry screening [24]. One of the perceived impediments in introducing a pulse oximetry screening program is the need for rapid access to cardiology services to perform an echocardiogram in the event of a failed screening test. In reality, these are babies likely to present to health care providers at some point, apart from the small number with transitional problems that will self-resolve. All health care facilities managing deliveries and newborn babies should already have existing referral and escalation pathways to deal with infants with suspected CHD. Pulse oximetry screening is simply a complement to the existing mechanisms whereby suspected CHD may be identified on physical examination in response to a member of staff reporting a 'dusky' baby or after a low saturation measure during an ad hoc pulse oximetry measure in a dusky appearing baby. These presentations are no different to a 'positive' pulse oximetry screen. In the published pulse oximetry studies, all babies with failed screens were referred for an echocardiogram to allow for full ascertainment of sensitivity and specificity in those babies with a low pulse oximetry reading. In fact, the AAP working group recommended that any newborn with a positive screen result first requires a comprehensive evaluation for causes of hypoxemia. In the absence of other findings to explain hypoxemia, CCHD needs to be excluded on the basis of a diagnostic echocardiogram (which would involve an echocardiogram within the hospital or birthing center or transport to another institution) [9]. The need for an echocardiogram should be determined on a case-by-case basis as it would be for other presentations of potential congenital heart disease (murmur, visible cyanosis). The actual number of infants requiring further investigation as a result of a failed pulse oximetry can be surprisingly small, and in particular the requirement for extra echocardiograms is minimal [18].

4. Pulse Oximetry of the Well Newborn versus Screening for CCHD

The dilemma that many countries are facing when introducing a program to identify hypoxic/borderline hypoxic infants is whether to mandate this as part of a formal national screening program or to introduce pulse oximetry as part of the routine observations performed on a newborn infant. There are pros and cons of each approach and these are summarized in Table 2. The introduction of pulse oximetry for all well newborns prior to discharge, by documenting SpO2 as the 5th vital sign, is appealing and relatively straight forward and the equipment and skills to measure it are already generally available. It is our opinion that delinking the term CCHD from the test allows for the documentation of SpO2 without needing to explain in detail about CCHD and complications that might occur from this, resulting in decreased parental anxiety, a reduced possibility of misinterpretation that CHD has been completely ruled out, false positives becoming less relevant such that earlier screening can be proposed, and a less likely implication of the need for a mandated echocardiogram in the event of a failed screen (Figure 1).

---

1. Consider a pulse oximetry measure as a standard vital sign that needs to be documented in all newborn babies.

2. Delink "Pulse Oximetry Screening" from "Screening for Critical Congenital Heart Diseases" – remove parental anxiety and the perception that CCHD is included / excluded by this test.

3. Measure in the first 24 hrs (allow first 4 hrs for transition). The 'false positives' are actually hypoxic babies warranting evaluation.

4. Do not delay pulse oximetry because an echocardiogram might be required in a false positive (for CCHD) baby.

5. Use existing assessment and referral pathways for a blue baby, heart murmur, and respiratory distress in the local hospital if there is a positive screen. A positive screen needs medical assessment, observation and sometimes a timely echocardiogram as a part of assessment but this is not mandated. We don't have to develop a whole new system.

6. Review the sensitivity and specificity of the current screening processes in place at your institution (antenatal ultrasound and newborn examination), they may be less accurate than introducing pulse oximetry screening

---

Figure 1. Pulse oximetry screening: A new paradigm.

Table 2. Formalised screening program versus vital sign documentation.

Screening Program	Hospital Led/5th Vital Sign
Meeting screening test criteria, Competing with other national screening programs for funding	More easily achievable without a complex application process
Research based: almost 500,000 babies tested	Harder to justify as not linked to CCHD research
Country-wide introduction, mandated, uniformity of coverage	Gaps in provision, Ad Hoc screening
Properly resourced and funded. Quality improvement more easily achieved	Resourcing is not excessive so achievable by most hospitals
CHD is a tested hard outcome	Importance of other diagnoses and timing of the test
Follows existing research based algorithms: reduced flexibility	Delink from CCHD terminology: reduces pressure from false positives and need for echocardiogram.

Importantly, the detailed requirements needed to satisfy inclusion as a formal country-wide screening test are not needed: these requirements can result in significant delays in the introduction of a screening program. The downside of this approach is that there may not be true nationwide screening, particularly at smaller, under-resourced hospitals. The approach may result in a less-uniform approach and lack of a formalized collection of results to understand the impact of screening. In contrast, a formal application to include pulse oximetry screening for CCHD as a part of a country screening program results in proper resourcing, oversight, and governance. It is more likely that all babies at all levels will be screened. However, the process takes time (5 years and still proceeding in the case of the United Kingdom) and will still suffer from all of the issues discussed above when pulse oximetry measures are linked to screening for CCHD. The Nordic countries have been successful in the approach of a hospital-by-hospital introduction of screening, resulting in an overall coverage of screening of close to 100% [26].

5. Conclusions

Currently in our part of the world, Australia has chosen to follow the introduction of screening on a hospital-by-hospital basis, adopting many of the tenants of the 5th vital sign approach, whilst New Zealand has signaled its intention to adopt a country-wide screening program due to some of the unique challenges of health care delivery they have [10]. It will be interesting to track how each country achieves the common aim of improving detection of CCHD and thus reducing deaths and neurodevelopmental injury associated with these significant congenital abnormalities. The body of research to date strongly supports the utility of screening all well newborn infants with pulse oximetry. However, the implementation of screening as performed in the research framework into the real life scenario has been impeded by many of the issues discussed in this paper. As more Units and countries describe their approach to screening and outcomes, a more balanced approach to the introduction of pulse oximetry screening is likely to be achieved.

References

1. Hoffman, J.I. It is time for routine neonatal screening by pulse oximetry. *Neonatology* **2011**, *99*, 1–9. [CrossRef] [PubMed]
2. Kuehl, K.S.; Loffredo, C.A.; Ferencz, C. Failure to diagnose congenital heart disease in infancy. *Pediatrics* **1999**, *103*, 743–747. [CrossRef] [PubMed]
3. Snookes, S.H.; Gunn, J.K.; Eldridge, B.J.; Donath, S.M.; Hunt, R.W.; Galea, M.P.; Shekerdemian, L. A systematic review of motor and cognitive outcomes after early surgery for congenital heart disease. *Pediatrics* **2010**, *125*, e818–e827. [CrossRef] [PubMed]
4. Sholler, G.F.; Kasparian, N.A.; Pye, V.E.; Cole, A.D.; Winlaw, D.S. Fetal and post-natal diagnosis of major congenital heart disease: Implications for medical and psychological care in the current era. *J. Paediatr. Child Health* **2011**, *47*, 717–722. [CrossRef] [PubMed]
5. Sharland, G. Fetal cardiac screening: Why bother? *Arch. Dis. Child. Fetal Neonatal Ed.* **2010**, *95*, F64–F68. [PubMed]
6. Mellander, M.; Sunnegardh, J. Failure to diagnose critical heart malformations in newborns before discharge—An increasing problem? *Acta Paediatr.* **2006**, *95*, 407–413. [CrossRef] [PubMed]
7. Ewer, A.K.; Middleton, L.J.; Furmston, A.T.; Bhoyar, A.; Daniels, J.P.; Thangaratinam, S.; Deeks, J.J.; Khan, K.S.; PulseOx Study Group. Pulse oximetry screening for congenital heart defects in newborn infants (pulseox): A test accuracy study. *Lancet* **2011**, *378*, 785–794. [CrossRef]
8. Thangaratinam, S.; Brown, K.; Zamora, J.; Khan, K.S.; Ewer, A.K. Pulse oximetry screening for critical congenital heart defects in asymptomatic newborn babies: A systematic review and meta-analysis. *Lancet* **2012**, *379*, 2459–2464. [CrossRef]
9. Kemper, A.R.; Mahle, W.T.; Martin, G.R.; Cooley, W.C.; Kumar, P.; Morrow, W.R.; Kelm, K.; Pearson, G.D.; Glidewell, J.; Grosse, S.D.; et al. Strategies for implementing screening for critical congenital heart disease. *Pediatrics* **2011**, *128*, e1259–e1267. [CrossRef] [PubMed]
10. Cloete, E.; Gentles, T.L.; Alsweiler, J.M.; Dixon, L.A.; Webster, D.R.; Rowe, D.L.; Bloomfield, F.H. Should new zealand introduce nationwide pulse oximetry screening for the detection of critical congenital heart disease in newborn infants? *N. Z. Med. J.* **2017**, *130*, 64–69. [PubMed]
11. Mikrou, P.; Singh, A.; Ewer, A.K. Pulse oximetry screening for critical congenital heart defects: A repeat UK national survey. *Arch. Dis. Child. Fetal Neonatal Ed.* **2017**, *102*, F558. [CrossRef] [PubMed]
12. Edwards, E.D.; Powell, C.V.; Mason, B.W.; Oliver, A. Prospective cohort study to test the predictability of the cardiff and vale paediatric early warning system. *Arch. Dis. Child.* **2009**, *94*, 602–606. [CrossRef] [PubMed]
13. Health, N. *Children and Infants—Recognition of a Sick Baby or Child in the Emergency Department*; NSW Health: Sydney, Australia, 2011.

14. Katzman, G.H. The newborn's spo2: A routine vital sign whose time has come? *Pediatrics* **1995**, *95*, 161–162. [PubMed]

15. Mower, W.R.; Sachs, C.; Nicklin, E.L.; Baraff, L.J. Pulse oximetry as a fifth pediatric vital sign. *Pediatrics* **1997**, *99*, 681–686. [CrossRef] [PubMed]

16. Powell, R.; Pattison, H.M.; Bhoyar, A.; Furmston, A.T.; Middleton, L.J.; Daniels, J.P.; Ewer, A.K. Pulse oximetry screening for congenital heart defects in newborn infants: An evaluation of acceptability to mothers. *Arch. Dis. Child. Fetal Neonatal Ed.* **2013**, *98*, F59–F63. [CrossRef] [PubMed]

17. Hom, L.A.; Silber, T.J.; Ennis-Durstine, K.; Hilliard, M.A.; Martin, G.R. Legal and ethical considerations in allowing parental exemptions from newborn critical congenital heart disease (cchd) screening. *Am. J. Bioeth.* **2016**, *16*, 11–17. [CrossRef] [PubMed]

18. Bhola, K.; Kluckow, M.; Evans, N. Post-implementation review of pulse oximetry screening of well newborns in an australian tertiary maternity hospital. *J. Paediatr. Child Health* **2014**, *50*, 920–925. [CrossRef] [PubMed]

19. Dawson, J.A.; Vento, M.; Finer, N.N.; Rich, W.; Saugstad, O.D.; Morley, C.J.; Davis, P.G. Managing oxygen therapy during delivery room stabilization of preterm infants. *J. Pediatr.* **2012**, *160*, 158–161. [CrossRef] [PubMed]

20. Narayen, I.C.; Blom, N.A.; Ewer, A.K.; Vento, M.; Manzoni, P.; te Pas, A.B. Aspects of pulse oximetry screening for critical congenital heart defects: When, how and why? *Arch. Dis. Child. Fetal Neonatal Ed.* **2016**, *101*, F162–F167. [CrossRef] [PubMed]

21. Meberg, A.; Brugmann-Pieper, S.; Due, R., Jr.; Eskedal, L.; Fagerli, I.; Farstad, T.; Froisland, D.H.; Sannes, C.H.; Johansen, O.J.; Keljalic, J.; et al. First day of life pulse oximetry screening to detect congenital heart defects. *J. Pediatr.* **2008**, *152*, 761–765. [CrossRef] [PubMed]

22. Arlettaz, R.; Bauschatz, A.S.; Monkhoff, M.; Essers, B.; Bauersfeld, U. The contribution of pulse oximetry to the early detection of congenital heart disease in newborns. *Eur. J. Pediatr.* **2006**, *165*, 94–98. [CrossRef] [PubMed]

23. de-Wahl Granelli, A.; Wennergren, M.; Sandberg, K.; Mellander, M.; Bejlum, C.; Inganas, L.; Eriksson, M.; Segerdahl, N.; Agren, A.; Ekman-Joelsson, B.M.; et al. Impact of pulse oximetry screening on the detection of duct dependent congenital heart disease: A swedish prospective screening study in 39,821 newborns. *Bmj* **2009**, *338*, a3037. [CrossRef] [PubMed]

24. Zhao, Q.M.; Ma, X.J.; Ge, X.L.; Liu, F.; Yan, W.L.; Wu, L.; Ye, M.; Liang, X.C.; Zhang, J.; Gao, Y.; et al. Pulse oximetry with clinical assessment to screen for congenital heart disease in neonates in china: A prospective study. *Lancet* **2014**, *384*, 747–754. [CrossRef]

25. Schultz, A.H.; Localio, A.R.; Clark, B.J.; Ravishankar, C.; Videon, N.; Kimmel, S.E. Epidemiologic features of the presentation of critical congenital heart disease: Implications for screening. *Pediatrics* **2008**, *121*, 751–757. [CrossRef] [PubMed]

26. de-Wahl Granelli, A.; Meberg, A.; Ojala, T.; Steensberg, J.; Oskarsson, G.; Mellander, M. Nordic pulse oximetry screening–implementation status and proposal for uniform guidelines. *Acta Paediatr.* **2014**, *103*, 1136–1142. [CrossRef] [PubMed]

9

At-Risk Testing for Pompe Disease Using Dried Blood Spots: Lessons Learned for Newborn Screening

Zoltan Lukacs [1], Petra Oliva [2,*], Paulina Nieves Cobos [1], Jacob Scott [2], Thomas P. Mechtler [2] and David C. Kasper [2]

[1] Newborn Screening and Metabolic Diagnostics Unit, Hamburg University Medical Center, 20251 Hamburg, Germany; lukacs@uke.de (Z.L.); acquim@hotmail.com (P.N.C.)

[2] ARCHIMED Life Science GmbH, 1110 Vienna, Austria; j.scott@archimedlife.com (J.S.); t.mechtler@archimedlife.com (T.P.M.); d.kasper@archimedlife.com (D.C.K.)

* Correspondence: p.oliva@archimedlife.com

Abstract: Pompe disease (GSD II) is an autosomal recessive disorder caused by deficiency of the lysosomal enzyme acid-α-glucosidase (GAA, EC 3.2.1.20), leading to generalized accumulation of lysosomal glycogen especially in the heart, skeletal, and smooth muscle, and the nervous system. It is generally classified based on the age of onset as infantile (IOPD) presenting during the first year of life, and late onset (LOPD) when it presents afterwards. In our study, a cohort of 13,627 samples were tested between January 2017 and December 2018 for acid-α-glucosidase (GAA, EC 3.2.1.20) deficiency either by fluorometry or tandem mass spectrometry (MS). Testing was performed for patients who displayed conditions of unknown etiology, e.g., CK elevations or cardiomyopathy, in the case of infantile patients. On average 8% of samples showed activity below the reference range and were further assessed by another enzyme activity measurement or molecular genetic analysis. Pre-analytical conditions, like proper drying, greatly affect enzyme activity, and should be assessed with measurement of reference enzyme(s). In conclusion, at-risk testing can provide a good first step for the future introduction of newborn screening for Pompe disease. It yields immediate benefits for the patients regarding the availability and timeliness of the diagnosis. In addition, the laboratory can introduce the required methodology and gain insights in the evaluation of results in a lower throughput environment. Finally, awareness of such a rare condition is increased tremendously among local physicians which can aid in the introduction newborn screening.

Keywords: newborn screening; Pompe disease; dried blood spots; Pompe disease diagnostics testing

1. Introduction

Pompe disease (GSD II) is an autosomal recessive disorder caused by deficiency of the lysosomal enzyme acid-α-glucosidase (GAA, EC 3.2.1.20), leading to a generalized accumulation of lysosomal glycogen especially in the heart, skeletal and smooth muscle, and the nervous system. It is generally classified based on the age of onset as infantile (IOPD) presenting during the first year of life, and late onset (LOPD) when it presents afterwards [1–3]. IOPD is usually associated with cardiomyopathy and then referred to as classic Pompe disease [1]. Infants with classic Pompe disease typically present during the first few weeks of life with hypotonia, progressive weakness, macroglossia, and hepatomegaly. Most of these infants die by their first birthday [4]. In the rare instances presenting without cardiomyopathy, it is referred to as non-classic Pompe disease [5–7].

The diagnosis of Pompe disease is usually made based on the typical clinical presentation followed by the demonstration of deficiency of GAA enzyme activity in muscle, skin fibroblasts or more recently dried blood spots (DBS) as well as GAA mutation analysis [2,8]. Diagnosis of Pompe disease through newborn screening (NBS) is also possible [9,10]. Prior to the initiation of enzyme replacement therapy, rapid determination of CRIM status [11,12] in patients with infantile onset Pompe disease is extremely important [13]. Depending on results immune-suppressive therapy may be initiated. Pompe disease is still considered to be a rare inborn error of metabolism with an estimated frequency of about 1/40,000 and a higher incidence in certain populations such as African Americans (1/14,000), Northern Europeans of Dutch origin and South East Asians [2]. Early results of newborn screening pilot studies from Taiwan [14] and the USA [15–17] indicated a higher general incidence, especially of LOPD cases which may be missed as clinical symptoms are less clear.

GAA catalyzes the hydrolysis of $\alpha1{\to}4$ glucosidic linkages in glycogen at acid pH [2]. Specificity for the natural substrate (glycogen) is gained during its maturation. The activity of mature (76/70-kDa) GAA for its natural (glycogen) substrate is considerably more robust than its activity towards the artificial substrate (4-methylumbelliferyl-α-D-glucoside; 4-MU), which is frequently used in in-vitro assays. However, 4-MU is also a substrate for several other enzymes including "leukocyte" neutral isoenzymes, glucosidase II (GANAB), neutral α-glucosidase C (GANC), and maltase glucoamylase (MGAM). Therefore, using maltose or, preferably, acarbose as an inhibitor of MGAM activity, allows for the measurement of GAA activity in DBS samples with minimal interference by other α-glucosidases. This assay serves as the basis for newborn screening and the non-invasive diagnosis of Pompe disease [18–20]. As a result, multiplex newborn screening assays for Pompe disease (based on GAA enzyme activity) and other lysosomal storage disorders using fluorometry, digital microfluidics or tandem mass spectrometry have been developed [10,21–23]. In addition for qualitative and quantitative assessments of the disease burden, and clinical measurement of the impact of Pompe disease on various affected systems, urinary glucose tetrasaccharide (Glc4), a biomarker of glycogen storage with 94% sensitivity and 84% specificity for Pompe disease, is frequently used in monitoring the response of patients to enzyme replacement therapy and as an adjunct to acid α-glucosidase activity measurements [24–26]. However, there is still no reliable biomarker to predict the natural course of the disease in an individual or the point of time when ERT should be administered for LOPD cases. This complicates the introduction of newborn screening in many areas. In contrast, diagnostic testing allows early detection of LOPD cases without ethical problems and may pave the way for a future introduction of whole population Pompe screening.

In this paper, we present the data from testing over 13,000 individuals suspected having of Pompe disease collected over a two-year period by two different centers in Europe (Hamburg, Germany and Vienna, Austria). At-risk testing is the use of the assay to determine whether an individual at increased risk of having Pompe disease (because they have family history or symptoms remotely associated with the disease but not pathognomic for the disease such as CK-elevations of unknown origin) has a deficiency of GAA. Further diagnostic testing will be required for individuals whose test is suggestive of the condition to confirm true deficiency of enzyme or for example a compromised sample, as sample quality and shipping conditions can affect the results.

2. Materials and Methods

A DBS kit containing a customized card (Whatman 903) for blood sampling and sampling instructions, and an envelope was provided to physicians upon request for α-glucosidase testing. Dried blood specimens were received with brief clinical details and an ICF (informed consent) between January 2017 through December 2018. DBS protocols used to measure α-glucosidase (EC:3.2.1.20) enzyme activities are given below.

2.1. Fluorometric Method

The method by Chamoles et al. [18] was slightly modified. A 3 mm DBS was eluted with 360 µL of demineralized water, then 40 µL aliquots transferred to a 96-well plate. The test was run using the artificial substrate 4-methylumbelliferyl-α-D-glucoside (1.4 mM, Sigma-Aldrich, Darmstadt, Germany) in 40 mM sodium acetate (CH3COONa) buffer at pH 3.8 (Merck, Darmstadt, Germany) with and without the addition of 10 µL of 80 µM acarbose solution (Toronto Research Chemicals, North York, ON, Canada).

The assay was also performed at pH 7.0 (40 mM CH3COONa buffer adjusted with hydrochloric acid/sodium hydroxide (HCl/NaOH) to pH 7.0), to assess the quality of the DBS. The α-glucosidase activity at pH 7.0 is a convenient tool for quality assessment because the same buffers adjusted to pH 7.0 can be used as for the target enzyme at pH 3.8. In addition, the enzyme activity at pH 7.0 is usually less stable than α-glucosidase activity at pH 3.8 when subjected to detrimental pre-analytical conditions, thereby being an early marker for specimen quality. All tests were run in duplicate. After incubation for 21 h at 37 °C, the reaction was stopped by the addition of 200 μL EDTA buffer (150 μM, pH 11.5; Sigma-Aldrich). The 40 μL of DBS eluate that had been stored at 4 °C overnight was added to specific wells that served as blanks. A standard curve of 4-methylumbelliferone (0 to 3 μM (Sigma-Aldrich)) run on each plate was used for the calculation of enzyme activities. The fluorescence was read on a Victor D instrument (Wallac Oy, Turku, Finland) or a BioTek Synergy H1 (Bad Friedrichshall, Germany). In addition to enzyme activity, the percent inhibition with acarbose and the ratio of α-glucosidase activities at pH 3.8 with inhibition to the activity at pH 7.0 were calculated to aid in the interpretation of results [27]. For samples from patients older than 1 year of age, a truncated assay which relied only on the measurement of α-glucosidase with acarbose inhibition was used. As a reference enzyme, β-galactosidase was run on these samples. Specimens from infants and those that showed diminished α-glucosidase activity in the truncated test, were analyzed using the test with and without acarbose. The calculation of additional ratios allowed for a better interpretation of results from samples with borderline values. Individuals from whom specimens with normal results in the truncated assay were considered not affected by Pompe disease and this assay allowed higher throughput testing and expedited reporting of results.

2.2. MS Method

The assay was based on previously published methods [9,28]. The samples were processed using the following steps. The activities of acid β-glucocerebrosidase (ABG; Gaucher disease), acid sphingomyelinase (ASM; Niemann-Pick A/B disease), α-glucosidase (GAA; Pompe disease) and α-galactosidase; GLA; Fabry disease) were measured in a multiplex assay. The extract from one 3.2 mm punch per DBS sample was combined with substrate and internal standard (S&IS) mixtures. Incubation was performed at 37 °C for 20–22 h. The reaction was stopped by adding 100 μL stopping solution (80% acetonitrile plus 0.2% formic acid in water). Aliquots were transferred to a new deep-well plate, covered with aluminum foil and centrifuged at 3000× g for 15 min prior to mass spectrometry analysis. Background activity of a blank blood collection paper spot was subtracted from the DBS activity. Two QC samples with previously established activity levels for each enzyme and heat inactivated samples were included in each plate as assay controls.

3. Results

Between January 2017 and December 2018 13,627 specimens were tested for GAA deficiency by fluorometry or tandem mass spectrometry (MS) using Dried Blood Spots (DBS) (Table 1). Specimens came from 51 different countries but most were from Germany, Poland, Turkey, Italy and Iran. Approximately 30% of all samples submitted were from infants. The median age was 17 years and the range 1–95 years. Specimens from individuals with family history of the condition were excluded.

Table 1. Number of samples tested between January 2017 and December 2018 at the specialized centers in Hamburg, Germany and Vienna, Austria.

	Fluorometry Method	MS Method
Number of tests	7340	6287
Normal enzyme activity	6921	5591
Enzyme activity below cut-off (positive)	419 (6%)	696 (11%)

Most of the tested samples (92%) showed normal enzyme activity. 8% of the samples showed enzyme activity below the respective cut-off. In most cases with decreased enzyme activity (419 from the fluorometric method and 696 from the MS method) genetic analysis was performed on the same bloodspot. 35–40% of the low enzyme samples screened by the MS method were genetically confirmed with two pathogenic variants, and similar confirmation rates have been obtained for the fluorometric method. Fluorometry has lower sensitivity in comparison to mass spectrometry [29].

Some positive results were obtained in specimens affected by detrimental pre-analytical conditions which did not necessarily reduce other enzyme activities. In those instances, a second card was requested for analysis.

Unfortunately, not all DBS came with a description of clinical symptoms. However, the major symptoms that were given are summarized in Table 2 grouped by analogous symptoms and sorted by severity. Cardiomyopathy was present almost exclusively in infant cases while CK-elevations of unknown origin or limb girdle muscle dystrophy of unknown origin were more prominent among LOPD cases in the Hamburg cohort.

Table 2. Clinical symptoms provided for samples submitted to the study centers in Hamburg and Vienna. Not all specimens contained such information.

	Clinical Presentation
1	Cardiomyopathy
2	Hypotonia—floppy baby, proximal and progressive muscle weakness, limb girdle muscle weakness, muscle pain, loss of strength and myalgia
3	Scoliosis myopathy, rigid spine, diffuse myopathy, myopathic syndrome, EMG: myogenic involvement, motor deficit of the belt
4	Elevated biomarkers—CK, myoglobin, transaminases

Statistical results of the GAA enzyme activity measurement using either fluorimetry or tandem mass spectrometry are listed in Table 3.

Table 3. Statistical results for both reference methods used in Hamburg (fluorometry) and Vienna (MS). For the normal values all specimens from individuals considered unaffected by Pompe disease have been included.

	Fluorometry Method [μmol/punch/h]		Tandem Mass Spectrometry Method [μmol/L/h] with Acarbose
	α-Glucosidase with Acarbose	α-Glucosidase without Acarbose	
Mean	7.43×10^{-8}	1.24×10^{-7}	9.24
Median	6.57×10^{-8}	1.05×10^{-7}	8.12
1st Percentile	2.14×10^{-8}	5.05×10^{-8}	4.69
99th Percentile	2.28×10^{-7}	3.75×10^{-7}	
99.9th Percentile	3.84×10^{-7}	5.42×10^{-7}	
Reference range	$4.29\text{–}34.29 \times 10^{-8}$	$7.14\text{–}47.62 \times 10^{-8}$	
Affected range	<0.4	n/a	3.3

The effect of drying conditions on GAA enzyme activity was studied. Duplicate specimens were collected. One was dried at room temperature overnight (dry) while the other remained in a plastic wrapping for 2 days to simulate transport without proper drying (wrapped). After this time period the sample was taken out of the plastic bag and dried overnight. Both were tested using the fluorometric method with and without addition of acarbose and as at pH 7.0 (reference enzyme). A significant decrease of enzyme activity (on average 50%) was observed if samples were not dried properly. In two cases (sample 2 and 3) it led to results that could be interpreted as consistent with Pompe disease or carrier status, while the interpretation of sample 5 changed from borderline positive into an unsuitable specimen. This observation is consistent with previously reported results [30]. Data are summarized in Table 4.

Table 4. Degradation study of GAA activities for five dried blood specimens that showed different index activities. Samples were either dried overnight after spotting (dry) or put into sealed plastic bags immediately, in order to simulate shipping without proper drying (wrapped). After 2 days the samples were taken out and allowed to dry overnight. Both specimens were tested in the same run in duplicates. All samples showed a significant decrease in activity when the specimen was not dried before shipping.

α-Glucosidase Activity [nmol/punch × 21 h] (Reference Range)	Sample 1		Sample 2		Sample 3		Sample 4		Sample 5	
	Wrapped	Dry	Wrapped	Dry	Wrapped	Dry	Wrapped	Dry	Wrapped	Dry
pH 3.8 (>1.5)	2.07	3.02	0.82	2.06	1.28	3.09	1.92	2.56	0.29	1.6
pH 7.0 (>1.8)	5.4	6.47	1.8	4.48	3.33	6.12	4.07	6.04	0.9	5.52
pH 3.8 with acarbose (>0.9)	1	1.72	0.54	1.19	0.72	1.86	1.12	1.35	0.18	0.58

4. Discussion

Newborn screening for Pompe disease can be performed by a variety of methods based on enzyme activity measurement. NBS provides early identification of both classic severe IOPD and less-severe LOPD patients. With early detection and ERT, there are benefits for classic severe IOPD patients, however current therapy has limitations, especially with respect to the neurologic manifestations of the disease. The combination of early detection, close monitoring, and early ERT may be beneficial to less-severe LOPD patients as well. However, in some countries and regions the identification of LOPD presents an ethical problem and whole population screening poses financial constraints on health care systems. In contrast, at-risk testing as presented here, may be a potential first step. It allows for earlier identification of IOPD cases and potentially also LOPD when performed with a targeted approach using nonspecific symptoms loosely associated with Pompe disease, such as CK elevations of unknown origin. Interestingly, usually mild to moderate CK elevations are observed in patients with Pompe disease, which do not improve under therapy. In our study we have received specimens from patients who presented with non-specific symptoms and thus, may have Pompe disease but may have had another disorder hence GAA measurement aids in the differential diagnosis. Among 13,627 samples tested, 8% had decreased enzyme activity. We have shown that detrimental pre-analytical conditions may also affect enzyme activities negatively, so further confirmation is necessary. For that purpose, another enzyme measurement can be performed, and a molecular genetic assay should also be carried out. Previously, we have demonstrated that about. 2% of patients tested are eventually confirmed with Pompe disease which is in agreement with other international studies [31,32]. This demonstrates the high efficacy of the at-risk testing approach. The time to diagnosis can be significantly shortened, especially for LOPD patients who present with less specific symptoms. For IOPD patients, testing may be helpful in regions that are not familiar with the specific symptoms however due to the first clear symptoms, in particular floppiness, which occurs around 2–3 months of age, an even earlier diagnosis remains restricted to newborn screening.

Interest in Pompe disease testing within NBS programs has increased substantially in recent years. Sample quality greatly affects results from Pompe testing and newborn screening in general. As previously described [30], the combination of humidity and heat has the greatest impact on enzyme stability. The authors also showed with their shipping study that when properly dried DBS were stored in either paper envelopes or plastic bags, enzyme activities remained essentially intact for nine days in the US postal setting [30]. In contrast, insufficient drying combined with shipping of the samples in sealed (plastic) containers leads to grossly reduced activity, especially of the acid α-glucosidase and may even result in erroneous interpretation of the results as the activity of the reference enzyme remains in the normal range.

For adequate samples, GAA levels in specimens from affected patients are well resolved from those observed in specimens from healthy subjects using either fluorometry or tandem mass spectrometry (Table 3). The strength of mass spectrometry lies especially in its ability to measure several enzyme activities simultaneously. This is beneficial for newborn screening when various different lysosomal storage disorders are included in a national panel. Furthermore, the different enzyme activities may aid in the evaluation of sample quality and thus differentiate the cause of low enzyme activity between deficiency in the individual and deficiency caused by inappropriate storage conditions or transport. Using the fluorometric method as described the activity of α-glucosidase at pH 7.0 can be measured. This is usually less stable than the acid α-glucosidase and therefore, is a good indicator of negative environmental influences. For α-glucosidase tests which only include the activity with inhibition, β-galactosidase may be an alternative reference enzyme to monitor sample quality. This additional fluorometric test is fast and inexpensive, however, it must be used with some caution. β-galactosidase in dried blood may be relatively stable, therefore, a low enzyme activity result for α-glucosidase may still be caused by pre-analytical conditions rather than an actual disease. This applies to reference enzymes in general, as different environmental conditions may affect these enzymes to varying degrees. Thus, despite problematic conditions prior to the arrival of the specimen in the laboratory, the reference enzyme(s) may still show normal activity levels in the DBS. Therefore, the assessment of another specimen, either again in DBS or in a different material should always be considered as a second step. For further confirmation, a molecular genetic assessment is necessary. In case of IOPD, it may replace the second enzyme assessment or can be carried out in parallel to save valuable time and initiate therapy more rapidly.

In conclusion, at-risk testing can provide a good first step for the future introduction of Pompe disease to a newborn screening program as the laboratory can introduce the required methodology and gain insights in the evaluation of results in a lower throughput environment. It yields immediate benefits for the patients regarding availability and timeliness of the diagnosis. Finally, awareness of this rare condition is increased tremendously among local physicians which can aid in the introduction of Pompe disease into a national newborn screening program.

Author Contributions: Conceptualization, Z.L. and D.C.K.; Data curation, Z.L., P.O., P.N.C., and T.P.M.; Investigation, T.P.M.; Project administration, Z.L.; Resources, D.C.K.; Validation, P.N.C. and J.S.; Writing—original draft, Z.L. and P.O.; Writing—review & editing, P.N.C., J.S., and D.C.K. All authors have read and agreed to the published version of the manuscript.

Acknowledgments: We thank our colleagues from ARCHIMEDlife and Hamburg University Medical Center, who provided insight and expertise that greatly assisted with all the interpretations and conclusions of this paper.

References

1. Chien, Y.-H.; Hwu, W.-L.; Lee, N.-C. Pompe disease: Early diagnosis and early treatment make a difference. *Pediatr. Neonatol.* **2013**, *54*, 219–227. [CrossRef]
2. Dasouki, M.; Jawdat, O.; Almadhoun, O.; Pasnoor, M.; McVey, A.L.; Abuzinadah, A.; Herbelin, L.; Barohn, R.J.; Dimachkie, M.M. Pompe disease: Literature review and case series. *Neurol. Clin.* **2014**, *32*, 751–776. [CrossRef]
3. Kohler, L.; Puertollano, R.; Raben, N. Pompe Disease: From Basic Science to Therapy. *Neurotherapeutics* **2018**, *15*, 928–942. [CrossRef]
4. Bay, L.B.; Denzler, I.; Durand, C.; Eiroa, H.; Frabasil, J.; Fainboim, A.; Maxit, C.; Schenone, A.; Spécola, N. Infantile-onset Pompe disease: Diagnosis and management TT—Enfermedad de Pompe infantil: Diagnóstico y tratamiento. *Arch. Argent. Pediatr.* **2019**, *117*, 271–278.
5. Van den Hout, H.M.P.; Hop, W.; van Diggelen, O.P.; Smeitink, J.A.M.; Smit, G.P.A.; Poll-The, B.-T.T.; Bakker, H.D.; Loonen, M.C.B.; de Klerk, J.B.C.; Reuser, A.J.J.; et al. The natural course of infantile Pompe's disease: 20 original cases compared with 133 cases from the literature. *Pediatrics* **2003**, *112*, 332–340. [CrossRef] [PubMed]

6. Case, L.E.; Beckemeyer, A.A.; Kishnani, P.S. Infantile Pompe disease on ERT: Update on clinical presentation, musculoskeletal management, and exercise considerations. *Am. J. Med. Genet. C Semin. Med. Genet.* **2012**, *160*, 69–79. [CrossRef]
7. Cupler, E.J.; Berger, K.I.; Leshner, R.T.; Wolfe, G.I.; Han, J.J.; Barohn, R.J.; Kissel, J.T.; AANEM Consensus Committee on Late-onset Pompe Disease. Consensus treatment recommendations for late-onset Pompe disease. *Muscle Nerve* **2012**, *45*, 319–333. [CrossRef] [PubMed]
8. Kishnani, P.S.; Hwu, W.-L.; Group, P.D.N.S.W. Introduction to the Newborn Screening, Diagnosis, and Treatment for Pompe Disease Guidance Supplement. *Pediatrics* **2017**, *140*, S1–S3. [CrossRef]
9. Metz, T.F.; Mechtler, T.P.; Orsini, J.J.; Martin, M.; Shushan, B.; Herman, J.L.; Ratschmann, R.; Item, C.B.; Streubel, B.; Herkner, K.R.; et al. Simplified newborn screening protocol for lysosomal storage disorders. *Clin. Chem.* **2011**, *57*, 1286–1294. [CrossRef]
10. Mechtler, T.P.; Stary, S.; Metz, T.F.; De Jesus, V.R.; Greber-Platzer, S.; Pollak, A.; Herkner, K.R.; Streubel, B.; Kasper, D.C. Neonatal screening for lysosomal storage disorders: Feasibility and incidence from a nationwide study in Austria. *Lancet* **2012**, *379*, 335–341. [CrossRef]
11. Bali, D.S.; Goldstein, J.L.; Banugaria, S.; Dai, J.; Mackey, J.; Rehder, C.; Kishnani, P.S. Predicting cross-reactive immunological material (CRIM) status in Pompe disease using GAA mutations: Lessons learned from 10 years of clinical laboratory testing experience. *Am. J. Med. Genet. C Semin. Med. Genet.* **2012**, *160C*, 40–49. [CrossRef]
12. Kishnani, P.S.; Corzo, D.; Leslie, N.D.; Gruskin, D.; Van der Ploeg, A.; Clancy, J.P.; Parini, R.; Morin, G.; Beck, M.; Bauer, M.S.; et al. Early treatment with alglucosidase alpha prolongs long-term survival of infants with Pompe disease. *Pediatr. Res.* **2009**, *66*, 329–335. [CrossRef]
13. Wang, Z.; Okamoto, P.; Keutzer, J. A new assay for fast, reliable CRIM status determination in infantile-onset Pompe disease. *Mol. Genet. Metab.* **2014**, *111*, 92–100. [CrossRef]
14. Chien, Y.-H.; Hwu, W.-L.; Lee, N.-C. Newborn screening: Taiwanese experience. *Ann. Transl. Med.* **2019**, *7*, 281. [CrossRef]
15. Elliott, S.; Buroker, N.; Cournoyer, J.J.; Potier, A.M.; Trometer, J.D.; Elbin, C.; Schermer, M.J.; Kantola, J.; Boyce, A.; Turecek, F.; et al. Pilot study of newborn screening for six lysosomal storage diseases using Tandem Mass Spectrometry. *Mol. Genet. Metab.* **2016**, *118*, 304–309. [CrossRef]
16. Bodamer, O.A.; Scott, C.R.; Giugliani, R.; Pompe Disease Newborn Screening Working Group. Newborn Screening for Pompe Disease. *Pediatrics* **2017**, *140*, S4–S13. [CrossRef]
17. Wasserstein, M.P.; Caggana, M.; Bailey, S.M.; Desnick, R.J.; Edelmann, L.; Estrella, L.; Holzman, I.; Kelly, N.R.; Kornreich, R.; Kupchik, S.G.; et al. The New York pilot newborn screening program for lysosomal storage diseases: Report of the first 65,000 infants. *Genet. Med.* **2019**, *21*, 631–640. [CrossRef]
18. Chamoles, N.A.; Niizawa, G.; Blanco, M.; Gaggioli, D.; Casentini, C. Glycogen storage disease type II: Enzymatic screening in dried blood spots on filter paper. *Clin. Chim. Acta* **2004**, *347*, 97–102. [CrossRef]
19. Zhang, H.; Kallwass, H.; Young, S.P.; Carr, C.; Dai, J.; Kishnani, P.S.; Millington, D.S.; Keutzer, J.; Chen, Y.-T.; Bali, D. Comparison of maltose and acarbose as inhibitors of maltase-glucoamylase activity in assaying acid alpha-glucosidase activity in dried blood spots for the diagnosis of infantile Pompe disease. *Genet. Med.* **2006**, *8*, 302–306. [CrossRef]
20. Niizawa, G.; Levin, C.; Aranda, C.; Blanco, M.; Chamoles, N.A. Retrospective diagnosis of glycogen storage disease type II by use of a newborn-screening card. *Clin. Chim. Acta* **2005**, *359*, 205–206. [CrossRef]
21. Sista, R.S.; Wang, T.; Wu, N.; Graham, C.; Eckhardt, A.; Winger, T.; Srinivasan, V.; Bali, D.; Millington, D.S.; Pamula, V.K. Multiplex newborn screening for Pompe, Fabry, Hunter, Gaucher, and Hurler diseases using a digital microfluidic platform. *Clin. Chim. Acta* **2013**, *424*, 12–18. [CrossRef]
22. Spáčil, Z.; Elliott, S.; Reeber, S.L.; Gelb, M.H.; Scott, C.R.; Tureček, F. Comparative triplex tandem mass spectrometry assays of lysosomal enzyme activities in dried blood spots using fast liquid chromatography: Application to newborn screening of Pompe, Fabry, and Hurler diseases. *Anal. Chem.* **2011**, *83*, 4822–4828. [CrossRef]
23. Mechtler, T.P.; Metz, T.F.; Muller, H.G.; Ostermann, K.; Ratschmann, R.; De Jesus, V.R.; Shushan, B.; Di Bussolo, J.M.; Herman, J.L.; Herkner, K.R.; et al. Short-incubation mass spectrometry assay for lysosomal storage disorders in newborn and high-risk population screening. *J. Chromatogr. B Anal. Technol. Biomed. Life Sci.* **2012**, *908*, 9–17. [CrossRef] [PubMed]

24. Xia, B.; Asif, G.; Arthur, L.; Pervaiz, M.A.; Li, X.; Liu, R.; Cummings, R.D.; He, M. Oligosaccharide analysis in urine by maldi-tof mass spectrometry for the diagnosis of lysosomal storage diseases. *Clin. Chem.* **2013**, *59*, 1357–1368. [CrossRef]

25. Young, S.P.; Piraud, M.; Goldstein, J.L.; Zhang, H.; Rehder, C.; Laforet, P.; Kishnani, P.S.; Millington, D.S.; Bashir, M.R.; Bali, D.S. Assessing disease severity in Pompe disease: The roles of a urinary glucose tetrasaccharide biomarker and imaging techniques. *Am. J. Med. Genet. C Semin. Med. Genet.* **2012**, *160C*, 50–58. [CrossRef]

26. Chien, Y.-H.; Goldstein, J.L.; Hwu, W.-L.; Smith, P.B.; Lee, N.-C.; Chiang, S.-C.; Tolun, A.A.; Zhang, H.; Vaisnins, A.E.; Millington, D.S.; et al. Baseline Urinary Glucose Tetrasaccharide Concentrations in Patients with Infantile- and Late-Onset Pompe Disease Identified by Newborn Screening. *JIMD Rep.* **2015**, *19*, 67–73. [PubMed]

27. Lukacs, Z.; Nieves Cobos, P.; Mengel, E.; Hartung, R.; Beck, M.; Deschauer, M.; Keil, A.; Santer, R. Diagnostic efficacy of the fluorometric determination of enzyme activity for Pompe disease from dried blood specimens compared with lymphocytes-possibility for newborn screening. *J. Inherit. Metab. Dis.* **2010**, *33*, 43–50. [CrossRef]

28. Verma, J.; Thomas, D.C.; Kasper, D.C.; Sharma, S.; Puri, R.D.; Bijarnia-Mahay, S.; Mistry, P.K.; Verma, I.C. Inherited Metabolic Disorders: Efficacy of Enzyme Assays on Dried Blood Spots for the Diagnosis of Lysosomal Storage Disorders. *JIMD Rep.* **2017**, *31*, 15–27.

29. Liao, H.-C.; Chiang, C.-C.; Niu, D.-M.; Wang, C.-H.; Kao, S.-M.; Tsai, F.-J.; Huang, Y.-H.; Liu, H.-C.; Huang, C.-K.; Gao, H.-J.; et al. Detecting multiple lysosomal storage diseases by tandem mass spectrometry— A national newborn screening program in Taiwan. *Clin. Chim. Acta* **2014**, *431*, 80–86. [CrossRef]

30. Elbin, C.S.; Olivova, P.; Marashio, C.A.; Cooper, S.K.; Cullen, E.; Keutzer, J.M.; Zhang, X.K. The effect of preparation, storage and shipping of dried blood spots on the activity of five lysosomal enzymes. *Clin. Chim. Acta* **2011**, *412*, 1207–1212. [CrossRef] [PubMed]

31. Lukacs, Z.; Cobos, P.N.; Wenninger, S.; Willis, T.A.; Guglieri, M.; Roberts, M.; Quinlivan, R.; Hilton-Jones, D.; Evangelista, T.; Zierz, S.; et al. Prevalence of Pompe disease in 3,076 patients with hyperCKemia and limb-girdle muscular weakness. *Neurology* **2016**, *87*, 295–298. [CrossRef] [PubMed]

32. Lukacs, Z.; Schoser, B. Meta-opinion: From screening to diagnosis of Pompe disease—A European perspective. *Expert Opin. Orphan Drugs* **2016**, *4*, 1075–1078. [CrossRef]

10

Evaluation of Technical Issues in a Pilot Multicenter Newborn Screening Program for Sickle Cell Disease

Maddalena Martella [1],*, Giampietro Viola [1], Silvia Azzena [1], Sara Schiavon [1], Andrea Biondi [2], Giuseppe Basso [1], Paola Corti [2], Raffaella Colombatti [1], Nicoletta Masera [2] and Laura Sainati [1]

[1] Dipartimento di Salute della Donna e del Bambino, Università di Padova, 35128 Padova, Italy; giampietro.viola.1@unipd.it (G.V.); azzena.silvia@yahoo.it (S.A.); schiavon_sara@libero.it (S.S.); giuseppe.basso@unipd.it (G.B.); rcolombatti@gmail.com (R.C.); laura.sainati@unipd.it (L.S.)

[2] Dipartimento di Pediatria, Università di Milano-Bicocca-Fondazione MBBM, San Gerardo Hospital, 20900 Monza, Italy; abiondi.unimib@gmail.com (A.B.); p.corti@hsgerardo.org (P.C.); n.masera@hsgerardo.org (N.M.)

* Correspondence: maddalena.martella@unipd.it;

Abstract: A multicenter pilot program for universal newborn screening of Sickle cell disease (SCD) was conducted in two centres of Northern Italy (Padova and Monza). High Performance Liquid Chromatography (HPLC) was performed as the first test on samples collected on Guthrie cards and molecular analysis of the β-globin gene (*HBB*) was the confirmatory test performed on the HPLC-positive or indeterminate samples. 5466 samples of newborns were evaluated. Of these, 5439/5466 were submitted to HPLC analysis and the molecular analysis always confirmed in all the alteration detected in HPLC (62/5439 newborns); 4/5439 (0.07%) were SCD affected, 37/5439 (0.68%) were HbAS carriers and 21/5439 (0.40%) showed other hemoglobinopathies. Stored dried blood spots were adequate for HPLC and β-globin gene molecular analysis. Samples were suitable for analysis until sixteen months old. A cut-off of A_1 percentage, in order to avoid false negative or unnecessary confirmation tests, was identified. Our experience showed that several technical issues need to be addressed and resolved while developing a multicenter NBS program for SCD in a country where there is no national neonatal screening (NBS) program for SCD and NBS programs occur on a regional basis.

Keywords: sickle cell disease; high performance liquid chromatography (HPLC); β-globin gene

1. Introduction

Neonatal screening (NBS) for Sickle cell disease (SCD) is an effective tool for the early detection of affected individuals, to direct them at the clinical programs to prevent complications and finally to offer genetic counseling to a family and is therefore highly recommended as the first step of comprehensive care [1–7]. In detail, early identification of affected SCD patients through a NBS program allows the introduction of penicillin prophylaxis from two months of age and performing of an adequate vaccination schedule with the reduction of mortality from infection, prompt enrolment in comprehensive care programs with timely parent health education, Trans Cranial Doppler (TCD) screening and prevention of acute events [1,2].

In Italy a national NBS program is not available and NBS programs are organized on a regional basis [8]. Haemoglobinopathies are included in the regional NBS program of only 1 out of the 20 regions [9], but some pilot programs have been conducted in the past years [10–12].

Padova and Monza, two towns located in the North of Italy, in the Veneto and Lombardia Regions respectively, have a high percentage of an immigrant population and an average of more than 3500 births every year, with 25% of them from immigrant parents [13]. We developed a pilot multicenter, multiregional universal NBS program for SCD [14].

The methods used and recommended for the SCD neonatal screening by International Guidelines can be qualitative, as IsoElectric Focusing (IEF), and quantitative, as Capillary Electrophoresis (CE), High Performance Liquid Chromatography (HPLC) and recently the Tandem Mass Spectrometry (MS/MS) [15], but the abnormal chromatogram must always have a confirmatory test with the different methodologies. Our protocol is an innovative way for SCD screening with the combination of HPLC analysis and molecular analysis. This type of approach has been used in very few studies [16,17].

The purpose of this manuscript is to highlight some of the technical challenges that we had to face in the development of our pilot screening. The objectives of this study were: (i) to define the sensitivity of our methods in order to establish a cut-off percentage for normality in the presence of low levels of β-globin chains, (ii) to maintain high-quality results to ensure the accurate interpretation of the analysis for immediate initiation of supportive care for affected newborns, (iii) to check the stability of the sample over time to ensure reliable measurements, a very important issue in a multicenter setting, (iv) to verify the organization and feasibility of a multiregional screening program. Finally, the flow chart for newborn screening for SCD is shown in Figure 1.

Flow chart for Newborn Screening for Sickle Cell Disease

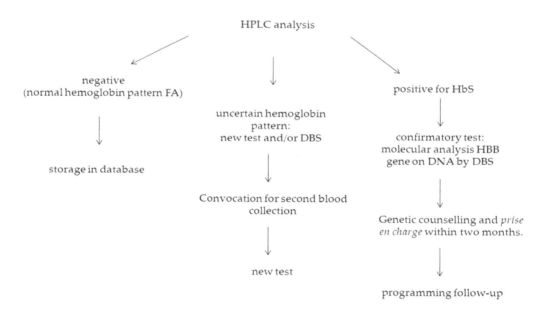

Figure 1. Flow chart for newborn screening for Sickle cell disease.

2. Materials and Methods

2.1. Study Design and Population

In Padova the NBS pilot program enrolled newborns from 2 May 2016 until 30 November 2017 while in Monza from 1 September 2016 until 31 August 2017. The screening was performed on all newborns from the 36th hour to the third day after birth. Blood collection was performed by pricking the heel of the newborn and collection on a Guthrie card (903 Whatman® in Padova and AHLSTROM® 226 in Monza) after informed consent from the parents was obtained.

Dried blood spots from Monza were sent to Padova through courier once a week and stored at room temperature and in a dark dry place in the NBS laboratory of Padova's Clinic of Pediatric Hematology-Oncology. The samples were analyzed after 7 days and the first test was performed with the VARIANT NBS Newborn Screening System (Bio-Rad Laboratories, Munich, Germany) and the confirmatory test, on the same sample, with molecular analysis of β-globin gene.

2.2. High Performance Liquid Chromatography (HPLC)

All specimens were first examined by High Performance Liquid Chromatography (HPLC) performed on a VARIANT NBS Newborn Screening System (Bio-Rad Laboratories) following the manufacturer's recommendations, within 7 days after blood spots had been taken. All chromatograms were automatically analyzed and visually inspected for absent Hemoglobin A and variant hemoglobins. The columns and all reagents such as buffers, primers, and hemoglobin standards were purchased from the manufacturer. Two or three disks (diameter of 3.2 mm) were punched out of the dried blood spot (DBS) and placed in a well of 96-well plate round bottom. In each well 280μL of distilled water was added and mixed with the pipette several times at room temperature. Two mixtures of hemoglobin standards FAES and FADC, respectively were analyzed in duplicate even if the run included more plates.

HPLC uses an ion exchange column with gradient elution. The presence of different hemoglobins is revealed through a UV-VIS detector settled at 415 nm. The time that passes from the injection of the sample to the output of the peak of hemoglobin type, is known as the retention time of that particular hemoglobin and represents a reproducible value for that column, at that gradient elution and at that temperature. For the different hemoglobins we have different retention times and characteristic chromatographic profiles, with the exception of HbE and HbA_2 that elute in the same peak, therefore making them indistinguishable from each other.

In addition, it is possible to quantify in a relative way the percentage of the different hemoglobins; the HPLC analysis helps to identify the differences between carrier individuals (HbS/HbA) and homozygous affected individuals (HbS/HbS) and also to differentiate heterozygous compounds such as HbS/HbC.

Moreover, the sensibility of the protocol has been verified with experiments of dilution on the SCD sample (HbSS) until 1:10.

2.3. Molecular Analysis of the β-globin Gene

Molecular analysis of the β-globin gene (HBB; MIM # 603903; NM_000518) represented the confirmatory test and was performed on all the following samples: those with an altered hemoglobin profile at HPLC, due to the presence of HbS or another hemoglobin variant; the specimens with HbA<5% or with HbA>30%, excluded transfusion anamnesis, were sent for molecular study. The samples with a red blood cell transfusion and HbA>30% were submitted for HPLC analysis three months later.

Genomic DNA, extracted using the Qiagen kit (QIAamp®DNA Mini and Blood), from blood spots allowed to air dry, were amplified by chain reaction of polymerase (PCR) at the exon level and at the intron-exon junctions with the primers below reported: HBB1 Fw5'-AAAAGTCAGGGCAGAGCCAT-3', HBB1 Rw5'-CCCAGTTTCTATTGGTCTCCTTAA-3', HBB2 Fw5'-GGGTTTCTGATAGGCACTGACTC-3', HBB2 Rw5'-AAAAGAAGGGGAAAGAAAACATCA-3', HBB3 Fw5'-TAGCAGCTACAATCCAGCTACCA-3', HBB3 Rw5'-GGACTTAGGGAACAAAGGACCT-3'.

Alterations of the coding sequence were analyzed and characterized by sequencing of the hemoglobin β chain coding HBB gene using an ABI Prism® 310 Genetic Analyzer Applied Biosystems. Sanger sequencing is the most comprehensive method of mutation detection and determines the exact sequence spanning the area of the primers used.

2.4. Management of Results

HPLC negative samples for abnormal hemoglobins didn't require further analysis. While, HPLC positive samples for abnormal chains underwent a confirmatory test with molecular analysis of the β-globin gene on the same sample collected at the nursery. Families with SCD children were called for a visit in the clinic within two months, while parents of HbS carriers were called for a visit and counselling within six months. Carriers of other hemoglobin variants received a letter, informing them of the results.

3. Results

In this study, 5466 samples of newborns from both birth centers were enrolled. Of these, 5439/5466 (2821/2826 of Padova, 99.8% and 2618/2640 of Monza 99.1%) were submitted for HPLC analysis. None of the samples collected were excluded from the analysis. Each sample was analyzed within 7 days after the blood had been spotted on the paper.

The results are summarized in Table 1. Molecular analysis always confirmed the abnormality detected in HPLC in 62/5466 newborns; other hemoglobin variants were also detected (HbC, HbD, HbE) in 0.5% of the cases in Monza and in 0.21% of those in Padova.

Table 1. Hemoglobin patterns observed in the pilot newborn screening.

Hb Pattern (HPLC)	HBB Genotype	Newborns (n.)
FAS	*HBB:* c.20A>T/wt	37 (0.68%)
FS	*HBB:* c.20A>T/c.20A>T	3 (0.055%)
FSC	*HBB:* c.20A>T/c.19A>T	1 (0.02%)
FAC	*HBB:* c.19A>T/wt	9 (0.16%)
FAD	*HBB:* c.364G>C/wt	8 (0.15%)
FAE	*HBB:* c.79C>T/wt	4 (0.07%)
Total		62 (1.14%)

n. = number of newborns.

28 samples (0.86%) of preterm infants, showed a value of HbA<5% at HPLC. Molecular analysis confirmed that 26/28 had genotype HbAA, while 2 samples with HbA values of 2.2% and 3.8%, respectively, had a genotype HbAD and a FAST value >10% (potential HbBart) and had been reported to the referring center. In an attempt to determine normal values for HbA and total HbF, the peak percentages of samples with a normal hemoglobin pattern were plotted against the gestational week. The results (see Figure 2) showed a correct Gaussian distribution for the HbA and HbF with a mean of 16.6% and 77.1% respectively as expected for at term newborns.

All dried blood spot cards collected and the storage methods turned out adequate both for HPLC analysis and β globin gene molecular analysis.

The experiments of dilution on the SCD sample (HbSS) detected low levels of HbS until 1:10.

In our experience we verified storage conditions and the reliability of the DBS a few months later [16] to understand if it was possible to identify the different hemoglobins according to our standard settings of the instrument. We repeated the HPLC analysis of different DBS series stored for sixteen months. In each series, the values of HbA peak area percentage identified in HPLC analysis, although reduced, allowed for the detection of the hemoglobin peaks; retention time was not modified by the samples aging: the HbA value was never <7% and never <800,000 μV*s, in terms of area under the curve (AUC) according to manufacturer instructions. HbS, when present was easily identified by HPLC analysis and similarly to HbA it was not influenced by sample aging [18]. The reduction of the HbA percentage should be attributed to physiological degradation of HbA and to the presence of cellulose particles removed from the Guthrie card together with the blood. In this study, the DBS up to sixteen months old provided satisfactory results (see Figure 3). The quality and the efficiency of the analysis was not affected by different types of Guthrie cards and the two different types of Guthrie cards gave the same performance.

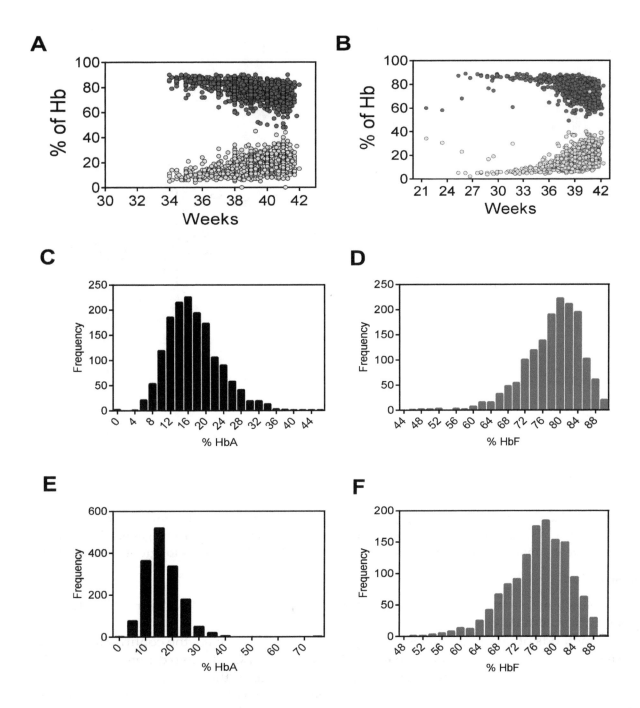

Figure 2. Percentages of HbF (red circles) and HbA (gray circles) according to the gestational age (weeks from conception to blood withdrawal) found in the cohort of Padova (**A**) and Monza (**B**). Distribution frequency of HbA and HbF in the cohort of Padova (**C,D**) and Monza (**E,F**).

Furthermore, we have noted in our experience that the needle restrains randomly, probably by electrostatic reasons, some blood spots that could cause not only the obstruction of the needle, but also the contamination of other wells. Thus, we recommend that the run must be always monitored and if necessary the run should be interrupted. At the end of every analysis session the instrument must be carefully cleaned.

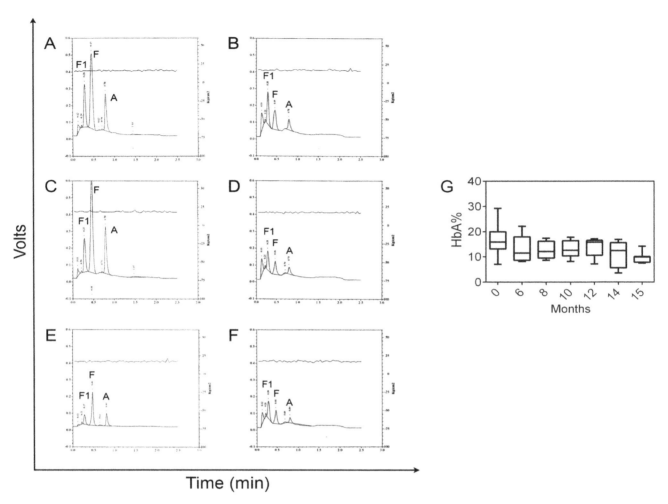

Figure 3. Representative chromatograms of a dried blood spot analyzed within 7 days from blood withdrawal (**A,C,E**) and after four (**B**), eight (**D**) and sixteen months (**F**). Percentages of HbA analyzed after different months from the blood withdrawal (**G**). At least five samples for group were analyzed.

4. Discussion

Our study represents the first multicenter pilot project of universal NBS for SCD in two different regions of Northern Italy.

The methods of investigation were adequate and highly specific, the confirmatory test always confirmed the abnormal hemoglobinopathies detected in HPLC. The two different types of Guthrie cards gave the same performances. The quality, the storage of the sample and the volume of the collected blood are very important factors that may affect the results in particular the retention time in HPLC of the different hemoglobins [19]. Our setting proved to be effective.

Moreover, in our experience we noted that it is very important for the setting of the 96-well plate for HPLC analysis to ensure the acquisition of the total area >800,000 µV*s, as recommended by the manufacture: The number of the spots, the volume of the water for Hb elution, mixed with the pipette several times at room temperature. The 96-well plate can be store at room temperature. This protocol ensures a homogeneous solution to detect the different hemoglobins. The sensitivity of the system can be considered optimal for all different hemoglobins in agreement with the hemoglobin standards FAES and FADC provided by the manufacturer. It is worthwhile to note that our data showed a normal distribution both for HbA and HbF in well agreement to that reported by Bouva et al. [20].

Finally, the sensibility of the protocol verified with experiments of dilution on the SCD sample (HbSS) until 1:10 guaranteed the possibility of detecting low levels of HbS.

Newborns born prematurely may yield misleading results. Premature infants may have very low levels of A_1 hemoglobin at birth; in the absence of a significant amount of A_1, β chains mutations can be undetectable. The cut-off of HbA<5% is efficient also for preterm newborns. The percentages of HbA and HbF were in agreement with previous reports [21,22], which found a great variability according to the maternal ethnic origin and the gestational age.

The VARIANT NBS Newborn Screening System for our experience has critical issues: the spots can remain attached to the needle causing obstruction or even the random fall of the spot. Therefore, caution is necessary and it is better to check the run and to wash frequently the needle and the instrument.

5. Conclusions

Our data demonstrate the feasibility of a multicentric SCD screening and indicate the robustness and reliability of the screening system. The data obtained from HPLC analysis were in excellent agreement with the large amount of data present in the literature. The sensitivity of the system can be considered optimal in conjunction with the molecular analysis of the β globin gene. A scaling up of the project to other areas of the two regions is now planned.

Author Contributions: Conceptualization, data curation, original draft preparation M.M. and G.V.; investigation, S.A. and S.S.; resources, G.B. and A.B.; project administration, N.M. and P.C.; L.S. and R.C. supervision, project administration and writing—review and editing.

References

1. Ware, R.E.; de Montalembert, M.; Tshilolo, L.; Abboud, M.R. Sickle cell disease. *Lancet* **2017**, *390*, 311–323. [CrossRef]
2. Piel, F.B.; Steinberg, M.H.; Rees, D.C. Sickle Cell Disease. *N. Engl. J. Med.* **2017**, *376*, 1561–1573. [CrossRef] [PubMed]
3. National Health System (NHS). Sicke Cell Disease in Childhood. Standard and Guidelines for clinical Care. 2nd Edition 2010. Available online: https://assets.publishing.service.gov.uk/government/uploads/system/uploads/attachment_data/file/408961/1332-SC-Clinical-Standards-WEB.pdf (accessed on 20 December 2018).
4. De Montalembert, M.; Ferster, A.; Colombatti, R.; Rees, D.C.; Gulbis, B. European Network for Rare and Congenital Anemias. ENERCA clinical recommendations for disease management and prevention of complications of sickle cell disease in children. *Am J. Hematol.* **2011**, *86*, 72–75. [CrossRef] [PubMed]
5. Colombatti, R.; Perrotta, S.; Samperi, P.; Casale, M.; Masera, N.; Palazzi, G.; Sainati, L.; Russo, G.; Italian Association of Pediatric Hematology-Oncology (AIEOP) Sickle Cell Disease Working Group. Organizing national responses for rare blood disorders: The Italian experience with sickle cell disease in childhood. *Orphanet J. Rare Dis.* **2013**, *8*, 169. [CrossRef] [PubMed]
6. De Franceschi, L.R.G.; Sainati, L.; Venturelli, D. SITE-AIEOP Recommendations for Sickle Cell Disease Neonatal Screening. Collana Scientifica Site n°5. Available online: http://www.site-italia.org/collana_scientifica.php (accessed on 20 December 2018).
7. Lobitz, S.; Telfer, P.; Cela, E.; Allaf, B.; Angastiniotis, M.; Backman, J.C.; Badens, C.; Bento, C.; Bouva, M.J.; Canatan, D.; et al. Newborn screening for sickle cell disease in Europe: Recommendations from a Pan-European Consensus Conference. *Br. J. Haematol.* **2018**, *183*, 648–660. [CrossRef] [PubMed]
8. Available online: http://www.aismme.org (accessed on 20 December 2018).
9. De Zen, L.; Dall'Amico, R.; Sainati, L.; Colombatti, R.; Testa, E.R.; Catapano, R.; Zanolli, F. Screening neonatale per le emoglobinopatie su Dried Blood Spot. In Proceedings of the XXXVI Congresso Nazionale Associazione Italiana Ematologia Oncologia Pediatrica (AIEOP), Pisa, Italy, 6–8 June 2010.
10. Rolla, R.; Castagno, M.; Zaffaroni, M.; Grigollo, B.; Colombo, S.; Piccotti, S.; Dellora, C.; Bona, G.; Bellomo, G. Neonatal screening for sickle cell disease and other hemoglobinopathies in "the changing Europe". *Clin. Lab.* **2014**, *60*, 2089–2093. [CrossRef] [PubMed]
11. Venturelli, D.; Lodi, M.; Palazzi, G.; Bergonzini, G.; Doretto, G.; Zini, A.; Monica, C.; Cano, M.C.; Ilaria, M.; Montagnani, G.; et al. Sickle cell disease in areas of immigration of high-risk populations: A low cost and reproducible method of screening in northern Italy. *Blood Transfus.* **2014**, *12*, 346–351. [PubMed]

12. Ballardini, E.; Tarocco, A.; Marsella, M.; Bernardoni, R.; Carandina, G.; Melandri, C.; Guerra, G.; Patella, A.; Zucchelli, M.; Ferlini, A.; et al. Universal neonatal screening for sickle cell disease and other haemoglobinopathies in Ferrara, Italy. *Blood Transfus.* **2013**, *11*, 245–249. [PubMed]

13. RapportoAnnuale ISTAT. 2017. Available online: https://www.istat.it/it/files//2017/05/RapportoAnnuale2017.pdf (accessed on 20 December 2018).

14. Martella, M.; Cattaneo, L.; Viola, G.; Azzena, S.; Cappellari, A.; Baraldi, E.; Zorloni, C.; Masera, N.; Biondi, A.; Basso, G.; et al. Universal Newborn Screening for Sickle Cell Disease: Preliminary Results of the First Year of a Multicentric Italian Project. In Proceedings of the 22nd Annual Congress of the European Hematology Association, Madrid, Spain, 22–25 June 2017.

15. Lobitz, S.; Klein, J.; Brose, A.; Blankenstein, O.; Frömmel, C. Newborn screening by tandem mass spectrometry confirms the high prevalence of sickle cell disease among German newborns. *Ann. Hematol.* **2017**, *23*, 1–6. [CrossRef] [PubMed]

16. Detemmerman, L.; Olivier, S.; Bours, V.; Boemer, F. Innovative PCR without DNA extraction for African sickle cell disease diagnosis. *Hematology* **2017**, *23*, 181–186. [CrossRef] [PubMed]

17. Kunz, J.B.; Awad, S.; Happich, M.; Muckenthaler, L.; Lindner, M.; Gramer, G.; Okun, J.G.; Hoffmann, G.F.; Bruckner, T.; Muckenthaler, M.U.; et al. Significant prevalence of sickle cell disease in Southwest Germany: Results from a birth cohort study indicate the necessity for newborn screening. *Ann. Hematol.* **2016**, *95*, 397–402. [CrossRef] [PubMed]

18. Martella, M.; Viola, G. Università di Padova, Padova, Italy. Chromatograms derived from HPLC analysis. Unpublish work, 2018.

19. Frömmel, C.; Brose, A.; Klein, J.; Blankenstein, O.; Lobitz, S. Newborn Screening for Sickle Cell Disease: Technical and Legal Aspects of a German Pilot Study with 38,220 Participants. *BioMed Res. Int.* **2014**, *2014*, 695828. [CrossRef] [PubMed]

20. Bouva, M.J.; Mohrmann, K.; Brinkman, H.B.J.M.; Kemper-Proper, E.A.; Elvers, B.; Loeber, J.G.; Verheul, F.E.A.M.; Giordano, P.C. Implementing neonatal screening for haemoglobinopathies in the Netherlands. *J. Med. Screen.* **2010**, *17*, 58–65. [CrossRef] [PubMed]

21. CorteÂs-Castell, E.; PalazoÂn-Bru, A.; Pla, C.; Goicoechea, M.; Rizo-Baeza, M.M.; Juste, M.; Gil-Guillen, V.F. Impact of prematurity and immigration on neonatal screening for sickle cell disease. *PLoS ONE* **2017**, *12*, e0171604. [CrossRef] [PubMed]

22. Allaf, B.; Patin, F.; Elion, J.; Couque, N. New approach to accurate interpretation of sickle cell disease newborn screening by applying multiple of median cutoffs and ratios. *Pediatr. Blood Cancer* **2018**, *65*, e27230. [CrossRef] [PubMed]

11

Neonatal Screening for Sickle Cell Disease in Belgium for More than 20 Years: An Experience for Comprehensive Care Improvement

Béatrice Gulbis [1,*], Phu-Quoc Lê [2], Olivier Ketelslegers [3], Marie-Françoise Dresse [4], Anne-Sophie Adam [1], Frédéric Cotton [1], François Boemer [5], Vincent Bours [5], Jean-Marc Minon [3] and Alina Ferster [2]

[1] Department of Clinical Chemistry, LHUB-ULB, Université Libre de Bruxelles (ULB) 322, Rue Haute, 1000 Brussels, Belgium; AnneSophie.Adam@LHUB-ULB.be (A.-S.A.); Frederic.Cotton@LHUB-ULB.be (F.C.)

[2] Department of Hemato-Oncology Hôpital Universitaire des Enfants Reine Fabiola, Université Libre de Bruxelles (ULB) 15, av. J.J. Crocq, 1020 Brussels, Belgium; phuquoc.le@huderf.be (P.-Q.L.); alina.ferster@huderf.be (A.F.)

[3] Department of Laboratory Medicine CHR de la Citadelle, 1, Boulevard de la 12ème Ligne, 4000 Liège, Belgium; olivier.ketelslegers@chrcitadelle.be (O.K.); jean.marc.minon@chrcitadelle.be (J.-M.M.)

[4] Department of Pediatric, University Hospital Liège, CHR de la Citadelle, 1, Boulevard de la 12ème Ligne, 4000 Liège, Belgium; marie.francoise.dresse@chrcitadelle.be

[5] Department of Human Genetics CHU Sart Tilman, Université de Liège (ULg) Domaine Universitaire du Sart Tilmant Bâtiment 35-B, 4000 Liège, Belgium; F.Boemer@chuliege.be (F.B.); vbours@chuliege.be (V.B.)

* Correspondence: Beatrice.Gulbis@LHUB-ULB.be;

Abstract: Our previous results reported that compared to sickle cell patients who were not screened at birth, those who benefited from it had a lower incidence of a first bacteremia and a reduced number and days of hospitalizations. In this context, this article reviews the Belgian experience on neonatal screening for sickle cell disease (SCD). It gives an update on the two regional neonatal screening programs for SCD in Belgium and their impact on initiatives to improve clinical care for sickle cell patients. Neonatal screening in Brussels and Liège Regions began in 1994 and 2002, respectively. Compiled results for the 2009 to 2017 period demonstrated a birth prevalence of sickle cell disorder above 1:2000. In parallel, to improve clinical care, (1) a committee of health care providers dedicated to non-malignant hematological diseases has been created within the Belgian Haematology Society; (2) a clinical registry was implemented in 2008 and has been updated in 2018; (3) a plan of action has been proposed to the Belgian national health authority. To date, neonatal screening is not integrated into the respective Belgian regional neonatal screening programs, the ongoing initiatives in Brussels and Liège Regions are not any further funded and better management of the disease through the implementation of specific actions is not yet perceived as a public health priority in Belgium.

Keywords: sickle cell disease; neonatal screening program; registry; birth prevalence

1. Introduction

At the World Health Organization, sickle cell disease has been recognized as a global public health problem [1]. The different migratory flows of recent decades have influenced the disease in European countries and in particular in Belgium [2]. According to our survey in 2007, there were approximately 400 patients (0.0036% of the total population) with sickle cell disease (SCD) living in Belgium. The implementation of a Belgian registry for SCD in 2008 allowed us to demonstrate that at the end of 2012, 469 SCD patients were regularly followed and registered by eight Belgian hospitals [3].

The benefit of neonatal screening for SCD has been established for many years [4]. Birth prevalence of this disease is not the only criterion for choosing to include sickle cell disease in the neonatal screening program, but in countries where birth prevalence of the condition is greater than 1:6000, this has been shown to be cost-effective [5]. However, in several European countries such as Belgium, neonatal screening for SCD is not part of the national neonatal screening program. Indeed, in Belgium, there are no national recommendations for sickle cell disease screening at birth and only local initiatives offer the benefit of early diagnosis to a small number of families. Following a successful Belgian screening in 2013 for two-thirds of neonates performed as part of a pilot study, it has been shown that the birth prevalence of SCD was 1:2329 [6].

In this context, this paper gives an update on the neonatal screening results for SCD and overall hemoglobinopathies in two different Belgian regions. In parallel with the increase in the number of sickle cell neonates born in Belgium, it also highlights the initiatives that have been conducted to improve the clinical care program.

2. Material and Methods

2.1. Neonatal Screening for Sickle Cell Disease

Neonatal screening for SCD began in five Brussels maternity wards in December 1994, but has been offered to all neonates in all maternity wards of the Brussels Region since 2004 (2004–2017: 310,053 neonates screened); screening began in one maternity ward in Liège Region in 2002 and was extended to 15 maternity wards in Liège Region in 2009 (East of Belgium; 2008–2017: 186,829 neonates screened). It is realized in three screening centers i.e., Brussels University Laboratory (LHUB-ULB), Centre Hospitalier Régional (CHR) de la Citadelle and Centre Hospitalier Universitaire (CHU) du Sart Tilman. The neonatal screening process is described in Table 1 and has been detailed previously [7–9]. Briefly, in LHUB-ULB and CHR de la Citadelle, liquid umbilical cord blood samples in EDTA were screened initially using an isoelectric focusing technique (IEF) (Perkin Elmer Life Sciences, Zaventem, Belgium) and since 2008, using a capillary zone electrophoresis (CZE) technique (Sebia Benelux, Vilvoorde, Belgium) [6]. In CHU du Sart Tilman, heel prick samples on filter paper were screened by tandem mass spectrometry (TMS) [7,8]. If a hemoglobin variant is detected, further analysis is performed on the same sample using high performance liquid chromatography (BioRad, Hercules, CA, USA) or DNA analysis [7–9]. If confirmed, a new sample is requested to use as a control.

Table 1. Neonatal screening process (offered to all neonates). CHR = Centre Hospitalier Régional. IEF = isoelectric focusing. CZE = capillary zone electrophoresis. TMS = tandem mass spectrometry.

Screening Centre	Sample	First Screening Test	Confirmation Test (Same Sample)	Report of Results	Ref.
Brussels Region	Umbilical cord blood liquid	IEF (<2008) CZE (≥2008)	HPLC	Any hemoglobinopathy detected	[7]
CHR Citadelle	Umbilical cord blood liquid	CZE	HPLC	Any hemoglobinopathy detected	[8]
Liège Region	Heel prick/filter paper	TMS	DNA	Any hemoglobinopathy detected	[9]

For the three screening centers, reports of results concern all SCD and all minor and major forms of hemoglobinopathy detected by the technique (Table 1). The screening of SCD in a neonate is reported immediately to the local coordinator and the medical staff of the maternity ward concerned. A new sample is requested for diagnosis.

For clarity, all results were also compiled in one period, i.e., 2009 to 2017, that allows us to report all results obtained from the three screening centers.

After confirmation of sickle cell disease on a new sample and, if feasible, before leaving the maternity ward, the families of an affected neonate received counselling and were referred to a specialized healthcare center where an initial visit was scheduled. The reference centers ensured the monitoring of affected children. The comprehensive care program includes the education of the patient and parents on subjects such as the prevention of complications, lifestyle, and management of fever and pain. The priority is to offer comprehensive and integrated care from neonatal screening throughout childhood and beyond to prevent acute complications, to delay the onset of chronic organ damage, and to treat acute complications for all neonates diagnosed with SCD. It is coordinated by a pediatrician who has acquired special skills in the care of patients with SCD.

2.2. Belgian Network of Health Care Providers and Registry for Sickle Cell Patients

In 2006, a red blood cell (RBC) disorders committee within a scientific society (the Belgian Haematology Society (BHS)) called the BHS RBC Committee was created. To date, it consists of 25 partners working in 14 different Belgian hospitals. The main objective of this network was to improve health care for patients affected by a non-malignant hematological disease, and in particular SCD. It does not currently benefit from any operating subsidy. It was supported on a temporary basis by grants. The main actors are pediatricians, adult hematologists, nurses and clinical biologists. To offer a unique tool to monitor the evolution of the population with SCD and to collect information on the main SCD complications (in particular for neonates screened at birth), a registry has been set up in 2008 by this committee. The objectives and implementation of the Belgian registry has been detailed previously [2]. Briefly, the BHS RBC Committee administers a centralized Belgian registry of patients with SCD. Eight centers participated with patient registration. Without national support, but thanks to a grant, in 2018, an updated registry has been launched and today, 12 centers participate. The items in the database were the subject of a consensus within the BHS RBC Committee. These data are updated annually. They make it possible to evaluate the benefit of neonatal screening and the follow-up of the patients screened at birth. For data privacy reasons, the information can only be accessed by healthcare professionals.

2.3. Comprehensive Care Improvement Plan

In 2014, to improve health care at a national level, the BHS RBC Committee proposed to define a plan of action. As part of the Belgian plan for rare diseases, this was submitted to the health authorities.

3. Results

3.1. Neonatal Screening for Sickle Cell Disease

During 2009 to 2017, 396,894 neonates were screened. This represents approximately 33% of births in Belgium. Screening coverage is almost 100%, except in two Brussels maternity wards where it is 85%. Birth prevalence of SCD and likely heterozygosity for hemoglobin (Hb) S are reported in Table 2. One sickle cell child born in one of the maternity wards where screening is performed was reported as not having been screened i.e., FSD^{Punjab}. The maternity ward has a screening coverage of around 85%. Most of the patients are homozygous for Hb S or compound heterozygous for Hb S and beta-thalassemia (210/246); 27/246 patients had a Hb SC disease.

Table 2. Distribution by year of neonates screened as having a sickle cell disease (SCD) i.e., homozygous for Hb S, compound heterozygous for Hb S and β-thalassemia, Hb C or another Hb variant; or likely heterozygous for hemoglobin S (FAS).

Year	Neonates Screened All Regions (*n*)	SCD Both Regions (*n*)	SCD Both Regions Birth Prevalence	FAS Brussels Region (*n*)	FAS Brussels Region Birth Prevalence	FAS Liège Region (*n*)	FAS Liège Region Birth Prevalence
2009	40,026	25	1:1601	421	1:54	159	1:109
2010	40,579	25	1:1561	449	1:52	150	1:115
2011	40,262	36	1:1088	458	1:50	112	1:154
2012	40,675	24	1:1768	460	1:51	175	1:98
2013	40,241	22	1:1829	520	1:45	161	1:104
2014	40,144	28	1:1487	447	1:52	192	1:87
2015	39,748	27	1:1529	449	1:52	174	1:94
2016	39,292	25	1:1572	504	1:46	200	1:82
2017	37,364	35	1:1068	503	1:42	193	1:83
Total	358,331	251	1:1427	4211	1:49	1516	1:100

The highest birth prevalence of neonates likely heterozygous for Hb S were observed for the two most recent years in both Brussels and Liège regions (Table 2). It is the most frequent hemoglobin variant observed in both regions that offer screening for SCD, with the most prevalent sickle cell disease being homozygosity for Hb S; β-thalassemia was observed only for two and seven neonates in the Brussels and Liège regions, respectively (Table 3).

Table 3. Neonatal screening for SCD by region: 2009–2017.

Type	Birth Prevalence Brussels Region *n* = 206,984	Birth Prevalence Liège Region *n* = 151,347
FS	1:1522	1:2481
FSC	1:7666	1:16,816
FSX	1:68,995	-
FE	-	1:151,347
FC	1:34,497	1:21,621
F-	1:103,492	1:21,621
FAS	1:49	1:100
FAC	1:394	1:655
FAE	1:2275	1:2259
FAD *	1:2587	1:7567
FAO *	1:4600	1:75,674

* Variant not screened by the method used in Centre Hospitalier Universitaire de Liège before 2014. Neonates homozygous for Hb S or compound heterozygous for Hb S and β-thalassemia (FS) or compound heterozygous for Hb S and C (FSC) or another Hb variant (FSX). Neonates homozygous for Hb C or compound heterozygous for Hb C and β-thalassemia (FC). Neonates homozygous for Hb E or compound heterozygous for Hb CE and β-thalassemia (FE). Neonates with absence of Hb A (F-). Neonates likely heterozygous for a hemoglobin variant i.e., Hb S (FAS), Hb C (FAC), Hb E (FAE), Hb D-Punjab (FAD), Hb O-Arab (FAO).

3.2. Belgian Network of Health Care Providers and Registry for Sickle Cell Patients

At the end of 2012, 469 patients were registered in the Belgian registry of patients with SCD. In September 2018, 538 patients had been registered in the updated database; 285 were born in Belgium, of which 64% (182/285) benefited from the neonatal screening program for SCD and 53 did not (i.e., born in other regions than those covered by neonatal screening and at least one born in the Brussels region). Compared to data in 2012, this means a longer follow-up and an increase in the number of affected patients screened at birth (or not).

3.3. Comprehensive Care Improvement Plan

A plan of action to improve health care for SCD patients has been proposed and submitted to the National Institute of Health in 2014 (Figure 1). To date, only the recognition of SCD as a rare disease in Belgium (Step 1) through the recognition of reference centers for hemoglobinopathies (Step 4) at the Belgian and European levels i.e., Cliniques Universitaires de Bruxelles Hôpital Erasme, and one related department i.e., Department of Hemato-Oncology, Immunology and Transplantation—Hôpital Universitaire des Enfants Reine Fabiola, has been effective.

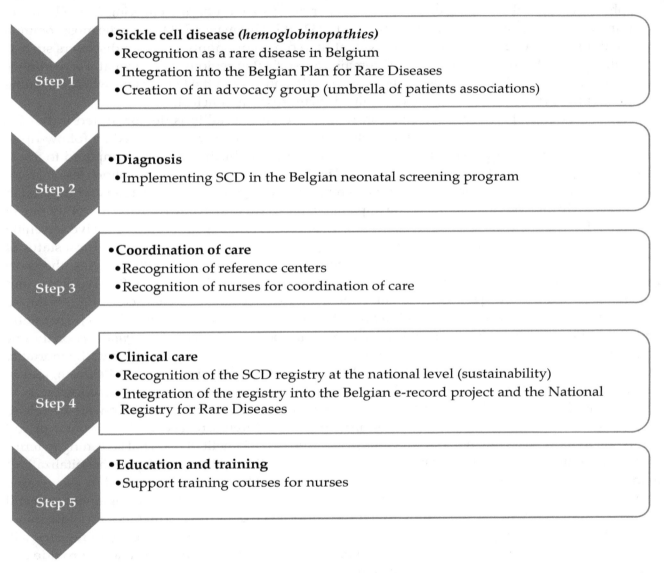

Figure 1. Plan of action to improve clinical care for SCD patients in Belgium.

The other steps of the plan (Figure 1) have not been debated or implemented. In particular, sickle cell disease has still not been included in the national neonatal screening program.

4. Discussion

Our study demonstrated that throughout the period of 2009 to 2017, the birth prevalence of sickle cell disease in two Belgian regions was higher than 1:2000 and heterozygosity for Hb S was the highest during the years 2016 and 2017 (>1:50 and >1:90 for Brussels and Liège Regions, respectively). To date, neonatal screening for SCD is not yet integrated into the national neonatal screening program. It also has no funding. Neonatal screening has been and is an important lever for providing health care improvements to sickle cell patients. In this respect, the creation of a Belgian network of health care professionals, particularly composed of many pediatricians, within a Belgian scientific society and the resulting initiatives (such as the implementation of a clinical registry of sickle cell patients) have been important steps. An action plan has also been proposed to the National Institute of Health in 2014.

In recent decades, as a result of migratory flows, the disease has spread throughout the world, particularly in Western Europe. It is therefore becoming a major concern of public health policies [10,11]. Belgium, with 20% of migrants including 12.5% of at-risk origin and its history of colonization in Africa and more particularly in the Democratic Republic of Congo, is also concerned [12]. During a pilot phase of neonatal screening extended over a period of six months and covering 2/3 of births in Belgium, the birth prevalence observed for SCD is 1/2329 [6]. This makes SCD one of the most common inherited diseases in Belgium, far more prevalent than other commonly screened disorders such as phenylketonuria. Birth prevalence of SCD remains at >1:2500 in regions were neonatal screening is performed. Despite the birth prevalence increases in 2016 and 2017 in the two regions where screening was performed, without national data, it is quite difficult to draw conclusions.

The advantage of neonatal screening in reducing early mortality is demonstrated in the US, various European countries and Jamaica. Vichinsky et al. showed that after a median follow-up of seven years, the overall mortality rate of patients diagnosed at birth was 1.8%, compared to 8% in children diagnosed after the age of three months [13]. Similarly, in the Jamaican cohort, less than 1% of children died in the first two years of life when preventive strategies were available, compared to 14% when early interventions could not be implemented [14]. In Brazil, however, the mortality rate of children with SCD remains high, at 7.4%, despite an effective, ongoing and comprehensive screening program. There are many reasons for this, including the low socio-economic and cultural status of affected families complicating regular clinical monitoring, long trips to health facilities, the short interval between onset of symptoms and death and inexperience of the health staff to recognize and manage SCD acute events [15]. Quinn et al. have demonstrated that neonatal screening minimizes morbidity and mortality through antibiotic prophylaxis and parental education [16,17]. Currently, with the addition of combined vaccination against pneumococcus and *Haemophilus influenzae* on the one hand, and integrated management that focuses on family education on the other hand, the mortality of newborns screened decreased to less than 1%. Screening is not widespread in Belgium, and in 2008, our BHS RBC Committee established a sickle cell registry. These two aspects allowed us to compare the future of SCD children that were screened (or not) at birth [18]. If we were unable to demonstrate a significant reduction in mortality among children screened in the neonatal period compared to those that were not, our previous results showed a benefit of neonatal screening in terms of decreasing the incidence of a first bacteremia and reducing the number and days of hospitalizations (expressed per 100 patient-years). Our only two deaths (in 1996 and 2000) occurred in very young patients, during a period marked by poor compliance and when integrated management was still immature [18]. Couque et al. also emphasized the importance of optimal adherence and integrated care on the prognosis of patients in 2016 [19]. The update of our cohort in the Belgian registry will allow us to monitor the effectiveness of the management of sickle cell patients and to provide any additional data regarding the benefit of screening.

The establishment of an integrated system for diagnosis and patient care is only beginning to emerge in Europe for several reasons. It concerns migrant minority communities of various origins, often isolated, disadvantaged and whose access to health care is not always easy; the perception of sickle cell disease in the communities concerned was not or is no longer adequate; and by lack of knowledge, the disease is often not recognized or trivialized by members of the medical community as well as by health managers [1]. In Belgium, a group of doctors involved in the management of sickle cell disease began in the early 2000s to reflect on the feasibility of an integrated care system initially in Brussels. This group wanted to focus on prevention while promoting health within a multidisciplinary group, as recommended by the World Health Organization [1]. This network aims to bring together all health professionals and patient associations concerned in a search for the best evidence of prevention, care and epidemiological data. It also aims to alert national health authorities to the real public health problems posed by SCD. This explains the approach that aims to propose an action plan for improving the management of SCD.

5. Conclusions

Neonatal screening for SCD performed in two Belgian regions demonstrated that its birth prevalence is higher than 1:2000. Those results pose the question of its integration into the regional neonatal screening program. In order to appreciate the benefit of neonatal screening in our care setting, a sickle cell registry has been set up and has been updated in 2018 with an increasing number of patients screened for ongoing evaluation. These initiatives have been one of the driving forces behind the creation of a Belgian network of healthcare professionals that aims to improve the management of all sickle cell patients.

Author Contributions: Methodology, B.G., O.K., F.B.; validation, P.-Q.L., A.F., F.C., F.B. and M.-F.D.; formal analysis, B.G., O.K., F.B., V.B., F.C., A.-S.A., P.-Q.L., A.F.; data curation, B.G., O.K., M.-F.D., J.-M.M., F.B., V.B., F.C., A.-S.A., P.-Q.L., A.F.; writing—original draft preparation, B.G.; writing—review and editing, P.-Q.L., O.K., M.-F.D., A.-S.A., F.C., F.B., V.B. and A.F.; funding acquisition, B.G., J.-M.M., V.B., A.F.

Acknowledgments: The authors would like to thank all caregivers who participated in the neonatal hemoglobinopathy screening program and the members of the Red Blood Cell Belgian Haematology Society committee for their fruitful collaboration.

References

1.   Sickle cell anemia. Available online: http://apps.who.int/gb/archive/pdf_files/wha59/a59_9-en.pdf (accessed on 11 November 2018).

2.   Aguilar Martinez, P.; Angastiniotis, M.; Eleftheriou, A.; Gulbis, B.; Mañú Pereira Mdel, M.; Petrova-Benedict, R.; Corrons, J.L. Haemoglobinopathies in Europe: Health & migration policy perspectives. *Orphanet J. Rare Dis.* **2014**, *9*, 97. [CrossRef] [PubMed]

3.   Lê, P.Q.; Gulbis, B.; Dedeken, L.; Dupont, S.; Vanderfaeillie, A.; Heijmans, C.; Huybrechts, S.; Devalck, C.; Efira, A.; Dresse, M.F.; et al. Survival among children and adults with sickle cell disease in belgium: Benefit from hydroxyurea treatment. *Pediatr. Blood Cancer* **2015**, *62*, 1956–1961. [CrossRef] [PubMed]

4.   Gaston, M.H.; Verter, J.I.; Woods, G.; Pegelow, C.; Kelleher, J.; Presbury, G.; Zarkowsky, H.; Vichinsky, E.; Iyer, R.; Lobel, J.S.; et al. For the Prophylactic Penicillin Study Group. Prophylaxis with oral penicillin in children with sickle cell anemia. A randomized trial. *N. Engl. J. Med.* **1986**, *314*, 1593–1599. [CrossRef] [PubMed]

5.   Castilla-Rodríguez, I.; Cela, E.; Vallejo-Torres, L.; Valcárcel-Nazco, C.; Dulín, E.; Espada, M.; Rausell, D.; Mar, J.; Serrano-Aguilar, P. Cost-effectiveness analysis of newborn screening for sickle-cell disease in Spain. *Exp. Opin. Orphan Drugs* **2016**, *4*, 567–575. [CrossRef]

6.   Ketelslegers, O.; Eyskens, F.; Boemer, F.; Bours, V.; Minon, J.M.; Gulbis, B. Epidemiological data on sickle cell disease in Belgium. *Belg. J. Hematol.* **2015**, *6*, 135–141.

7.   Wolff, F.; Cotton, F.; Gulbis, B. Screening for haemoglobinopathies on cord blood: Laboratory and clinical experience. *J. Med. Screen.* **2012**, *19*, 116–122. [CrossRef] [PubMed]

8.   Gulbis, B.; Cotton, F.; Ferster, A.; Ketelslegers, O.; Dresse, M.F.; Rongé-Collard, E.; Minon, J.M.; Lê, P.Q.; Vertongen, F. Neonatal haemoglobinopathy screening in Belgium. *J. Clin. Pathol.* **2009**, *62*, 49–52. [CrossRef] [PubMed]

9.   Boemer, F.; Cornet, Y.; Libioulle, C.; Segers, A.; Bours, V.; Schoos, R. 3-Years experience review of neonatal screening for hemoglobin disorders using tandem mass spectrometry. *Clin. Chim. Acta* **2011**, *412*, 1476–1479. [CrossRef] [PubMed]

10. Weatherall, D.J. The inherited diseases of hemoglobin are an emerging global health burden. *Blood* **2010**, *115*, 4331–4436. [CrossRef] [PubMed]

11. Piel, F.B.; Tatem, A.J.; Huang, Z.; Gupta, S.; Williams, T.N.; Weatherall, D.J. Global migration and the changing distribution of sickle haemoglobin: A quantitative study of temporal trends between 1960 and 2000. *Lancet Glob. Health* **2014**, *2*, 80–89. [CrossRef]

12. Migrations en Belgique: Données statistiques. Available online: www.myria.be/files/Migration-rapport-2015-C2.pdf (accessed on 7 October 2018).

13. Vichinsky, E.; Hurst, D.; Earles, A.; Kleman, K.; Lubin, B. Newborn screening for sickle cell disease: Effect on mortality. *Pediatrics* **1988**, *81*, 749–755. [PubMed]

14. King, L.; Fraser, R.; Forbes, M.; Grindley, M.; Ali, S.; Reid, M. Newborn sickle cell disease screening: The Jamaican experience (1995–2006). *J. Med. Screen.* **2007**, *14*, 117–122. [CrossRef] [PubMed]

15. Sabarense, A.P.; Lima, G.O.; Silva, L.M.; Viana, M.B. Survival of children with sickle cell disease in the comprehensive newborn screening programme in Minas Gerais, Brazil. *Paediatr. Int. Child Health* **2015**, *35*, 329–332. [CrossRef] [PubMed]

16. Quinn, C.T.; Rogers, Z.R.; Buchanan, G.R. Survival of children with sickle cell disease. *Blood* **2004**, *103*, 4023–4027. [CrossRef] [PubMed]

17. Quinn, C.T.; Rogers, Z.R.; McCavit, T.L.; Buchanan, G.R. Improved survival of children and adolescents with sickle cell disease. *Blood* **2010**, *115*, 3447–3452. [CrossRef] [PubMed]

18. Lê, P.Q.; Ferster, A.; Dedeken, L.; Vermylen, C.; Vanderfaeillie, A.; Rozen, L.; Heijmans, C.; Huybrechts, S.; Devalck, C.; Efira, A.; et al. Neonatal screening improves sickle cell disease clinical outcome in Belgium. *J. Med. Screen* **2018**, *25*, 57–63. [CrossRef] [PubMed]

19. Couque, N.; Girard, D.; Ducrocq, R.; Boizeau, P.; Haouari, Z.; Misud, F.; Holvoet, L.; Ithier, G.; Belloy, M.; Odièvre, M.H.; et al. Improvement of medical care in a cohort of newborns with sickle-cell disease in North Paris: Impact of national guidelines. *Br. J. Haematol.* **2016**, *173*, 927–937. [CrossRef] [PubMed]

12

Newborn Screening for Pompe Disease

Takaaki Sawada, Jun Kido * and Kimitoshi Nakamura

Department of Pediatrics, Graduate School of Medical Sciences, Kumamoto University, Kumamoto 860-8556, Japan; sawada.takaki@kuh.kumamoto-u.ac.jp (T.S.); nakamura@kumamoto-u.ac.jp (K.N.)
* Correspondence: kidojun@kuh.kumamoto-u.ac.jp;

Abstract: Glycogen storage disease type II (also known as Pompe disease (PD)) is an autosomal recessive disorder caused by defects in α-glucosidase (AαGlu), resulting in lysosomal glycogen accumulation in skeletal and heart muscles. Accumulation and tissue damage rates depend on residual enzyme activity. Enzyme replacement therapy (ERT) should be started before symptoms are apparent in order to achieve optimal outcomes. Early initiation of ERT in infantile-onset PD improves survival, reduces the need for ventilation, results in earlier independent walking, and enhances patient quality of life. Newborn screening (NBS) is the optimal approach for early diagnosis and treatment of PD. In NBS for PD, measurement of AαGlu enzyme activity in dried blood spots (DBSs) is conducted using fluorometry, tandem mass spectrometry, or digital microfluidic fluorometry. The presence of pseudodeficiency alleles, which are frequent in Asian populations, interferes with NBS for PD, and current NBS systems cannot discriminate between pseudodeficiency and cases with PD or potential PD. The combination of *GAA* gene analysis with NBS is essential for definitive diagnoses of PD. In this review, we introduce our experiences and discuss NBS programs for PD implemented in various countries.

Keywords: Pompe disease; newborn screening; pseudodeficiency; genotype-phenotype correlation; treatment and follow-up

1. Introduction

Glycogen storage disease type II (OMIM 232300), also known as Pompe disease (PD), is an autosomal recessive disorder caused by a defect in α-glucosidase (AαGlu; EC 3.2.1.20/3), resulting in the accumulation of lysosomal glycogen in skeletal and heart muscles [1]. The rates of accumulation and tissue damage depend on the residual enzyme activity. Patients with infantile-onset PD (IOPD) exhibit nearly complete absence of AαGlu activity and develop hypotonia and hypertrophic cardiomyopathy during infancy. Patients with IOPD eventually die of cardiorespiratory failure because massive amounts of glycogen accumulate in their skeletal and heart muscles. Patients with late-onset PD (LOPD) who exhibit marked reductions in AαGlu activity exhibit skeletal muscle dysfunction but rarely present with cardiac muscle disorders. The onset time and phenotypes of LOPD are variable, and patients are likely to exhibit manifestations in the fifth decade or later in life [2]. Enzyme replacement therapy (ERT) is essential for the treatment of IOPD [3,4]. ERT should be started before symptoms are clearly present, prior to the development of irreversible damage, to achieve optimal outcomes [5]. Early initiation of ERT can improve survival rates and quality of life in patients with IOPD, reducing the need for ventilation and leading to earlier independent walking [6].

Newborn screening (NBS) is an optimal approach for early diagnosis and treatment of IOPD. NBS, including pilot studies, is currently being carried out in several countries worldwide. Here, we describe NBS programs for PD, the diagnostic algorithm for PD, AαGlu enzyme assays using dried blood spots (DBSs) and fibroblasts, *GAA* gene analysis, and pseudodeficiency in *GAA*. Additionally, we discuss optimal treatments for PD, the current status of NBS worldwide, and future challenges in the development of NBS programs.

2. NBS Program for PD

NBS for PD is currently performed in Taiwan, Japan, and several states in the United States of America (USA). Current NBS systems measure AαGlu enzyme activity in DBSs.

In Japan, DBSs are prepared at maternity clinics or obstetrics departments using standard procedures at 4–6 days after birth for newborn mass screening according to public health system guidelines. After dropping blood spots onto filter papers (Toyo Roshi Kaisha, Ltd., Tokyo, Japan), DBSs are dried for at least 4 h at room temperature and sent to the Newborn Screening Center in Kumamoto within 1 week after preparation. The AαGlu activity in DBSs is then analyzed. The cutoff values in the AαGlu activity assay using DBSs differ for each research group but are set between 0.1 and 0.5 percentile values for the population or 20% to 30% of the mean value of the population. For newborns with values less than the cutoff values, a second AαGlu activity assay and *GAA* gene analysis are then performed [7].

At our institution, NBS for PD is performed in three steps (Figure 1). In the first step, newborns with AαGlu activity under the cutoff value of 6.5 pmol/h/disk (10% of the median value in the population) are recalled, and their DBSs are evaluated again. In the second step, using the Ba/Zn method, newborns with AαGlu activity under the cutoff value of 5.5 pmol/h/disk are called to the hospital within 2 months for a clinical examination. The infants are examined using physical and biochemical assays to confirm symptomatic signs of IOPD, and a third AαGlu assay is also performed. Finally, *GAA* gene analysis is performed in newborns with AαGlu activity under the cutoff value of 4.0 pmol/h/disk. The period after birth until the result of the first AαGlu assay is acquired is 1–2 weeks, and the period until the result of the second AαGlu assay is acquired is within 4 weeks. Thereafter, the period from birth until clinical examination is within 2 months, and the period from birth until *GAA* gene analysis and final diagnosis is up to 6 months [7].

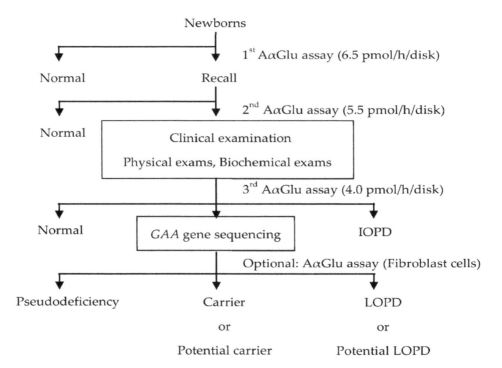

Figure 1. Flow chart of newborn screening (NBS) for Pompe disease (PD) in Japan. IOPD: infant-onset Pompe disease; LOPD: late-onset Pompe disease.

A definitive diagnosis of PD is achieved in patients harboring two known pathogenic *GAA* variants with decreased AαGlu activity in the blood (leukocytes, DBSs, isolated lymphocytes) or another tissue, such as fibroblast. A probable diagnosis for PD can be made in patients with decreased enzyme activity but ambiguous *GAA* gene analysis owing to the presence of molecular variants of unknown significance (VOUS). Moreover, the prevalence of pseudodeficiency alleles is high in Asian populations.

Figure 2 shows the diagnostic algorithm for PD. Clinicians can definitively diagnose patients with IOPD if they present with certain clinical manifestations, including heart or skeletal muscle deficiencies. Patients with LOPD definitively diagnosed by *GAA* gene analysis will need to be regularly followed up for the development of signs or symptoms related to PD, even if their *GAA* gene variants are known, because there is considerable variation in how and when patients will present symptoms. Patients with one or no known variants exhibiting decreased enzymatic activity should receive additional tests, including physical examinations, cardiac evaluations, AαGlu activity assays in fibroblasts, urinary glucotetrasaccharide (HEX4) and blood creatine kinase (CK) analyses, and/or parental DNA analyses. Through these additional tests, patients with one or no known variants may be diagnosed with LOPD, potential LOPD, or non-LOPD (carrier or pseudodeficiency) [8].

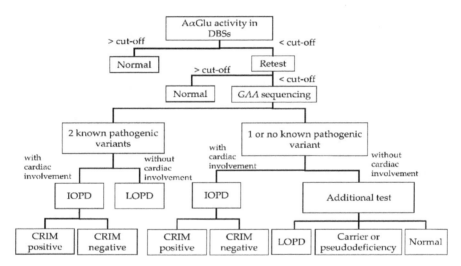

Figure 2. Flow chart of diagnosis for PD (modified from the Pompe Disease Newborn Screening Working Group [8]). DBS: dried blood spot; CRIM: cross-reactive immunological material.

3. AαGlu Enzyme Assay

In NBS for PD, AαGlu activity in DBSs is measured. Conventionally, the AαGlu activities in lymphocytes, fibroblasts, and skeletal muscles are analyzed for the diagnosis of PD [9]. Neutrophils in the blood contain maltase glucoamylase, another type of α-glucosidase. Because the pH at which this enzyme functions is consistent with that of AαGlu, the AαGlu activity assays in the blood are likely to result in false-negative results for defects in AαGlu [9]. However, large-scale NBS using DBSs has become possible owing to the use of acarbose, which inhibits the activity of maltase glucoamylase [10,11].

Measurement of AαGlu enzyme activity in DBSs can be carried out using fluorometry with the fluorogenic substrates of 4-methylumbelliferyl α-D-glucopyranoside (4MU-αGlc) [12], tandem mass spectrometry (MS/MS) [11], or digital microfluidic fluorometry [13]. Tandem mass spectrometry using mass-differentiated internal standards can quantify the corresponding enzymatic products and enables multiplex assays of a set of corresponding enzymes that cause lysosomal storage disorders (LSDs), such as PD, mucopolysaccharidosis (MPS), Fabry disease (FD), Gaucher disease (GD), Krabbe disease, and Niemann–Pick A/B disease. Additionally, digital microfluidics, a type of fluorometry, can be used to perform multiple assays of enzymes in the lysosome [14]. Tandem mass spectrometry is considered superior to fluorometry in terms of sensitivity, and some reports have shown that tandem mass spectrometry can distinguish pseudodeficiencies, which cannot be identified in patients with PD using fluorometry [15]. However, this is controversial because no reports have compared the outcomes of tandem mass spectrometry with those of fluorometry in the same samples. Moreover, the cutoff values used in NBS differ according to institution and region owing to factors such as differences in samples, measurement instruments, and humidity.

4. *GAA* **Gene Analysis**

GAA gene analysis is essential for definitive diagnosis of PD. The *GAA* gene is located on chromosome 17q25. It is 18.3 kb long, contains 20 exons, and encodes 952 amino acids. At present, more than 900 variants are registered in the ClinVar [16] or Pompe disease *GAA* variant databases [17], and the numbers are increasing. About two-thirds of these variants are classified by clinical significance and the other third of the variants are VOUS. Although bioinformatic tools such as Polyphen-2 [18], Human Splicing Finder [19], and Mutation Tester [20] are useful to estimate the pathogenicity of VOUS, these tools are insufficient for making the diagnosis. The progression of symptoms, treatment, and its outcomes are most important. Follow-up studies on the patients or potential patients with PD are essential and will help clinicians to diagnosis and determine proper treatment of patients with VOUS.

5. **Pseudodeficiency**

A pseudodeficiency allele is a change in the *GAA* gene sequence that results in AαGlu enzyme activity reduction, but is not enough to cause PD [21,22]. In our previous pilot program, the presence of pseudodeficiency alleles was shown to interfere with NBS for PD [23]. This suggests that NBS for PD must be able to distinguish PD cases and those with pseudodeficiency alleles in the *GAA* gene sequence. Asian patients are frequently homozygous or heterozygous for these pseudodeficiency alleles c.[1726G>A; 2965G>A] (p.[G576S; E689K]). Moreover, pseudodeficiency variants such as c. 1726G>A (p. G576S) are modifiers of pathogenic variants, which can result in greater reductions in GAA enzyme activity than with only the pathogenic variants [24]. Therefore, evaluation of pseudodeficiency in the *GAA* gene is essential in NBS.

Attempts have been made to distinguish cases with pseudodeficiency from patients with PD by methods other than *GAA* gene analysis; however, no reports have described a successful approach to achieve this goal.

6. **AαGlu Activity in Fibroblasts**

The measurement of AαGlu activity in fibroblasts was previously the gold standard for the diagnosis of PD [9]. This method can exclude the contribution of maltase glucoamylase activity. However, AαGlu assays in fibroblasts are difficult to perform as an NBS approach because acquiring fibroblasts for use in the AαGlu assay requires a skin biopsy, which is invasive and requires lengthy fibroblast culturing times. Despite this, AαGlu assays in fibroblasts are thought to be useful as additional tests for definitive diagnosis, even if *GAA* gene analysis cannot be used for the diagnosis of PD due to the presence of VOUS or only one known pathogenic variant for PD.

7. **Cross-Reactive Immunological Material (CRIM)**

Patients with IOPD should receive early ERT immediately after diagnosis of PD. Moreover, patients should undergo evaluation of CRIM before receiving ERT [25]. Patients with IOPD exhibiting residual AαGlu enzyme activity are CRIM-positive, and patients with IOPD exhibiting no residual AαGlu enzyme activity are CRIM-negative. CRIM-negative patients develop neutralizing antibodies for recombinant human lysosomal α-glucosidase (rhGAA) when receiving ERT, which impairs the effects of ERT [25,26].

In previous approaches for the evaluation of CRIM, residual AαGlu enzyme activity in fibroblasts was measured using an invasive method that required a long time to obtain results. Currently, the outcomes of *GAA* gene analysis contribute to estimations of the outcomes of CRIM [27].

8. ERT

ERT for patients with IOPD should be initiated as early as possible before irreversible damage occurs. Yang et al. indicated that early identification of patients with IOPD allows for very early initiation of ERT. Starting ERT even a few days earlier may lead to better patient outcomes [28]. Starting ERT early is effective in patients with LOPD as well; however, early ERT before presentation of signs or symptoms in patients with LOPD is generally not recommended [29]. Administration of ERT in the absence of symptoms of LOPD, even when blood CK and urine HEX4 are elevated, is avoided. The recommendation of ERT for patients with LOPD remains controversial.

Patients with LOPD should receive regular follow-ups, and levels of markers, such as blood CK and urine HEX4, should be monitored [30]. If patients with LOPD presenting symptoms of PD did not undergo NBS, their diagnosis and treatment are often delayed [31]. However, patients with LOPD diagnosed using NBS can be followed up and receive therapy immediately after presentation of the symptoms of PD [32]; treatment of these patients should not be delayed.

9. Immunomodulation to ERT

A variety of immunomodulation therapies have been developed to prevent the generation of neutralizing antibodies to rhGAA that would impair the effect of ERT. The immunomodulation therapies are elimination therapy for the neutralizing antibodies to rhGAA that have already been generated or prevention therapy for avoiding generation of the neutralizing antibodies before ERT. Rituximab, methotrexate, and intravenous immunoglobulins are often used for the immunomodulation therapies.

Prevention therapy has higher cost benefit than elimination therapy. Therefore, it is beneficial to identify CRIM-negative patients with IOPD before ERT in order to prevent generating neutralizing antibodies. Even some CRIM-positive IOPD patients are likely to develop neutralizing antibodies. The individualized T cell epitope measure scoring method, using a combination of individualized Human Leukocyte Antigen (HLA)-binding predictions and GAA genotype, may predict patient-specific risk of developing neutralizing antibodies to rhGAA [33].

Most patients with LOPD develop IgG antibodies to rhGAA, typically within 3 months of initiation of treatment [4]. Moreover, some patients who develop high, sustained antibody titers may have poorer clinical responses to treatment. Patients with IOPD or LOPD receiving ERT should routinely undergo tests for neutralizing antibodies for rhGAA. In rare cases in which high neutralizing antibodies interfere with the effects of ERT in patients with PD, we should consider the administration of immunosuppressants with ERT as well as discontinuing ERT.

10. The Follow-Up Period

Patients with IOPD who were diagnosed by NBS and received ERT should undergo regular follow-ups to assess treatment efficacy, onset of new symptoms, and deterioration of symptoms every month for the first 6 months or more [9,30]. In particular, cardiac evaluation is essential every month in the first 4 months of life and every 1–2 months thereafter. Clinicians should measure anti-rhGAA antibodies regardless of the state of CRIM. Patients with IOPD require immunosuppressants when they develop high titers of anti-rhGAA antibodies [34].

Patients with asymptomatic LOPD should undergo regular follow-up every 3 months during the first year after diagnosis. If they remain free of symptoms for 12 months, follow-ups every 3–12 months is required. Patients should receive ERT if they present signs or symptoms of PD.

Patients with symptomatic LOPD receiving ERT should undergo regular follow-ups monthly for 4 months after receiving ERT and then every 3 months thereafter, including monitoring for antibodies [30]. Because blood CK, aspartate aminotransferase (AST), alanine aminotransferase (ALT) levels, and urine HEX4 levels may increase before the onset of PD symptoms, these markers should be assessed regularly.

11. NBS Programs for PD Worldwide

The Newborn Screening Center at the National Taiwan University Hospital initiated an NBS program for PD in 2005. The outcomes of this large-scale NBS for PD in Taiwan demonstrated that the survival rates and ventilation-free rates of patients who were diagnosed with IOPD by NBS and received early ERT were higher than those of patients with IOPD who received ERT after presenting symptoms for IOPD [6,24]. Several regions in Japan also started NBS for PD in April, 2013 [7]. Moreover, the USA added PD to the Recommended Uniform Screening Panel (RUSP) and started NBS for PD in 2015. Currently, several countries worldwide have started pilot or regular NBS programs for PD (Table 1). The number and frequency of pseudodeficiencies and carriers between Japan and Taiwan are shown in Table 2 [35]; those in each country are displayed in Table 3.

Table 1. Summary of NBS programs for Pompe disease.

	Country (No. of Newborns)	No. of Recalls (%)	No. of Patients (Prevalence)		Screening Method	Frequently Detected Pathogenic Variants	Reference
			IOPD	LOPD			
	Taiwan (473,738)	2210 (0.47)	9 (1/52,638)	19 (1/24,934)	fluorometric assay	c.1935C>A, c.2238G>C	Chiang et al. (2012) [36]
	Taiwan (191,786)	874 (0.46)	5 (1/38,357)	11 (1/17,435)	MS/MS	c.1935C>A, c.[752C>T; 761C>T]	Liao et al. (2014) [37]
	Taiwan (64,148)	92 (0.14)	1 (1/64,148)	5 (1/12,830)	MS/MS	NA	Chiang et al. (2018) [38]
	Japan (103,204)	225 (0.24)	0	3 (1/34,401)	fluorometric assay	c.[752C>T; 761C>T], c.317G>A	Momosaki et al. (2019) [7]
USA	Washington (111,554)	17 (0.02)	0	4 (1/27,889)	MS/MS	c.-32-13T>G	Scott et al. (2013) [39]
	Washington (44,047)	9 (0.02)	0	1 (1/44,047)	MS/MS	c.2168del13ins10	Elliott et al. (2016) [40]
	Missouri (43,701)	18 (0.04)	3 (1/14,567)	5 (1/8740)	DMF	NA	Hopkins et al. (2015) [41]
	Illinois (219,973)	139 (0.06)	2 (1/149,987)	8 (1/37,497)	MS/MS	c.-32-13T>G	Burton et al. (2017) [42]
	New York (18,105)	6 (0.03)	0	1 (1/18,105)	MS/MS	c.-32-13T>G	Wasserstein et al. (2019) [43]
	Austria (34,736)	5 (0.01)	0	4 (1/8684)	MS/MS	c.896T>C, c.-32-13T>G	Mechtler et al. (2012) [44]
	Hungary (40,024)	163 (0.41)	0	9 (1/4447)	MS/MS	c.664G>A, c.-32-13T>G	Wittmann et al. (2012) [45]
	Italy (44,411)	8 (0.02)	2 (1/22,206)	0	MS/MS	c.-32-13T>G, c.236_246del	Burlina et al. (2018) [46]
	Mexico (20,018)	19 (0.09)	0	1 (1/ 20,018)	MS/MS	c.1375G>A	Navarrete-Martínez et al. (2017) [47]
	Brazil (103,204)	NA	0	0	DMF	-	Bravo et al. (2017) [48]

NA: not available.

Table 2. The distribution of pseudodeficiency alleles and PD-associated variants in newborns who were detected by NBS for PD.

Country/ Reference	Pseudodeficiency Alleles	No. of PD-Associated Variants			Prevalence (%)
		0	1	2	
Japan (n = 103,204)/ Momosaki, et al. (2019) [7]	Homozygous	24	8	0	32/71 (45.1%)
	Heterozygous	0	35	3	38/71 (53.5%)
	None	0	0	1	1/71 (1.5%)
	Diagnosis	Pseudodeficiency 24/71 (33.8%)	Carrier or potential carrier 43/71 (60.6%)	Patient or potential patient 4/71 (5.6%)	
Taiwan (n = 132,538)/ Labrousse et al. (2009) [35]	Homozygous	36	32	0	68/104 (65.4%)
	Heterozygous	0	27	7	34/104 (32.7%)
	None	0	0	2	2/104 (1.9%)
	Diagnosis	Pseudodeficiency 36/104 (34.6%)	Carrier or potential carrier 59/104 (56.7%)	Patient or potential patient 9/104 (8.7%)	

Table 3. Number of pseudodeficiencies and carriers in each country.

Country (No. of Newborns)		Pseudodeficiency (with 0 PD-Associated Variants)		Carrier or Potential Carrier (with 1 PD-Associated Variant)		Reference
		No.	Genotype	No.	Genotype	
USA	Washington (111,554)	6	pseudodeficiency allele/wt. (n = 6)	7	pathogenic allele/wt. (n = 4) pathogenic allele/pseudodeficiency allele (n = 3)	Scott et al. (2013) [39]
	Washington (44,047)	0		0		Elliott et al. (2016) [40]
	Missouri (43,701)	2	NA	3	NA	Hopkins et al. (2015) [41]
	Illinois (219,973)	15	NA	19	NA	Burton et al. (2017) [42]
	New York (18,105)	3	c.[1726G>A; 2065G>A]/c.[1726G>A; 2065G>A] (n = 2) c.[1726G>A; 2065G>A]/wt.	2	c.2560C>T(VOUS)/c.858+20_85 8+26del*(Predicted Benign) c.[1726G>A; 2065G>A]/c.-32-13T>G	Wasserstein et al. (2019) [43]
	Austria (34,736)	0		0		Mechtler et al. (2012) [44]
	Hungary (40,024)	0		17	NA	Wittmann et al. (2012) [45]
	Italy (44,411)	0		2	c.[1726G>A; 2065G>A]/c.-32-13T>G c.1726G>A/c.-32-13T>G	Burlina et al. (2018) [46]
	Mexico (20,018)	8	c.[1726G>A; 2065G>A]/c.[1726G>A; 2065G>A] (n = 6) c.[1726G>A;2065G>A]/wt. (n = 2)	2	c.[1726G>A; 2065G>A]/c.-32-13T>G (n = 2)	Navarrete-Martínez et al. (2017) [47]
	Brazil (103,204)	0		1	c.[1726G>A; 2065G>A]/c.-32-13T>G	Bravo et al. (2017) [48]

NA: not available.

11.1. Taiwan

Chien et al. performed the first large pilot NBS program to detect PD in newborns in Taiwan using a fluorometric enzymatic assay to determine AαGlu activity in DBSs. They conducted a pilot NBS of 132,538 newborns, accounting for almost 45% of newborns in Taiwan, between October 2005 and March 2007. Of the 132,538 newborns screened, 1093 (0.82%) underwent repeated DBS sampling, and 121 (0.091%) newborns were recalled for additional evaluation. PD was identified in 4 newborns (3 IOPD and 1 LOPD) [49]. Owing to this outcome, NBS for PD is now regularly conducted in Taiwan. Moreover, they identified 9 patients with IOPD and 19 patients with LOPD among 473,738 newborns by NBS for PD between October 2005 and December 2011 [36]. They launched a four-plex MS/MS LSD newborn screening test also including AαGlu (PD), acid α-galactosidase (FD), acid α-glucocerebrosidase (GD), and acid α-L-iduronidase (MPSI) in 2015. Through 2017, 64,148 newborns were screened for these four LSDs using their system. The cutoff levels in this new NBS system were established as 0.1 percentile of the population, or 13–15% of the normal mean. This NBS detected 20 infants with less than the cutoff value, and 1 patient with IOPD, 5 patients with LOPD, and 14 infants with false-positive results were identified [38].

Liao et al. reported the results of 191,786 newborns evaluated in an NBS program for PD using a system that could detect multiple LSDs by MS/MS from February 2010 to January 2013. After the initial DBS screening, 9 newborns were referred to hospitals directly with AαGlu values lower than the critical cutoff value (0.20 μmol/L/h) or combined with some clinical symptoms. In total, 874 (0.46%) newborns were recalled for second DBSs, 225 (0.12%) suspected newborns with decreased AαGlu activity were referred to hospitals, and 16 newborns were confirmed to have PD. In *GAA* gene analysis, 5 newborns were classified as IOPD and 11 newborns as LOPD. *GAA* gene analysis demonstrated that c.1935C>A (p.D645E) was detected in all cases of IOPD, c.[752C>T; 761C>T] (p.[S251L; S254L]) was detected in 8 cases of LOPD, and the c.1726G>A (p.G576S) pseudodeficiency variant was detected in 2 cases of IOPD and 5 cases of LOPD. The variants c.1840A>G (p.614A), c.2647-23delT, c.1054C>T (p.Q352*), IVS7+2T>C, and IVS17-5T>C were identified as novel variants. The false-positive rate in the tandem mass method was similar to that in fluorometric assays [37].

11.2. Japan

We started a pilot study of NBS for FD using 4-methylumbelliferyl-α-d-galactopyranoside (4MU-αGlc) in August 2006 and have conducted NBS of 5 LSDs, including PD, FD, GD, MPSI, and MPSII [50,51].

We reported the results of NBS for PD using 4MU-αGlc in 103,204 newborns [7]. Among these newborns, 225 newborns were retested using a second AαGlu assay, and 111 newborns with low AαGlu activities under the cutoff in the second AαGlu assay were evaluated for IOPD detection using physical and biochemical examinations (CK, ALT, AST, and lactate dehydrogenase), echocardiogram assessments, and a third AαGlu assay. For the 71 newborns with low AαGlu activity under the cutoff in the third AαGlu assay, *GAA* gene sequencing was performed using NGS. The AαGlu activities in fibroblasts were measured in 32 of the 71 newborns. In this study, no newborns developed IOPD, and 50 variants were detected. Eight variants were novel: c.547-67C>G, c.692+38C>T, c.1082C>A (p.P361Q), c.1244C>T (p.T415M), c.1552-52C>A, c.1638+43G>T, c.2003A>G (p.Y668C), and c.2055C>G (p.Y685*). The most common mutation was c.[752C>T;761C>T] (p.[S251L; S254L]), accounting for 20 alleles (14.1%, 20/142). The pseudodeficiency alleles c.1726G>A (p.G576S) and c.2065G>A (p.E689K) were detected in 71.8% (102/142) and 72.5% (103/142) of all newborns with low AαGlu activity, respectively.

This study identified 3 newborns with potential LOPD but without IOPD detection. Although these 3 patients developed no symptoms related to PD and received no treatment, the c.317G>A (p.R106H), c.1244C>T (p.T415M), and c.2003A>G (p.Y668C) mutations in these 3 patients were considered novel mutations. The prevalence of potential PD was 1 per 34,401 births. Newborns with both pseudodeficiency alleles and PD-associated pathogenic variants were detected in Japan as well as in Taiwan (Table 2). Table S1 displays the distribution of mutations and predictably pathogenic variants in NBS for PD in Japan.

11.3. USA

In 2008, the Advisory Committee on Heritable Disorders in Newborns and Children (ACHDNC) evaluated the NBS system for PD. The committee found significant evidence gaps related to the accuracy of screening and to the benefits and harms of presymptomatic diagnosis and precluded recommendation of NBS of PD for the Recommended Uniform Screening Panel (RUSP). In 2013, the ACHDNC reconsidered PD after it was nominated again. Based in part on new information presented to the ACHDNC by the external condition review workgroup, NBS for PD was recommended for addition to the RUSP and was added in March 2015. Prosser et al. estimated that screening 4 million babies born each year in the United States would detect 134 cases with PD including 40 cases with IOPD, compared with 36 cases detected clinically without screening [52]. NBS would also identify 94 cases of LOPD that might not become symptomatic for decades. By identifying 40 cases with IOPD, NBS would avert 13 deaths and identify 26 individuals requiring mechanical ventilation by the age of 36 months.

11.3.1. Washington

In 2013, Scott et al. reported screening results for more than 110,000 newborns in Washington. They detected PD, FD, GD, MPSI, MPSII (α-l-iduronide-2-sulfatase), Niemann–Pick A/B disease (acid sphingomyelinase), MPSIV-A (galactose-6-sulfate sulfatase), MPSVI (N-acetylgalactosamine-4-sulfatase), and Krabbe disease (galactocerebrosidase) using a technology which simultaneously measured multiple enzyme activities by MS/MS [39]. AαGlu activity in DBSs was measured in 111,544 cases. A cutoff value was established as 15% of the mean value. Seventeen samples had enzyme activities with less than the cutoff value. Four cases (2 cases with the homozygous IVS1-13T>G variant, 1 case with the compound heterozygous c.365T>A/c.1925T>A variant, and 1 case with the compound heterozygous IVS1-13T>G/c.1-17C>T variant) were confirmed to be patients with LOPD or potential LOPD, 4 cases had a single nucleotide change on one allele (carrier of PD), 3 cases were identified as carriers with an additional pseudodeficiency allele, and 6 cases were heterozygotes for a pseudodeficiency allele only. The prevalence of infants with LOPD or potential LOPD was 1 per 27,800 births.

Elliott et al. evaluated 43,000 newborns in NBS using a multiplex MS/MS enzymatic activity assay of 6 lysosomal enzymes for PD, FD, GD MPSI, Niemann–Pick A/B disease, and Krabbe disease. The cutoff value was established as 10% of the mean value. A newborn with p.G576S/p.T602I (a probable low activity variant) and a newborn with the homozygous c.2168del13ins10 (p.A724Gfs*44) variant (a frameshift variant leading to a nearby stop codon) were identified [40].

11.3.2. Missouri

A full-population pilot study of 43,701 newborns using DBSs in a multiplex fluorometric enzymatic assay for detecting PD, FD, GD, and MPSI was performed in Missouri on January 11, 2013 [41]. The cutoff values for AαGlu activities were set at the 0.17 percentile in the pilot study. Of the 18 cases that screened positive for AαGlu deficiency, 3 were diagnosed with IOPD, 3 were classified as LOPD, 2 were classified as potential LOPD or VOUS, 2 had pseudodeficiencies, and 3 were carriers. The prevalence of PD was 1 per 8740 births.

11.3.3. Illinois

The Newborn Screening Laboratory of Illinois performed NBS for 5 LSD-associated enzymes, including PD, FD, MPSI, and Niemann–Pick A/B disease, among 219,973 newborn DBSs using MS/MS from November 1, 2014 to August 31, 2016 [42]. In total, 139 (0.06%) had a positive or borderline test result in PD, necessitating additional testing. The cutoff values for AαGlu activities were defined as follows: positive = less than or equal to 18% of the daily median value, and borderline = greater than 18% and less than or equal to 22% of the daily median value. Ten cases of PD (two cases of IOPD and eight cases of LOPD) were detected. The frequency of PD was 1 per 21,997 births. Two infants diagnosed with IOPD developed elevated CK levels and clear evidence of cardiomyopathy at the time of initial evaluation which included chest radiography, electrocardiography, and echocardiography. These patients are regularly receiving ERT. Eight infants diagnosed with LOPD had either homozygous or compound heterozygous variants of the common splicing mutation c.-32-13T>G observed in patients with LOPD. *GAA* pseudodeficiency was detected in 15 infants, including 14 identified as Asian (4 Chinese, 3 Filipino, 2 Korean, 2 Indian, 1 Japanese, and 2 others). There were four infants with an undetermined classification or "potential PD."

11.3.4. New York

A pilot NBS study for 18,105 newborns was performed through October 1, 2014 [43]. Six cases were positive in the screen (1 case of LOPD, 3 cases of pseudodeficiency, and 2 carriers) with a mean AαGlu activity of less than or equal to 15% of the daily mean activity, yielding a referral rate of 0.033%. One case with LOPD had the homozygous c.-32-13T>G variant and low leukocyte AαGlu activity; however, examination results and laboratory values were normal and HEX4 testing was negative. Two cases were homozygous for the common pseudodeficiency allele, and another case carried one copy of the pseudodeficiency allele; leukocyte AαGlu activity in these infants ranged from low to normal. One case was found to have c.2560C>T (p.R854*) and an intronic variant believed to be benign. This infant was diagnosed as being a carrier because AαGlu activity was high.

11.4. Austria

DBSs of 34,736 newborns were collected consecutively in the national routine Austrian NBS program from January 2010 to July 2010 and analyzed for enzyme activities of acid β-glucocerebrosidase, α-galactosidase, α-glucosidase, and acid sphingomyelinase by electrospray ionization MS/MS [44]. The cutoff value for AαGlu was based on the 0.1 percentile value from 5000 cases of AαGlu activity. This first-line screening for low AαGlu activity detected 25 cases, and retests showed 5 cases with low

AαGlu activities. Sequence analyses of the *GAA* gene identified 4 cases with PD presenting homozygous c.896T>C (p.L299P), homozygous c.-32-13T>G, or compound heterozygous c.-32-13T>G/c.1551+1G>A (V480_I517del) variants. The prevalence of PD was 1 per 8684 births.

11.5. Hungary

In the Hungarian NBS program, 40,024 newborns were screened for PD, FD, GD, and Niemann–Pick A/B disease using MS/MS [45]. The 0.25th–0.5th percentile of AαGlu activities from 1000 cases were defined as the cutoff values; 663 cases (1.66%) were submitted for retesting. Among them, 163 cases (0.41%) had abnormal AαGlu activities in DBSs. After retesting, *GAA* gene analysis was performed in 64 (0.160%) cases with low AαGlu activity. *GAA* gene analysis detected 9 cases with PD and 25 carriers for PD. Three cases remained uncertain owing to inclusive *GAA* variants. Five cases had c.664G>A (p.V222M)/c.664G>A (p.V222M), and the other cases had c.-32-13T>G/c.-32-13T>G, c.664G>A (p.V222M)/c.2174G>A (p.R725Q), c.1216G>A (p.D406N)/c.1409A>C (p.N470T), and c.1552-3C>G/c.1552-3C>G. The 25 carriers had *GAA* gene variants related to PD, including -32-13T>G, c.307T>G (p.C103G), c.664G>A (p.V222M), c.763C>T (p.Q255X), c.841C>T (p.R281W), c.875A>G, c.1437+1G>A, c.1468 T>C (p.F490L), c.1552-3C>G, c.1903A>G (p.N635D), c.2237G>T (p.W746L), and c.2482-2A>G. The prevalence of PD was 1 per 20,012 births.

11.6. Italy

NBS programs for PD, FD, GD, and MPSI were performed using DBSs from 44,411 newborns by multiplexed MS/MS with the NeoLSD assay system in northeastern Italy from September 2015 to January 2017 [46]. Among the 44,411 newborns screened for the four LSDs, 40 cases (0.09%) had enzyme activity below 0.2 multiples of the median and were recalled for collection of a second DBS. Eight cases showed low AαGlu activities. Five patients underwent *GAA* gene analysis, and 2 cases were identified as juvenile types of PD because of the presence of the compound heterozygote of c.-32-13T>G (IVS1-13T>G)/c.236_246del (p.P79Rfs*12); elevated blood CK, AST, and ALT levels; and slightly enlarged heart findings. These patients underwent ERT immediately after diagnosis of PD. One case was classified as VOUS, and 2 cases were carriers for *GAA* variants. The frequency of PD was 1 per 22,205 births.

A total of 3403 newborns (1702 males and 1701 females) in the Umbria area of central Italy were screened for PD, FD, GD, and MPSI using DBSs [53]. The cutoff value was established as 35% of the normal median AαGlu activity. Although 3 cases showed AαGlu activities with less than the cutoff value in DBSs, none of these cases showed abnormal lymphocyte AαGlu activities. This pilot study identified no infants with PD.

11.7. Mexico

NBS for 6 LSDs, including PD, FD, GD MPSI, Niemann–Pick A/B disease, and Krabbe disease, using a multiplex MS/MS enzymatic assay was performed in 20,018 newborns (10,241 males and 9777 females) from July 1, 2012 to April 30, 2016 [47]. Nineteen presumptive positive infants showed low AαGlu activity in the first DBS. In the second AαGlu activity test, 16 infants were positive. Among these infants, 11 showed low leukocyte AαGlu activity. Five infants could not complete the protocol, three of whom lost healthcare insurance and 2 of whom refused to continue the protocol. In 11 infants with low leukocyte AαGlu activity, 10 infants harbored a pseudodeficiency variant associated with low AαGlu enzyme activity, but without signs of PD (homozygous or heterozygous for c.[1726G>A; 2065G>A] (p.[G576S; E689K])). Moreover, 2 infants harbored a compound heterozygous variant for the pseudodeficiency allele and the -32-13 T> G variant. The patient with potential LOPD presented with the c.1375G>A (p.D459N) variant, which was reported as an LOPD variant, and the VOUS c.1220A>G (p.Y407C) variant, which was predicted to be pathogenic.

11.8. Brazil

A pilot NBS study used a digital microfluidic platform to simultaneously measure the activities of AαGlu, acid β-glucosidase, α-galactosidase, and iduronidase to screen for PD, GD, FD, and MPSI in DBSs, respectively [54]. The cutoff value for AαGlu was defined as less than 30% of the mean enzyme activity in samples from 1000 unaffected babies. One case was identified to be pseudodeficiency, and no infants were identified with PD [48,55].

12. Genotype–Phenotype Correlation

Known variants in PD are registered in PD variant databases, including the Pompe Center (http://www.pompevariantdatabase.nl/pompe_mutations_list.php?orderby=aMut_ID1) and ClinVar (http://www.ncbi.nlm.nih.gov/clinvar). Moreover, in PolyPhen-2 (http://genetics.bwh.harvard.edu/pph2), the impact of missense variants on amino acid substitutions is evaluated. Human Splicing Finder (http://www.umd.be/HSF3/) can predict the impact of splicing abnormalities.

c.525delT (p.E176Rfs*45), a common frameshift variant in the Netherlands [56], c.1935C>A (p.D645E), a common missense variant in Taiwan [6], and c.2560C>T (p.R854*), a common nonsense variant in Africa [57], are considered variants for IOPD. c.-32-13T>G is commonly detected in Caucasian patients with LOPD, and patients with the homozygous c.-32-13T>G variant rarely develop cardiac manifestations as infants [58]. c.-32-13T>G is considered a variant in LOPD. However, because even patients with the same variants can develop both IOPD and LOPD phenotypes, the phenotype cannot be predicted from gene analysis alone. Moreover, the distribution of gene variants differs in each region. In the future, the accumulation of genetic information for patients in each region will be essential for predicting phenotypes.

13. Potential Concern of Screening for PD

NBS not only detects patients with IOPD but also patients with LOPD and potential LOPD. The effectiveness of NBS for identification of patients with LOPD and potential LOPD is controversial. Patients with LOPD who would present with PD symptoms within 2–3 years can receive medication before the progression of the symptoms, due to early diagnosis of LOPD through NBS. However, the demerits of NBS for patients with LOPD and potential LOPD should be considered because the time from diagnosis to presentation of PD symptoms may be more than 10 years, and some patients with LOPD or potential LOPD may not ever develop PD symptoms. Therefore, problems such as the psychological stress for the family due to LOPD and potential LOPD diagnosis [59], the cost and time of visiting hospitals and receiving medical examinations, and the potential of receiving overtreatment are issues likely to occur.

As shown in the guidelines for PD promulgated by the Pompe Disease Newborn Screening Working Group [30], clinicians should consider the need for psychosocial support for families during follow-ups for presymptomatic patients with LOPD. As more patients or potential patients with LOPD are diagnosed and followed up, it has been demonstrated that LOPD causes more symptoms than proximal myopathy or respiratory failure; it is a multiorgan disorder involving muscular, respiratory, musculoskeletal, peripheral nervous, vascular, cardiac, and gastrointestinal systems. Common symptoms reported in LOPD are proximal muscle weakness, trunk muscle weakness, exercise intolerance, shortness of breath, impaired cough, and gait difficulties. Because LOPD is a multisystemic disease, clinicians should be aware of all known symptoms and indicators in order to prevent delayed diagnoses and misdiagnoses. The understanding of the natural history of LOPD is advanced in the use of ERT. In the future, the disease concept of LOPD as well as IOPD will be more established.

14. Future Challenges

NBS programs for PD can contribute to early detection and early intervention in patients with IOPD and LOPD. Early ERT can change the natural clinical course and result in better outcomes in patients with IOPD. Because of changes in the natural clinical course, neurological manifestations, which had not previously been discussed, have become apparent [60]. For example, some patients with IOPD receiving ERT present with learning disorders as neurological manifestations. Currently available rhGAA therapy cannot cross the blood–brain barrier [61,62]. Moreover, patients with LOPD detected in NBS can receive follow-up and early intervention before exhibiting deterioration of PD symptoms [32].

Nevertheless, currently available NBS programs that evaluate AαGlu activity in DBSs, even those using tandem mass spectrometry, cannot discriminate pseudodeficiency from cases of PD or potential PD. Because families of newborns with pseudodeficiency have anxiety related to the results of NBS, new NBS programs, such as those using a combination of AαGlu enzyme assays and *GAA* gene analysis from DBS, can be used to distinguish pseudodeficiency from PD or VOUS. Such approaches are urgently needed.

In the future, next-generation treatments, including chaperon therapy [63] and gene therapy for PD [64,65], are expected to have favorable outcomes. Therefore, many researchers should contribute to the development of novel, improved NBS programs and the spread of such NBS programs to more regions around the world.

Author Contributions: Conceptualization, T.S., J.K. and K.N.; writing—original draft preparation, T.S. and J.K.; writing—review and editing, J.K. and K.N.; visualization, T.S. and J.K.; supervision, J.K. and K.N.; project administration, J.K. and K.N.; funding acquisition, K.N. All authors have read and agreed to the published version of the manuscript.

Acknowledgments: We are grateful to Fumiko Nozaki, Naomi Yano, Ayuko Tateishi, Emi Harakawa, Yasuyo Sakamoto, Hiroko Nasu, and Matsumi Harada for their technical support in the NBS for PD in Japan. Special thanks for Keishin Sugawara for his expert advice.

References

1. Martiniuk, F.; Mehler, M.; Pellicer, A.; Tzall, S.; La Badie, G.; Hobart, C.; Ellenbogen, A.; Hirschhorn, R. Isolation of a cDNA for human acid α-glucosidase and detection of genetic heterogeneity for mRNA in three α-glucosidase-deficient patients. *Proc. Natl. Acad. Sci. USA* **1986**, *83*, 9641–9644. [CrossRef] [PubMed]
2. Hagemans, M.L.C.; Winkel, L.P.F.; Hop, W.C.J.; Reuser, A.J.J.; Van Doorn, P.A.; van der Ploeg, A.T. Disease severity in children and adults with Pompe disease related to age and disease duration. *Neurology* **2005**, *64*, 2139–2141. [CrossRef] [PubMed]
3. Kishnani, P.S.; Corzo, D.; Nicolino, M.; Byrne, B.; Mandel, H.; Hwu, W.L.; Leslie, N.; Levine, J.; Spencer, C.; McDonald, M.; et al. Recombinant human acid α-glucosidase: Major clinical benefits in infantile-onset Pompe disease. *Neurology* **2007**, *68*, 99–109. [CrossRef] [PubMed]
4. van der Ploeg, A.T.; Clemens, P.R.; Corzo, D.; Escolar, D.M.; Florence, J.; Groeneveld, G.J.; Herson, S.; Kishnani, P.S.; Laforet, P.; Lake, S.L.; et al. A Randomized Study of Alglucosidase Alfa in Late-Onset Pompe's Disease. *N. Engl. J. Med.* **2010**, *362*, 1396–1406. [CrossRef]
5. Kishnani, P.S.; Corzo, D.; Leslie, N.D.; Gruskin, D.; Van Der Ploeg, A.; Clancy, J.P.; Parini, R.; Morin, G.; Beck, M.; Bauer, M.S.; et al. Early treatment with alglucosidase alfa prolongs long-term survival of infants with pompe disease. *Pediatr. Res.* **2009**, *66*, 329–335. [CrossRef]

6. Chien, Y.-H.; Lee, N.-C.; Thurberg, B.L.; Chiang, S.-C.; Zhang, X.K.; Keutzer, J.; Huang, A.-C.; Wu, M.-H.; Huang, P.-H.; Tsai, F.-J.; et al. Pompe disease in infants: Improving the prognosis by newborn screening and early treatment. *Pediatrics* **2009**, *124*, e1116–e1125. [CrossRef]

7. Momosaki, K.; Kido, J.; Yoshida, S.; Sugawara, K.; Miyamoto, T.; Inoue, T.; Okumiya, T.; Matsumoto, S.; Endo, F.; Hirose, S.; et al. Newborn screening for Pompe disease in Japan: Report and literature review of mutations in the *GAA* gene in Japanese and Asian patients. *J. Hum. Genet.* **2019**, *64*, 741–755. [CrossRef]

8. Burton, B.K.; Kronn, D.F.; Hwu, W.-L.; Kishnani, P.S.; Pompe Disease Newborn Screening Working Group. The Initial Evaluation of Patients after Positive Newborn Screening: Recommended Algorithms Leading to a Confirmed Diagnosis of Pompe Disease. *Pediatrics* **2017**, *140*, S14–S23. [CrossRef]

9. Kishnani, P.S.; Steiner, R.D.; Bali, D.; Berger, K.; Byrne, B.J.; Case, L.E.; Crowley, J.F.; Downs, S.; Howell, R.R.; Kravitz, R.M.; et al. Pompe disease diagnosis and management guideline. *Genet. Med.* **2006**, *8*, 267–288. [CrossRef]

10. Jack, R.M.; Gordon, C.; Scott, C.R.; Kishnani, P.S.; Bali, D. The use of acarbose inhibition in the measurement of acid alpha-glucosidase activity in blood lymphocytes for the diagnosis of Pompe disease. *Genet. Med.* **2006**, *8*, 307–312. [CrossRef]

11. Li, Y.; Scott, C.R.; Chamoles, N.A.; Ghavami, A.; Pinto, B.M.; Turecek, F.; Gelb, M.H. Direct multiplex assay of lysosomal enzymes in dried blood spots for newborn screening. *Clin. Chem.* **2004**, *50*, 1785–1796. [CrossRef] [PubMed]

12. Chamoles, N.A.; Niizawa, G.; Blanco, M.; Gaggioli, D.; Casentini, C. Glycogen storage disease type II: Enzymatic screening in dried blood spots on filter paper. *Clin. Chim. Acta* **2004**, *347*, 97–102. [CrossRef] [PubMed]

13. Sista, R.S.; Wang, T.; Wu, N.; Graham, C.; Eckhardt, A.; Winger, T.; Srinivasan, V.; Bali, D.; Millington, D.S.; Pamula, V.K. Multiplex newborn screening for Pompe, Fabry, Hunter, Gaucher, and Hurler diseases using a digital microfluidic platform. *Clin. Chim. Acta* **2013**, *424*, 12–18. [CrossRef] [PubMed]

14. Graham, C.; Sista, R.S.; Kleinert, J.; Wu, N.; Eckhardt, A.; Bali, D.; Millington, D.S.; Pamula, V.K. Novel application of digital microfluidics for the detection of biotinidase deficiency in newborns. *Clin. Biochem.* **2013**, *46*, 1889–1891. [CrossRef]

15. Liao, H.-C.; Chan, M.-J.; Yang, C.-F.; Chiang, C.-C.; Niu, D.-M.; Huang, C.-K.; Gelb, M.H. Mass Spectrometry but Not Fluorimetry Distinguishes Affected and Pseudodeficiency Patients in Newborn Screening for Pompe Disease. *Clin. Chem.* **2017**, *63*, 1271–1277. [CrossRef]

16. Landrum, M.J.; Chitipiralla, S.; Brown, G.R.; Chen, C.; Gu, B.; Hart, J.; Hoffman, D.; Jang, W.; Kaur, K.; Liu, C.; et al. ClinVar: Improvements to accessing data. *Nucleic Acids Res.* **2020**, *48*, D835–D844. [CrossRef]

17. Niño, M.Y.; in 't Groen, S.L.M.; Bergsma, A.J.; Beek, N.A.M.E.; Kroos, M.; Hoogeveen-Westerveld, M.; Ploeg, A.T.; Pijnappel, W.W.M.P. Extension of the Pompe mutation database by linking disease-associated variants to clinical severity. *Hum. Mutat.* **2019**, *40*, 1954–1967. [CrossRef]

18. Adzhubei, I.; Jordan, D.M.; Sunyaev, S.R. Predicting Functional Effect of Human Missense Mutations Using PolyPhen-2. *Curr. Protoc. Hum. Genet.* **2013**. [CrossRef]

19. Desmet, F.-O.; Hamroun, D.; Lalande, M.; Collod-Béroud, G.; Claustres, M.; Béroud, C. Human Splicing Finder: An online bioinformatics tool to predict splicing signals. *Nucleic Acids Res.* **2009**, *37*, e67. [CrossRef]

20. Schwarz, J.M.; Cooper, D.N.; Schuelke, M.; Seelow, D. Mutationtaster2: Mutation prediction for the deep-sequencing age. *Nat. Methods* **2014**, *11*, 361–362. [CrossRef]

21. Kroos, M.A.; Mullaart, R.A.; Van Vliet, L.; Pomponio, R.J.; Amartino, H.; Kolodny, E.H.; Pastores, G.M.; Wevers, R.A.; Van der Ploeg, A.T.; Halley, D.J.J.J.; et al. p.[G576S; E689K]: Pathogenic combination or polymorphism in Pompe disease? *Eur. J. Hum. Genet.* **2008**, *16*, 875–879. [CrossRef] [PubMed]

22. Tajima, Y.; Matsuzawa, F.; Aikawa, S.; Okumiya, T.; Yoshimizu, M.; Tsukimura, T.; Ikekita, M.; Tsujino, S.; Tsuji, A.; Edmunds, T.; et al. Structural and biochemical studies on Pompe disease and a "pseudodeficiency of acid α-glucosidase". *J. Hum. Genet.* **2007**, *52*, 898–906. [CrossRef] [PubMed]

23. Kumamoto, S.; Katafuchi, T.; Nakamura, K.; Endo, F.; Oda, E.; Okuyama, T.; Kroos, M.A.; Reuser, A.J.J.; Okumiya, T. High frequency of acid α-glucosidase pseudodeficiency complicates newborn screening for glycogen storage disease type II in the Japanese population. *Mol. Genet. Metab.* **2009**, *97*, 190–195. [CrossRef] [PubMed]

24. Chien, Y.-H.; Hwu, W.-L.; Lee, N.-C. Pompe Disease: Early Diagnosis and Early Treatment Make a Difference. *Pediatr. Neonatol.* **2013**, *54*, 219–227. [CrossRef]

25. Kishnani, P.S.; Goldenberg, P.C.; DeArmey, S.L.; Heller, J.; Benjamin, D.; Young, S.; Bali, D.; Smith, S.A.; Li, J.S.; Mandel, H.; et al. Cross-reactive immunologic material status affects treatment outcomes in Pompe disease infants. *Mol. Genet. Metab.* **2010**, *99*, 26–33. [CrossRef]

26. Banugaria, S.G.; Prater, S.N.; Ng, Y.K.; Kobori, J.A.; Finkel, R.S.; Ladda, R.L.; Chen, Y.T.; Rosenberg, A.S.; Kishnani, P.S. The impact of antibodies on clinical outcomes in diseases treated with therapeutic protein: Lessons learned from infantile Pompe disease. *Genet. Med.* **2011**, *13*, 729–736. [CrossRef]

27. Desai, A.K.; Kazi, Z.B.; Bali, D.S.; Kishnani, P.S. Characterization of immune response in Cross-Reactive Immunological Material (CRIM)-positive infantile Pompe disease patients treated with enzyme replacement therapy. *Mol. Genet. Metab. Rep.* **2019**, *20*, 100475. [CrossRef]

28. Yang, C.F.; Yang, C.C.; Liao, H.C.; Huang, L.Y.; Chiang, C.C.; Ho, H.C.; Lai, C.J.; Chu, T.H.; Yang, T.F.; Hsu, T.R.; et al. Very Early Treatment for Infantile-Onset Pompe Disease Contributes to Better Outcomes. *J. Pediatr.* **2016**, *169*, 174–180.e1. [CrossRef]

29. Hundsberger, T.; Schoser, B.; Leupold, D.; Rösler, K.M.; Putora, P.M. Comparison of recent pivotal recommendations for the diagnosis and treatment of late-onset Pompe disease using diagnostic nodes—the Pompe disease burden scale. *J. Neurol.* **2019**, *266*, 2010–2017. [CrossRef]

30. Kronn, D.F.; Day-Salvatore, D.; Hwu, W.-L.L.; Jones, S.A.; Nakamura, K.; Okuyama, T.; Swoboda, K.J.; Kishnani, P.S.; Pompe Disease Newborn Screening Working Group. Management of confirmed newborn-screened patients with pompe disease across the disease spectrum. *Pediatrics* **2017**, *140*, S24–S45. [CrossRef]

31. Lagler, F.B.; Moder, A.; Rohrbach, M.; Hennermann, J.; Mengel, E.; Gökce, S.; Hundsberger, T.; Rösler, K.M.; Karabul, N.; Huemer, M. Extent, impact, and predictors of diagnostic delay in Pompe disease: A combined survey approach to unveil the diagnostic odyssey. *JIMD Rep.* **2019**, *49*, 89–95. [CrossRef]

32. Chien, Y.H.; Lee, N.C.; Huang, H.J.; Thurberg, B.L.; Tsai, F.J.; Hwu, W.L. Later-onset pompe disease: Early detection and early treatment initiation enabled by newborn screening. *J. Pediatr.* **2011**, *158*, 1023–1027.e1. [CrossRef]

33. De Groot, A.S.; Kazi, Z.B.; Martin, R.F.; Terry, F.E.; Desai, A.K.; Martin, W.D.; Kishnani, P.S. HLA- and genotype-based risk assessment model to identify infantile onset pompe disease patients at high-risk of developing significant anti-drug antibodies (ADA). *Clin. Immunol.* **2019**, *200*, 66–70. [CrossRef] [PubMed]

34. Desai, A.K.; Li, C.; Rosenberg, A.S.; Kishnani, P.S. Immunological challenges and approaches to immunomodulation in Pompe disease: A literature review. *Ann. Transl. Med.* **2019**, *7*, 285. [CrossRef]

35. Labrousse, P.; Chien, Y.-H.H.; Pomponio, R.J.; Keutzer, J.; Lee, N.-C.C.; Akmaev, V.R.; Scholl, T.; Hwu, W.-L.L. Genetic heterozygosity and pseudodeficiency in the Pompe disease newborn screening pilot program. *Mol. Genet. Metab.* **2010**, *99*, 379–383. [CrossRef] [PubMed]

36. Chiang, S.-C.C.; Hwu, W.-L.L.; Lee, N.-C.C.; Hsu, L.-W.W.; Chien, Y.-H.H. Algorithm for Pompe disease newborn screening: Results from the Taiwan screening program. *Mol. Genet. Metab.* **2012**, *106*, 281–286. [CrossRef]

37. Liao, H.-C.; Chiang, C.-C.; Niu, D.-M.; Wang, C.-H.; Kao, S.-M.; Tsai, F.-J.; Huang, Y.-H.; Liu, H.-C.; Huang, C.-K.; Gao, H.-J.; et al. Detecting multiple lysosomal storage diseases by tandem mass spectrometry—A national newborn screening program in Taiwan. *Clin. Chim. Acta* **2014**, *431*, 80–86. [CrossRef] [PubMed]

38. Chiang, S.-C.; Chen, P.-W.; Hwu, W.-L.; Lee, A.-J.; Chen, L.-C.; Lee, N.-C.; Chiou, L.-Y.; Chien, Y.-H. Performance of the four-plex tandem mass spectrometry lysosomal storage disease newborn screening test: The necessity of adding a 2nd tier test for Pompe disease. *Int. J. Neonatal Screen.* **2018**, *4*, 41. [CrossRef]

39. Scott, C.R.; Elliott, S.; Buroker, N.; Thomas, L.I.; Keutzer, J.; Glass, M.; Gelb, M.H.; Turecek, F. Identification of infants at risk for developing Fabry, Pompe, or mucopolysaccharidosis-I from newborn blood spots by tandem mass spectrometry. *J. Pediatr.* **2013**, *163*, 498–503. [CrossRef]

40. Elliott, S.; Buroker, N.; Cournoyer, J.J.; Potier, A.M.; Trometer, J.D.; Elbin, C.; Schermer, M.J.; Kantola, J.; Boyce, A.; Turecek, F.; et al. Pilot study of newborn screening for six lysosomal storage diseases using Tandem Mass Spectrometry. *Mol. Genet. Metab.* **2016**, *118*, 304–309. [CrossRef] [PubMed]

41. Hopkins, P.V.; Campbell, C.; Klug, T.; Rogers, S.; Raburn-Miller, J.; Kiesling, J. Lysosomal Storage Disorder Screening Implementation: Findings from the First Six Months of Full Population Pilot Testing in Missouri. *J. Pediatr.* **2015**, *166*, 172–177. [CrossRef] [PubMed]

42. Burton, B.K.; Charrow, J.; Hoganson, G.E.; Waggoner, D.; Tinkle, B.; Braddock, S.R.; Schneider, M.; Grange, D.K.; Nash, C.; Shryock, H.; et al. Newborn Screening for Lysosomal Storage Disorders in Illinois: The Initial 15-Month Experience. *J. Pediatr.* **2017**, *190*, 130–135. [CrossRef] [PubMed]

43. Wasserstein, M.P.; Caggana, M.; Bailey, S.M.; Desnick, R.J.; Edelmann, L.; Estrella, L.; Holzman, I.; Kelly, N.R.; Kornreich, R.; Kupchik, S.G.; et al. The New York pilot newborn screening program for lysosomal storage diseases: Report of the First 65,000 Infants. *Genet. Med.* **2019**, *21*, 631–640. [CrossRef] [PubMed]

44. Mechtler, T.P.; Stary, S.; Metz, T.F.; De Jesús, V.R.; Greber-Platzer, S.; Pollak, A.; Herkner, K.R.; Streubel, B.; Kasper, D.C. Neonatal screening for lysosomal storage disorders: Feasibility and incidence from a nationwide study in Austria. *Lancet* **2012**, *379*, 335–341. [CrossRef]

45. Wittmann, J.; Karg, E.; Turi, S.; Legnini, E.; Wittmann, G.; Giese, A.-K.; Lukas, J.; Gölnitz, U.; Klingenhäger, M.; Bodamer, O.; et al. Newborn screening for lysosomal storage disorders in hungary. *JIMD Rep.* **2012**, *6*, 117–125.

46. Burlina, A.B.; Polo, G.; Salviati, L.; Duro, G.; Zizzo, C.; Dardis, A.; Bembi, B.; Cazzorla, C.; Rubert, L.; Zordan, R.; et al. Newborn screening for lysosomal storage disorders by tandem mass spectrometry in North East Italy. *J. Inherit. Metab. Dis.* **2018**, *41*, 209–219. [CrossRef]

47. Navarrete-Martínez, J.I.; Limón-Rojas, A.E.; de Jesús Gaytán-García, M.; Reyna-Figueroa, J.; Wakida-Kusunoki, G.; del Rocío Delgado-Calvillo, M.; Cantú-Reyna, C.; Cruz-Camino, H.; Cervantes-Barragán, D.E. Newborn screening for six lysosomal storage disorders in a cohort of Mexican patients: Three-year findings from a screening program in a closed Mexican health system. *Mol. Genet. Metab.* **2017**, *121*, 16–21.

48. Bravo, H.; Neto, E.C.; Schulte, J.; Pereira, J.; Filho, C.S.; Bittencourt, F.; Sebastião, F.; Bender, F.; de Magalhães, A.P.S.; Guidobono, R.; et al. Investigation of newborns with abnormal results in a newborn screening program for four lysosomal storage diseases in Brazil. *Mol. Genet. Metab. Rep.* **2017**, *12*, 92–97. [CrossRef]

49. Chien, Y.-H.; Chiang, S.-C.; Zhang, X.K.; Keutzer, J.; Lee, N.-C.; Huang, A.-C.; Chen, C.-A.; Wu, M.-H.; Huang, P.-H.; Tsai, F.-J.; et al. Early Detection of Pompe Disease by Newborn Screening Is Feasible: Results from the Taiwan Screening Program. *Pediatrics* **2008**, *122*, e39–e45. [CrossRef]

50. Nakamura, K.; Hattori, K.; Endo, F. Newborn screening for lysosomal storage disorders. *Am. J. Med. Genet. Part C Semin. Med. Genet.* **2011**, *157*, 63–71. [CrossRef]

51. Sawada, T.; Kido, J.; Yoshida, S.; Sugawara, K.; Momosaki, K.; Inoue, T.; Tajima, G.; Sawada, H.; Mastumoto, S.; Endo, F.; et al. Newborn screening for Fabry disease in the western region of Japan. *Mol. Genet. Metab. Rep.* **2020**, *22*, 100562. [CrossRef] [PubMed]

52. Prosser, L.A.; Lam, K.K.; Grosse, S.D.; Casale, M.; Kemper, A.R. Using Decision Analysis to Support Newborn Screening Policy Decisions: A Case Study for Pompe Disease. *MDM Policy Pract.* **2018**, *3*. [CrossRef] [PubMed]

53. Paciotti, S.; Persichetti, E.; Pagliardini, S.; Deganuto, M.; Rosano, C.; Balducci, C.; Codini, M.; Filocamo, M.; Menghini, A.R.; Pagliardini, V.; et al. First pilot newborn screening for four lysosomal storage diseases in an Italian region: Identification and analysis of a putative causative mutation in the *GBA* gene. *Clin. Chim. Acta* **2012**, *413*, 1827–1831. [CrossRef] [PubMed]

54. Camargo Neto, E.; Schulte, J.; Pereira, J.; Bravo, H.; Sampaio-Filho, C.; Giugliani, R. Neonatal screening for four lysosomal storage diseases with a digital microfluidics platform: Initial results in Brazil. *Genet. Mol. Biol.* **2018**, *41*, 414–416. [CrossRef]

55. Rojas Málaga, D.; Brusius-Facchin, A.C.; Michelin-Tirelli, K.; Félix, T.M.; Schulte, J.; Pereira, J.; Camargo Neto, E.; Sampaio Filho, C.; Giugliani, R. Pseudo deficiency of acid α-glucosidase: A challenge in the newborn screening for Pompe disease. *Genet. Mol. Res.* **2017**, *16*, 16039844.

56. Ausems, M.G.E.M.; Verbiest, J.; Hermans, M.M.P.; Kroos, M.A.; Beemer, F.A.; Wokke, J.H.J.; Sandkuijl, L.A.; Reuser, A.J.J.; Van Der Ploeg, A.T. Frequency of glycogen storage disease type II in The Netherlands: Implications for diagnosis and genetic counselling. *Eur. J. Hum. Genet.* **1999**, *7*, 713–716. [CrossRef]

57. Becker, J.A.; Vlach, J.; Raben, N.; Nagaraju, K.; Adams, E.M.; Hermans, M.M.; Reuser, A.J.; Brooks, S.S.; Tifft, C.J.; Hirschhorn, R.; et al. The African origin of the common mutation in African American patients with glycogen-storage disease type II. *Am. J. Hum. Genet.* **1998**, *62*, 991–994. [CrossRef]

58. Herbert, M.; Cope, H.; Li, J.S.; Kishnani, P.S. Severe Cardiac Involvement Is Rare in Patients with Late-Onset Pompe Disease and the Common c.-32-13T>G Variant: Implications for Newborn Screening. *J. Pediatr.* **2018**, *198*, 308–312. [CrossRef]

59. Pruniski, B.; Lisi, E.; Ali, N. Newborn screening for Pompe disease: Impact on families. *J. Inherit. Metab. Dis.* **2018**, *41*, 1189–1203. [CrossRef]

60. Prater, S.N.; Banugaria, S.G.; Dearmey, S.M.; Botha, E.G.; Stege, E.M.; Case, L.E.; Jones, H.N.; Phornphutkul, C.; Wang, R.Y.; Young, S.P.; et al. The emerging phenotype of long-term survivors with infantile Pompe disease. *Genet. Med.* **2012**, *14*, 800–810. [CrossRef]

61. Chien, Y.H.; Lee, N.C.; Peng, S.F.; Hwu, W.L. Brain development in infantile-onset pompe disease treated by enzyme replacement therapy. *Pediatr. Res.* **2006**, *60*, 349–352. [CrossRef]

62. Spiridigliozzi, G.A.; Keeling, L.A.; Stefanescu, M.; Li, C.; Austin, S.; Kishnani, P.S. Cognitive and academic outcomes in long-term survivors of infantile-onset Pompe disease: A longitudinal follow-up. *Mol. Genet. Metab.* **2017**, *121*, 127–137. [CrossRef] [PubMed]

63. Roig-Zamboni, V.; Cobucci-Ponzano, B.; Iacono, R.; Ferrara, M.C.; Germany, S.; Bourne, Y.; Parenti, G.; Moracci, M.; Sulzenbacher, G. Structure of human lysosomal acid α-glucosidase—A guide for the treatment of Pompe disease. *Nat. Commun.* **2017**, *8*, 1111. [CrossRef] [PubMed]

64. Lim, J.-A.; Yi, H.; Gao, F.; Raben, N.; Kishnani, P.S.; Sun, B. Intravenous Injection of an AAV-PHP.B Vector Encoding Human Acid α-Glucosidase Rescues Both Muscle and CNS Defects in Murine Pompe Disease. *Mol. Ther. Methods Clin. Dev.* **2019**, *12*, 233–245. [CrossRef] [PubMed]

65. Byrne, B.J.; Fuller, D.D.; Smith, B.K.; Clement, N.; Coleman, K.; Cleaver, B.; Vaught, L.; Falk, D.J.; McCall, A.; Corti, M. Pompe disease gene therapy: Neural manifestations require consideration of CNS directed therapy. *Ann. Transl. Med.* **2019**, *7*, 290. [CrossRef] [PubMed]

13

Psychological Impact of NBS for CF

Jane Chudleigh [1],* and Holly Chinnery [2]

[1]   School of Health Sciences, City, University of London, London EC1V 0HB, UK
[2]   Faculty of Sports, Health and Applied Science, St Mary's University, London TW1 4SX, UK;
     holly.chinnery@stmarys.ac.uk
*   Correspondence: j.chudleigh@city.ac.uk

Abstract: Newborn screening for cystic fibrosis has resulted in diagnosis often before symptoms are recognised, leading to benefits including reduced disease severity, decreased burden of care, and lower costs. The psychological impact of this often unsought diagnosis on the parents of seemingly well children is less well understood. The time during which the screening result is communicated to families but before the confirmatory test results are available is recognised as a period of uncertainty and it is this uncertainty that can impact most on parents. Evidence suggests this may be mitigated against by ensuring the time between communication and confirmatory testing is minimized and health professionals involved in communicating positive newborn screening results and diagnostic results for cystic fibrosis to families are knowledgeable and able to provide appropriate reassurance. This is particularly important in the case of false positive results or when the child is given a Cystic Fibrosis Screen Positive, Inconclusive Diagnosis designation. However, to date, there are no formal mechanisms in place to support health professionals undertaking this challenging role, which would enable them to meet the expectations set out in specific guidance.

Keywords: newborn bloodspot screening; cystic fibrosis; psychological impact

---

1. Introduction

The increased use globally of newborn bloodspot screening (NBS) for cystic fibrosis (CF) has resulted in diagnosis often before symptoms are recognised. Benefits include reduced disease severity, decreased burden of care, and lower costs [1–5]. Without NBS, the diagnosis of CF relies on the recognition of particular clinical signs and symptoms, which often results in delayed diagnosis. This can lead to an arduous journey for parents characterised by uncertainty and anxiety as they seek answers and are referred to a number of different clinical specialities before the correct, definitive diagnosis is made [6].

NBS for CF may pose different challenges when compared to other conditions included in NBS programmes, such as sickle cell disease (SCD) which commonly includes antenatal screening, meaning that parents are aware of their own carrier status and the theoretical risk to their unborn child [7]. For CF, parents are often unaware and have not sought information regarding their own carrier status [8]. However, other challenges, such as the method and content of communication, may be similar between conditions.

Despite the undisputed clinical and fiscal benefits of CF NBS, several challenges have been noted, one of which being the potential psychological impact on the child's family. One small study consisting of qualitative interviews with the parents of children diagnosed with CF either via NBS, prenatally, or after the development of symptoms suggested that for those diagnosed via NBS, the early, unsought diagnosis had the potential to deeply affect parents in many ways. These included questioning their competence to care for their baby and their sense of who the baby is. In addition, early diagnosis led to the disease taking centre stage during the child's early weeks and months and caused health professionals to loom very large in the family's life at this formative time [9]. Another study in the US, which explored the parental experiences associated with receiving a positive NBS result for one of the metabolic conditions, supported these findings and suggested that the methods used to communicate the NBS result and the condition specific knowledge of the individual imparting the result influenced parental dissatisfaction, anxiety, and distress [10]. The similarities between the findings of these studies perhaps reflect the fact that CF and the metabolic conditions have a genetic origin and therefore staff knowledge and understanding about the cause and immediate and longer term implications of these are vital.

Like all conditions, it is important that careful consideration is given to how positive CF NBS results are communicated to parents as this is often unexpected, represents a life limiting diagnosis for the child and often a life changing event for the parents. As for many conditions, it may not be possible to remove parental anguish completely from what is an upsetting time. However, it is important for health professionals to communicate positive CF NBS results in a manner that minimises potential distress and does not detrimentally affect parents' relationships with their child and other family members. This chapter will focus on the psychological impact of CF, with implications not always limited to CF, and will explore the current guidance regarding communication strategies, the impact of poor communication practices, and information giving in times of uncertainty, and make recommendations for future practice.

2. Guidance Regarding Communication of Positive NBS Results for CF

Internationally, detailed guidelines exist for the processing of positive CF NBS results [11,12]. However, these primarily focus on laboratory processes and subsequent clinical management; less attention is given to how positive CF NBS results should be communicated to families to minimise potential distress. The European best practice guidelines for CF neonatal screening [3] recognise the time period during which the screening result is communicated to families but before the confirmatory test results are available, as a "period of maximal uncertainty." It is therefore suggested that during this time, information should be provided to families in a format that will be easy for them to digest, using language the family can understand. In addition, information should be structured, clarified, and summarised appropriately and parental understanding should be checked and questions encouraged. These guidelines also suggest the health professional communicating the NBS result should explore the families' beliefs, concerns, and expectations in order to tailor information and the conversation style for the needs of the parent(s). Moreover, in anticipation of further communication needs, the health professional should encourage parental participation in decisions and enlist resources and appropriate support. Finally, health professionals informing parents of their child's positive CF NBS result should be knowledgeable about CF, NBS principles, basic CF genetics, and the psychosocial pitfalls that some parents may experience [3].

More specific guidance from the United Kingdom states that families should be informed by an initial structured telephone call undertaken by a well-informed health professional with appropriate experience and support to give bad news [13]. European guidelines recognise the importance of CF team members possessing compassionate communication and effective information giving skills and the ability to recognise and respond to emotional distress. In addition, these guidelines suggest that some CF team members may require training in more specific skills, such as breaking bad news, recognising significant psychopathology, and appropriate referral should such instances occur. The advantages of the inclusion of specialist mental health professionals in CF teams, such as clinical psychologists or psychiatrists, is also recognised [12].

3. Impact of Communicating Positive NBS Results to Families

In 2015, a systematic review summarised if, and how, information provision has been included in economic evaluations of NBS programmes [14]. This review highlighted that only three studies included an estimate of the cost of information provision in their analysis and none of the studies captured the impact of information provision after screening [14]. One study in the systematic review [14] referred to costs related to the impact of poor information provision specifically related to false positive results rather than poor information provision at the time of communicating the initial NBS+ result per se [15]. This review concluded that evidence existed to support the notion that poor information provision in relation to NBS does impact on parents but there have been few attempts to quantify the impact of information provision in economic evaluations of NBS to date. Importantly, this review confirmed that there are no current data on the long-term impact of poor information provision and subsequent use of healthcare resources and impact on parents' health and well-being. This is interesting since the provision of adequate information and therefore good parental knowledge about their child's false positive CF NBS result, meant that the number of visits to the child's General Practitioner did not differ significantly between the false positive and the negative NBS groups [16]. Therefore, there is clearly a need to explore the role of information provision on the subsequent healthcare resource use.

Studies that have focused on CF NBS have identified adverse outcomes associated with the approaches and methods used to communicate CF NBS results to families. Interviews with the mothers ($n = 106$) and fathers ($n = 97$) of children with a confirmed diagnosis of congenital hypothyroidism (CHT) ($n = 37$), CF-carrier ($n = 43$), or CF ($n = 26$) in the United States (US) found that the majority of parents across all groups reported strong initial emotional reactions such as shock, panic, and anxiety about what results meant. The responses are likely related to the fact that currently, antenatal screening for CHT and CF is not routinely undertaken, therefore parents are unaware of the potential risk of their unborn baby being affected by these conditions. Responses related to positive CF NBS results included fears of the child dying, parental somatic symptoms, such as nausea and suffocation, difficulty bonding with their infant, marital discord, and changed reproductive plans [17]. These differences may reflect the fact that while CHT is treatable with a very good prognosis when diagnosed and treated in infancy, CF continues to be a life-limiting condition with no cure. In addition, in the majority of cases, CHT does not have a genetic origin and therefore does not have the same reproductive implications as CF. A similar study conducted in the US explored factors affecting parent–child relationships one year after positive NBS with 131 mothers and 118 fathers of 131 infants who had a positive NBS result for CF ($n = 23$), CF carrier ($n = 38$), CHT ($n = 35$), or normal NBS ($n = 35$). The parents of children with CF reported higher perceptions of child vulnerability and fathers of children who were CF carriers, viewed their children as more attached. The findings also indicated that infant feeding problems, particularly in the presence of a serious health condition like CF, could represent an important sign of more deeply rooted concerns regarding the parent–child relationship [18].

A study in the UK to explore parents' experience of receiving a positive NBS result used semi-structured interviews with 12 mothers (five with a child with CF and seven with a child with SCD and 10 fathers (five each with a child with CF or SCD) of children diagnosed via NBS [19]. The mothers of infants with a positive NBS for CF found being alone when they received their child's positive CF NBS result upsetting and fathers expressed distress at not being able to support their partner during this time. This also reportedly had the potential to impact on parental relationships as the mother then became responsible for informing the baby's father of the positive CF NBS result. These findings were not reported by the parents of babies who had received a positive NBS for SCD who described being aware of their 'risk' due to the results of antenatal screening [19]. Therefore they were less shocked by the result but were more concerned with the stigma associated with a diagnosis of SCD, which has been commonly cited in the literature [20]. Conversely, the parents of babies with a positive NBS results for CF did not report feeling stigma associated with the condition. CF NBS results also impacted on parental relationships in other ways, including parents questioning their choice of partner and feelings of confusion and guilt at having passed the defective gene on to their child. This was similar to the responses of parents whose baby had received a positive NBS for SCD and perhaps reflects the genetic implications of both conditions.

Receiving the CF NBS result from a health professional perceived to be less informed and therefore unable to answer parental questions about CF was also undesirable and had the potential to impact on future relationships with that health professional [19]. It should be noted that the sample size in this study was small but reflects the findings of other studies. A prospective questionnaire survey of 138 parents who had received a positive CF NBS in Switzerland indicated that most parents ($n = 122$; 88%) were satisfied with screening, four (3%) were not, and 12 (9%) were unsure. The parents received their child's positive CF NBS result over the telephone from a CF physician and were invited for diagnostic testing during the same conversation; 100 (74%) of the parents found the information provided satisfactory. This supports the importance of the person reporting the NBS result having condition specific knowledgeable. The remaining parents who were unsatisfied stated the caller had not explained the test result and the disease or had provided superficial information and instead focused on arranging the appointment [21].

A study in Germany evaluating CF NBS since its introduction in 2016 found that of the 105 (54.7%) families involved in the study (out of 192 who had gone through diagnostic testing after a positive CF NBS result), only 30 parents obtained information about the newborn screening by a physician despite this being mandatory in Germany. Despite this, parents being informed about the positive CF NBS result by a CF specialist were more satisfied with the given information than those informed by the maternity ward. Furthermore, waiting for more than 3 days between the information about the CF NBS result and the diagnostic testing was too long for 77.7% of the families [22]. These findings and those of the study in Switzerland [21] highlight the importance of ensuring that diagnostic testing is undertaken in a timely manner to reduce the parental anxiety and uncertainty associated with the positive NBS result.

Evidence also exists regarding the impact of communicating practices specifically for NBS carrier results. Semi-structured face-to-face interviews conducted with 49 mothers, 16 fathers and 2 grandparents of 51 infants identified CF NBS as carriers of CF ($n = 27$) and SCD ($n = 24$), in England demonstrated untoward anxiety or distress among parents was influenced by how results were conveyed rather than the carrier result per se [23].

In summary, communication of positive CF NBS can influence outcomes in the short term [17,19,21,23] but may also have a longer term impact on children and families [18]. Evidence suggests that the distress caused can manifest in several ways, including arguments between couples, including the apportioning of blame [19,23], the alteration of life plans, an inability to conduct the tasks of daily living, such as going to work or socializing [23], long-term alterations in parent–child relationships [18], and mistrust and lack of confidence affecting ongoing relationships with staff [19].

4. Dealing with Uncertainty: False Positives and CF Screen Positive, Inconclusive Diagnosis (CFSPID)

It has already been highlighted that the time period during which the NBS result is communicated to families but before the confirmatory test results are available, is a "period of maximal uncertainty" [3]. The impact of uncertainty associated with NBS results has been considered extensively in the literature and similar issues have been identified for many of the conditions included in NBS programmes. This is an important consideration that is by no means exclusive to the CF community but may be more prevalent in conditions with a genetic origin such as CF, SCD, and the metabolic conditions due to the longer term implications such as the effect on future reproductive decisions [24–26].

False positive NBS results have the potential to lead to ongoing uncertainty for parents. However, engaging the parents of children who have received a false positive results for any of the conditions included in NBS programmes in research, is notoriously difficult. Studies that have managed to capture this study population have produced conflicting information regarding the potential for false positive results to have a detrimental effect on the family system.

In France, a prospective study conducted with 86 families at 3, 12, and 24 months after receiving a false positive CF NBS result using the Perceived Stress Scale, and the Vulnerable Child Scale found that although 96.5% of parents said they had been anxious at the time of the sweat test, 86% felt entirely reassured 3 months afterwards. The mean perceived stress scale scores did not differ from the French population and the mean vulnerable child scale indicated a low parental perception of child vulnerability. These scores were not found to differ at 12 and 24 months after receiving the false positive CF NBS result. Indeed, 86% to 100% of families no longer worried about CF and all parents stated that they would have the test performed again for another child [27].

Similarly, in the Netherlands, 62 parents (59%) who had received a false positive CF NBS result, and 146 parents (46%) who had received a negative CF NBS result, returned questionnaires to assess long-term effects of false positive results on parental anxiety and stress. In addition, 24 mothers and three fathers participated in 25 semi-structured interviews. Parents showed strong negative feelings after being informed about the positive CF NBS screening result and satisfaction with time of referral was negatively associated with the number of days between being informed and the appointment at the hospital ($r = 0.402$; $p = 0.001$), indicating the importance of timely confirmatory testing. After confirmation that their child was healthy and not affected by CF, most parents felt reassured. Indeed, parental concern about their baby's health or the number of visits to their General Practitioner did not differ significantly between the false positive and the negative NBS groups. After six months, no difference in anxiety levels between both groups of parents was found. Only 6% (4/62) of parents who received a false positive CF NBS result said they would not participate in NBS in the future, while 16% (10/62) were not sure [16].

Likewise, a study in Canada that included 134 mothers who had received a false positive CF NBS for their child and 411 controls who completed questionnaires when their infant was 2 and 12 months old and 54 mothers who had received a false positive CF NBS for their child who were interviewed found that mean anxiety, distress, and vulnerability scores did not differ between the two groups. Of those who received a false positive CF NBS result, 61% were informed by their primary care physician and 39% by a genetic counsellor. The majority (87%) of mothers stated the time between being notified of the positive screen and learning the final results was the "scariest time of their lives", stating that having been home from hospital with an apparently healthy infant, it was alarming to learn that their child might have a chronic illness. Mothers placed tremendous value on the fact that time to confirmatory testing was quick (generally ≤48 h) and valued the excellent coordination of care, particularly being given a time and location to attend for confirmatory testing. Mothers in this study valued the screening system of care in mitigating concerns [28].

Conversely, interviews with 87 parents of 44 infants in the US who had been identified as CF carriers following a false positive CF NBS result found that this resulted in poor intra and interpersonal relationships within the family system and more widely. The parents expressed concerns about test accuracy, the child's health, especially in those who had exhibited signs of respiratory illness, and the future. Parents described the period of uncertainty ending in the child being a carrier rather than being affected by CF, enabling them to gain new perspectives and strengthen their relationship. For one father in the study, the false positive result led to him questioning the child's paternity. The authors also describe extended family members searching for the source of the genetic defect that had led to the child's carrier status; wondering if other relatives had CF and/or were carriers. Parents also talked about their support for NBS and feeling empathy for parents of affected children [29]. Interestingly, this study does not mention the time between parents receiving the NBS results and confirmatory testing, which may have mitigated against these negative outcomes [16,27,28].

The relatively recent new designation of CF Screen Positive, Inconclusive Diagnosis (CFSPID) [30] provides another layer of uncertainty for CF NBS. However, there is very little available evidence about the psychological impact of a CFSPID designation on families. A secondary analysis of interview data obtained from a small subset of five couples when their infants were 2 to 6 months old and later at 12 months of age who participated in a larger project demonstrated that uncertainty emerged as the central dimension of parents' experience when given a CFPSID designation for their child.

This uncertainty was linked to the fact that the screening and diagnostic test results were perceived as being contradictory; the presence of two CF mutations from the screening result, usually resulting in an abnormal diagnostic test, CF symptoms, and a CF diagnosis, was confusing to parents, as their child had a normal or borderline sweat test result and were asymptomatic. Moreover, the lack of existing knowledge about the prognostic implications of the identified mutations left health professionals and parents with little certainty about the implications for the infants' future health trajectory [31]. A more recent study with eight parents (three couples and two mothers) supported these initial findings and suggested that CFSPID results caused parental distress, initiated with the first communication of the result and persisting thereafter, but that approaches to the delivery of CFSPID results might reduce the impact [32]. This supports the findings of studies discussed above regarding the importance of the approach used to deliver positive NBS results for other conditions but, perhaps more importantly, the knowledge of the person delivering an uncertain result and their ability to alleviate the parental anxiety associated with this uncertainty [10,19,21,22].

Whilst being confusing for parents, the unknown longer term implications of certain NBS outcomes can also be challenging for health professionals. For instance, borderline CHT results can be challenging to manage to ensure best outcomes for the child in the longer term [33]. Similarly, a Canadian study identified uncertainty associated with the diagnostic as well as the prognostic outcomes for infants with certain metabolic conditions. Health care providers in this study also described transferring some of the uncertainty to parents while involving them in the ongoing monitoring of their child for signs and symptoms that may indicate a more serious prognostic outcome than initially suspected. Finally, the importance of being honest about uncertainty rather than seeing it as a weakness was also viewed as being important by health care providers [34]. These studies highlight the difficulties faced by parents trying to understand the NBS outcomes of uncertain long-term significance as well as the importance of health professionals have adequate knowledge and skills to manage these conditions and parental expectations.

5. Conclusions

The findings of the studies presented above demonstrate the importance of carefully considered information provision to reduce psychological impact when imparting positive CF NBS to parents. The method of delivery of information would seem to be far less important than the knowledge of the person responsible and their ability to answer parents' questions and provide reassurance [19,21–23], particularly if a degree of uncertainty is present, such as with CFSPID results [32]. Despite this, the findings of a recent study found that the CF NBS result is communicated by a range of health professionals internationally and that this may not always be the most appropriate or knowledgeable person but is influenced by many factors, including geographical/logistical, legal, financial and cultural constraints [35]. Additionally, a study in the UK found that specific training for professionals involved in communicating positive NBS results is lacking [36] but is clearly needed to ensure they are adequately prepared to undertake this challenging task. This would also help to meet the suggestions contained within the European guidelines regarding the skills CF team members should possess [12].

Ensuring the most appropriate person communicates a positive CF NBS result is particularly important in cases where there may be a degree of uncertainty, such as for false positive CF NBS results or a CFSPID designation [31,32]. Evidence suggests that good information provision and timely confirmatory testing can mitigate against the long-term psychological distress that has previously been considered to be associated with a false positive CF NBS result [16,27,28].

References

1. Bush, A. Newborn screening for cystic fibrosis—Benefit or bane? *Paediatr. Respir. Rev.* **2008**, *9*, 301–302. [CrossRef] [PubMed]
2. Castellani, C.; Massie, J.; Sontag, M.; Southern, K.W. Newborn screening for cystic fibrosis. *Lancet Respir. Med.* **2016**, *4*, 653–661. [CrossRef]
3. Castellani, C.; Southern, K.W.; Brownlee, K.; Dankert Roelse, J.; Duff, A.; Farrell, M.; Mehta, A.; Munck, A.; Pollitt, R.; Sermet-Gaudelus, I.; et al. European best practice guidelines for cystic fibrosis neonatal screening. *J. Cyst. Fibros.* **2009**, *8*, 153–173. [CrossRef] [PubMed]
4. Farrell, P.M.; White, T.B.; Derichs, N.; Castellani, C.; Rosenstein, B.J. Cystic Fibrosis Diagnostic Challenges over 4 Decades: Historical Perspectives and Lessons Learned. *J. Pediatr.* **2017**, *181*, S16–S26. [CrossRef]
5. Southern, K.W.; Merelle, M.M.; Dankert-Roelse, J.E.; Nagelkerke, A.D. Newborn screening for cystic fibrosis. *Cochrane Database Syst. Rev.* **2009**, CD001402. [CrossRef]
6. Merelle, M.E.; Huisman, J.; Alderden-van der Vecht, A.; Taat, F.; Bezemer, D.; Griffioen, R.W.; Brinkhorst, G.; Dankert-Roelse, J.E. Early versus late diagnosis: Psychological impact on parents of children with cystic fibrosis. *Pediatrics* **2003**, *111*, 346–350. [CrossRef]
7. Weil, L.G.; Charlton, M.R.; Coppinger, C.; Daniel, Y.; Streetly, A. Sickle cell disease and thalassaemia antenatal screening programme in England over 10 years: A review from 2007/2008 to 2016/2017. *J. Clin. Pathol.* **2020**, *73*, 183–190. [CrossRef]
8. De Boeck, K. Cystic fibrosis in the year 2020: A disease with a new face. *Acta Paediatr.* **2020**. [CrossRef]
9. Grob, R. Is my sick child healthy? Is my healthy child sick? Changing parental experiences of cystic fibrosis in the age of expanded newborn screening. *Soc. Sci. Med.* **2008**, *67*, 1056–1064. [CrossRef]
10. Buchbinder, M.; Timmermans, S. Newborn screening for metabolic disorders: Parental perceptions of the initial communication of results. *Clin. Pediatr.* **2012**, *51*, 739–744. [CrossRef]
11. Farrell, P.M.; White, T.B.; Ren, C.L.; Hempstead, S.E.; Accurso, F.; Derichs, N.; Howenstine, M.; McColley, S.A.; Rock, M.; Rosenfeld, M.; et al. Diagnosis of Cystic Fibrosis: Consensus Guidelines from the Cystic Fibrosis Foundation. *J. Pediatr.* **2017**, *181*, S4–S15. [CrossRef] [PubMed]
12. Castellani, C.; Duff, A.J.A.; Bell, S.C.; Heijerman, H.G.M.; Munck, A.; Ratjen, F.; Sermet-Gaudelus, I.; Southern, K.W.; Barben, J.; Flume, P.A.; et al. ECFS best practice guidelines: The 2018 revision. *J. Cyst. Fibros.* **2018**, *17*, 153–178. [CrossRef] [PubMed]
13. Public Health England. *NHS Newborn Blood Spot Screening Programme: Managing Positive Results from Cystic Fibrosis Screening*; Public Health England: London, UK, 2017; pp. 1–20.
14. Wright, S.J.; Jones, C.; Payne, K.; Dharni, N.; Ulph, F. The Role of Information Provision in Economic Evaluations of Newborn Bloodspot Screening: A Systematic Review. *Appl. Health Econ. Health Policy* **2015**, *13*, 615–626. [CrossRef] [PubMed]
15. Schoen, E.J.; Baker, J.C.; Colby, C.J.; To, T.T. Cost-benefit analysis of universal tandem mass spectrometry for newborn screening. *Pediatrics* **2002**, *110*, 781–786. [CrossRef]
16. Vernooij-van Langen, A.M.; van der Pal, S.M.; Reijntjens, A.J.; Loeber, J.G.; Dompeling, E.; Dankert-Roelse, J.E. Parental knowledge reduces long term anxiety induced by false-positive test results after newborn screening for cystic fibrosis. *Mol. Genet. Metab. Rep.* **2014**, *1*, 334–344. [CrossRef]
17. Salm, A.; Yetter, E.; Tluczek, A. Informing parents about positive newborn screening results: Parents' recommendations. *J. Child Health Care* **2012**, *16*, 367–381. [CrossRef]
18. Tluczek, A.; Clark, R.; McKechnie, A.C.; Brown, R.L. Factors affecting parent-child relationships one year after positive newborn screening for cystic fibrosis or congenital hypothyroidism. *J. Dev. Behav. Pediatr.* **2015**, *36*, 24–34. [CrossRef]
19. Chudleigh, J.; Buckingham, S.; Dignan, J.; O'Driscoll, S.; Johnson, K.; Rees, D.; Wyatt, H.; Metcalfe, A. Parents' Experiences of Receiving the Initial Positive Newborn Screening (NBS) Result for Cystic Fibrosis and Sickle Cell Disease. *J. Genet. Couns.* **2016**, *25*, 1215–1226. [CrossRef]
20. Marsh, V.M.; Kamuya, D.M.; Molyneux, S.S. All her children are born that way': Gendered experiences of stigma in families affected by sickle cell disorder in rural Kenya. *Ethn. Health* **2011**, *16*, 343–359. [CrossRef]
21. Rueegg, C.S.; Barben, J.; Hafen, G.M.; Moeller, A.; Jurca, M.; Fingerhut, R.; Kuehni, C.E.; The Swiss Cystic Fibrosis Screening Group. Newborn screening for cystic fibrosis—The parent perspective. *J. Cyst. Fibros.* **2016**, *15*, 443–451. [CrossRef]

22. Brockow, I.; Nennstiel, U. Parents' experience with positive newborn screening results for cystic fibrosis. *Eur. J. Pediatr.* **2019**, *178*, 803–809. [CrossRef]

23. Ulph, F.; Cullinan, T.; Qureshi, N.; Kai, J. Parents' responses to receiving sickle cell or cystic fibrosis carrier results for their child following newborn screening. *Eur. J. Hum. Genet.* **2015**, *23*, 459–465. [CrossRef]

24. Wilkie, D.J.; Gallo, A.M.; Yao, Y.; Molokie, R.E.; Stahl, C.; Hershberger, P.E.; Zhao, Z.; Suarez, M.L.; Labotka, R.J.; Johnson, B.; et al. Reproductive health choices for young adults with sickle cell disease or trait: Randomized controlled trial immediate posttest effects. *Nurs. Res.* **2013**, *62*, 352–361. [CrossRef]

25. Plumridge, G.; Metcalfe, A.; Coad, J.; Gill, P. The role of support groups in facilitating families in coping with a genetic condition and in discussion of genetic risk information. *Health Expect. Int. J. Public Particip. Health Care Health Policy* **2012**, *15*, 255–266. [CrossRef]

26. The Socio-Psychological Research in Genomics (SPRinG) Collaboration; Eisler, I.; Ellison, M.; Flinter, F.; Grey, J.; Hutchison, S.; Jackson, C.; Longworth, L.; MacLeod, R.; McAllister, M.; et al. Developing an intervention to facilitate family communication about inherited genetic conditions, and training genetic counsellors in its delivery. *Eur. J. Hum. Genet.* **2015**, *24*, 794–802. [CrossRef]

27. Beucher, J.; Leray, E.; Deneuville, E.; Roblin, M.; Pin, I.; Bremont, F.; Turck, D.; Ginies, J.L.; Foucaud, P.; Rault, G.; et al. Psychological effects of false-positive results in cystic fibrosis newborn screening: A two-year follow-up. *J. Pediatr.* **2010**, *156*, 771–776. [CrossRef]

28. Hayeems, R.Z.; Miller, F.A.; Barg, C.J.; Bombard, Y.; Kerr, E.; Tam, K.; Carroll, J.C.; Potter, B.K.; Chakraborty, P.; Davies, C.; et al. Parent Experience with False-Positive Newborn Screening Results for Cystic Fibrosis. *Pediatrics* **2016**, *138*, e20161052. [CrossRef]

29. Tluczek, A.; Orland, K.M.; Cavanagh, L. Psychosocial consequences of false-positive newborn screens for cystic fibrosis. *Qual. Health Res.* **2011**, *21*, 174–186. [CrossRef]

30. Munck, A.; Mayell, S.J.; Winters, V.; Shawcross, A.; Derichs, N.; Parad, R.; Barben, J.; Southern, K.W. Cystic Fibrosis Screen Positive, Inconclusive Diagnosis (CFSPID): A new designation and management recommendations for infants with an inconclusive diagnosis following newborn screening. *J. Cyst. Fibros.* **2015**, *14*, 706–713. [CrossRef]

31. Tluczek, A.; Chevalier McKechnie, A.; Lynam, P.A. When the cystic fibrosis label does not fit: A modified uncertainty theory. *Qual. Health Res.* **2010**, *20*, 209–223. [CrossRef]

32. Johnson, F.; Southern, K.W.; Ulph, F. Psychological Impact on Parents of an Inconclusive Diagnosis Following Newborn Bloodspot Screening. *Int. J. Neonatal Screen.* **2019**, *5*, 23. [CrossRef]

33. Lain, S.J.; Bentley, J.P.; Wiley, V.; Roberts, C.L.; Jack, M.; Wilcken, B.; Nassar, N. Association between borderline neonatal thyroid-stimulating hormone concentrations and educational and developmental outcomes: A population-based record-linkage study. *Lancet Diabetes Endocrinol.* **2016**, *4*, 756–765. [CrossRef]

34. Azzopardi, P.J.; Upshur, R.E.G.; Luca, S.; Venkataramanan, V.; Potter, B.K.; Chakraborty, P.K.; Hayeems, R.Z. Health-care providers' perspectives on uncertainty generated by variant forms of newborn screening targets. *Genet. Med.* **2019**, 1–8. [CrossRef]

35. Chudleigh, J.; Ren, C.L.; Barben, J.; Southern, K.W. International approaches for delivery of positive newborn bloodspot screening results for CF. *J. Cyst. Fibros.* **2019**, *18*, 614–621. [CrossRef]

36. Chudleigh, J.; Chinnery, H.; Bonham, J.R.; Olander, E.K.; Moody, L.; Simpson, A.; Morris, S.; Ulph, F.; Bryon, M.; Southern, K.W. A qualitative exploration of health professionals' experiences of communicating positive newborn bloodspot screening results for nine conditions in England. *BMJ Open* **2020**, in press.

14

The First Year Experience of Newborn Screening for Pompe Disease in California

Hao Tang *, Lisa Feuchtbaum, Stanley Sciortino, Jamie Matteson, Deepika Mathur, Tracey Bishop and Richard S. Olney

Genetic Disease Screening Program, California Department of Public Health, 850 Marina Bay Parkway, MS 8200, USA; lisa.feuchtbaum@cdph.ca.gov (L.F.); stanley.sciortino@cdph.ca.gov (S.S.); jamie.matteson@cdph.ca.gov (J.M.); deepika.mathur@cdph.ca.gov (D.M.); tracey.bishop@cdph.ca.gov (T.B.); richard.olney@cdph.ca.gov (R.S.O.)
* Correspondence: hao.tang@cdph.ca.gov

Abstract: The California Department of Public Health started universal newborn screening for Pompe disease in August 2018 with a two-tier process including: (1) acid alpha-glucosidase (GAA) enzyme activity assay followed by, (2) *GAA* gene sequencing analysis. This study examines results from the first year of screening in a large and diverse screening population. With 453,152 screened newborns, the birth prevalence and GAA enzyme activity associated with various types of Pompe disease classifications are described. The frequency of *GAA* gene mutations and allele variants are reported. Of 88 screen positives, 18 newborns were resolved as Pompe disease, including 2 classic infantile-onset and 16 suspected late-onset form. The c.-32-13T>G variant was the most common pathogenic mutation reported. African American and Asian/Pacific Islander newborns had higher allele frequencies for both pathogenic and pseudodeficiency variants. After the first year of Pompe disease screening in California, the disease distribution in the population is now better understood. With the ongoing long-term follow-up system currently in place, our understanding of the complex genotype-phenotype relationships will become more evident in the future, and this should help us better understand the clinical significance of identified cases.

Keywords: Pompe disease; newborn screening; California

---

1. Introduction

Pompe disease is a sometimes-fatal inherited lysosomal storage disorder caused by the abnormal accumulation of glycogen in cells, which can result in progressive dysfunction of the heart and other muscles. Also known as glycogen storage disease type II, Pompe disease is caused by a deficiency of the acid alpha-glucosidase (GAA) enzyme that breaks down a type of complex sugar, lysosomal glycogen. The birth prevalence of Pompe disease has been estimated to be 1 in 40,000 [1,2], or 25 per 1 million births, although studies from Israel, Taiwan and some parts of the United States reported higher prevalence rates [3–5].

The severity, age of onset, and rate of progression of Pompe disease vary among individuals, who have been generally categorized into three types. The classic infantile-onset Pompe disease (IOPD) shows symptoms within a few months of birth, characterized by fatal cardiomyopathy if untreated. The non-classic infantile-onset form begins before age one, typically with no heart complications. The late-onset Pompe disease (LOPD) appears later in childhood, adolescence, or adulthood [6–8]. The variance in phenotypes has been linked to different *GAA* gene variants, which are the cause for GAA enzyme deficiency. Certain pathogenic variants on both *GAA* alleles severely reduce GAA activity and usually lead to IOPD. On the other hand, some variants of the *GAA* gene exhibit low levels of GAA activity, leading to more moderate forms of Pompe disease [1,9]. To date, enzyme replacement therapy

(ERT) has been the only direct medical treatment for all forms of Pompe disease by reducing GAA deficiency. Treatment beginning as soon as the disease is detected, or as early as possible, can generate the most benefit for patients [10–14].

The clinical work-up of Pompe disease usually involves measuring GAA enzyme activity and molecular analysis to confirm the diagnosis [5,15]. Recent studies have shown that a tandem mass spectrometry (MS/MS)-based GAA enzyme activity assay could be a functional laboratory method for Pompe disease detection [16,17]. The option of multiplex testing for Pompe disease, along with other MS/MS disorders using the same dried blood spot (DBS), helped promote Pompe disease as a viable disorder to add to newborn screening panels [18,19]. The first newborn screening program for Pompe disease was implemented in Taiwan as early as 2005 [20]. Since then, several other countries and U.S. states have conducted pilot screening studies with promising results [5,21–23]. Subsequently, an external condition review workgroup commissioned by the Health Resources and Services Administration examined the evidence for including Pompe disease on the federal Recommended Uniform Screening Panel (RUSP) in 2013 [24]. In 2013, the Advisory Committee on Heritable Disorders in Newborns and Children voted to recommend that the United States Secretary of Health and Human Services add the disorder to the RUSP, which occurred in March 2015 [25]. As of November 2019, 22 states are screening for Pompe disease [26].

The addition of Pompe disease to California's Newborn Screening (NBS) panel followed passage of SB 1095 in the California legislature in 2016 that amended the Health and Safety Code [27,28]. This required the Genetic Disease Screening Program (GDSP) of the California Department of Public Health to add Pompe disease in order to be compliant with the RUSP, and this process has been described in more detail by Bronstein et al. [29]. On August 29, 2018, California began universal screening for Pompe disease.

This paper reports the findings from the first year of population-based Pompe disease screening. We describe our screening and follow-up algorithm as well as epidemiological and clinical outcomes of screening, including disease and variant classification and other characteristics of the Pompe cases identified to date.

2. Materials and Methods

In California, Pompe disease screening is a two-tier process as shown in Figure 1. DBSs are analyzed using flow injection analysis-tandem mass spectrometry (FIA-MS/MS) to measure GAA enzyme activity. Specimens whose GAA enzyme activity levels are below 18% of the daily median are separated into two groups. Those with very low levels, below 10% of the daily median, are immediately called out as screen positive and sent for *GAA* gene sequencing and clinical follow-up, while those with intermediate GAA enzyme levels, between 10% and 18% of the daily median await *GAA* gene sequencing results before the final interpretation is made. The specimens with intermediate GAA enzyme levels are only referred for clinical follow-up if at least one pathogenic variant, likely pathogenic variant or variant of uncertain significance (VUS) is found.

Clinical follow-up is conducted in one of fifteen metabolic specialty care centers across California. The specialty care centers provide genetic counseling, confirmatory testing, diagnosis, and long-term clinical care when appropriate.

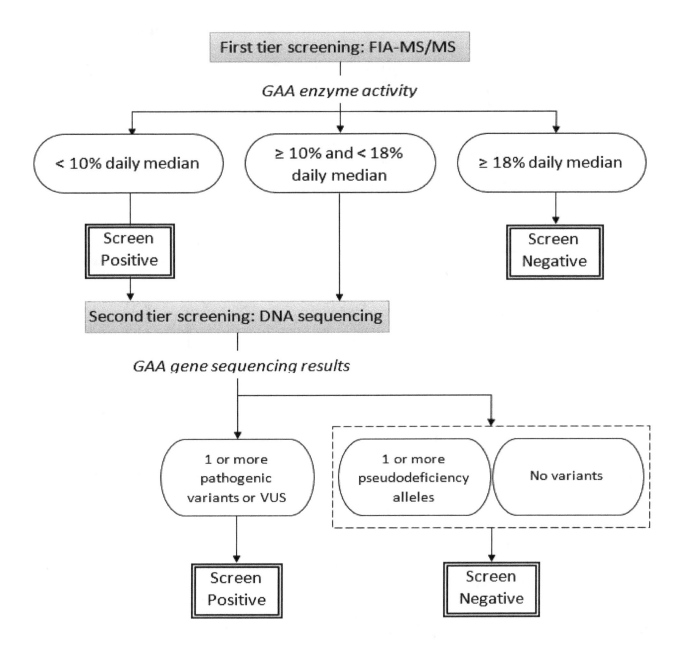

Figure 1. California Pompe disease newborn screening algorithm.

All testing results (biochemical and DNA sequencing), along with demographic information and follow-up reports (short-term follow-up to diagnosis and long-term follow-up for five years), associated with the referred newborns are entered and stored in GDSP's web-based Screening Information System (SIS), including a newborn screening registry that houses all clinically confirmed Pompe disease cases. The categories of the California Pompe disease case resolutions include: (1) classic infantile-onset Pompe disease (with cardiac involvement), (2) non-classic infantile-onset Pompe disease (without cardiac involvement), (3) late-onset Pompe disease, and (4) not-otherwise-specified Pompe disease. After referral, metabolic specialists make the diagnostic decision following established case definitions [30] and general guidelines (Table 1). Newborns who are carriers or who only have pseudodeficiency alleles are also recorded in the registry for reference, but these newborns are not referred for additional clinical follow-up. Variant classification of pathogenic, likely pathogenic, uncertain significance, and pseudodeficiency allele are based on established guidelines with published *GAA* mutations [31–33]. For some of the analyses, we combined late-onset and not-otherwise-specified Pompe disease cases into a "suspected late-onset" category due to the similarities of their diagnostic characteristics (both had no symptoms and had similar GAA levels and variants).

Table 1. California newborn screening Pompe disease diagnosis guideline.

Diagnosis	Mutation Status	Symptoms	Long-Term Follow-Up
Pompe–classic infant onset (with cardiac involvement) *	Pathogenic/likely pathogenic/VUS alleles ** ≥ 2	Yes, with positive cardiac involvement	Yes
Pompe–non-classic infant onset (without cardiac involvement) *	Pathogenic/likely pathogenic/VUS alleles ** ≥ 2	Yes, without positive cardiac involvement	Yes
Pompe–late onset Pompe disease *	Pathogenic/likely pathogenic/VUS alleles ** ≥ 2	No	Yes
Pompe–not otherwise specified *	Pathogenic/likely pathogenic/VUS alleles ** ≥ 2	No	Yes
Pompe–carrier	Pathogenic/likely pathogenic/VUS alleles = 1	No	No
Pompe–pseudodeficiency	Pseudodeficiency alleles	No	No
No disorder	No mutation found	No	No

* Regardless of the presence of pseudodeficiency allele, ** Any combination of pathogenic-pathogenic, pathogenic-likely pathogenic, pathogenic-VUS, likely pathogenic-VUS, and VUS-VUS.

We used California newborn screening data collected from 29 August 2018 through 31 August 2019. We described neonatal characteristics of all screen-positives by disease category. Demographic characteristics included newborns' sex (female, male), nursery type (Neonatal Intensive Care Unit (NICU), non-NICU), and maturity at birth (premature/<37 weeks, term/≥37 weeks). GAA enzyme activity was measured as µmol/L per hour, and the distribution of its percentage of the daily median was examined by Pompe disease categories using a box and whisker plot. We tabulated variant classification distribution across race/ethnicity groups. Race/ethnicity of each newborn was recorded as a multiple-choice check box on the GDSP Test Request Form (TRF). Single ethnic choices on the TRF were recoded to African American, Asian/Pacific Islander (API), Hispanic, non-Hispanic (NH) White, and Other. If multiple categories were reported for a newborn, we used a hierarchy to recode race/ethnicity to a single group following the order of (1) African American, (2) Hispanic, (3) API, (4) NH White, and (5) Other. Native Americans were included in the 'other' category. Variant classification information was reported for all diagnosed cases. Case notes and follow-up reports were abstracted and reviewed for the two classic IOPD patients.

All analyses were performed with SAS/STAT software version 9.4 of the SAS system for Windows (SAS Institute, Cary, NC, USA).

3. Results

3.1. Birth Prevalence

During the study period, 453,152 newborns received genetic disease screening from GDSP. Based on the GAA enzyme activity cutoff (percentage of daily median <18%), 88 newborns were screen positive for Pompe disease and received *GAA* gene sequencing to analyze mutations. Among those referred, two were diagnosed with classic IOPD, and 16 had case resolution of LOPD including 11 late-onset and five not-otherwise-specified Pompe disease, indicating an overall birth prevalence of 1 in 25,200. As of the time of this reporting, we have yet to observe a non-classic IOPD case.

Table 2 shows selected characteristics of 88 Pompe disease screen positives that have a case resolution. Male infants were more likely to be called out as screen positive. Nearly 40% of Pompe disease positive infants were in the NICU when the blood specimens were drawn, while in general, around 10% of infants were in the NICU statewide. Both classic IOPD newborns were in the NICU, and only two suspected LOPD infants needed intensive care. Interestingly, 11 out of 20 pseudodeficiency newborns and 14 of 16 false positive (no mutations found) newborns were in NICUs, suggesting other neonatal factors might play a role in reducing GAA enzyme activity in the absence of a pathogenic *GAA* gene variant. For example, eight out of 20 pseudodeficiency newborns were born prematurely.

Table 2. California Pompe disease screening results (among screen positives) by neonatal factors.

	Classic Infantile-Onset	Suspected Late-Onset	Carrier	Pseudo-Deficiency	No Disorder	Overall
Sex						
Female	1	5	14	11	6	37
Male	1	11	20	9	10	51
Nursery						
NICU	2	1	4	11	14	32
Non-NICU	0	15	30	9	2	56
Maturity						
Premature	1	2	4	8	2	17
Full term	1	14	30	12	14	71
Total	2	16	34	20	16	88
Birth prevalence	5/1,000,000	36/1,000,000	75/1,000,000	45/1,000,000		
	(1 in 226,600)	(1 in 28,300)	(1 in 13,300)	(1 in 22,700)		

3.2. GAA Activities and Pompe Disease Diagnosis

A potential link between GAA activities and forms of Pompe disease was observed. GAA values for the two patients diagnosed as classic IOPD had GAA activity significantly lower than LOPD cases and other non-disease categories (Figure 2). This observation was expected based on the pathogenesis of Pompe disease. Suspected LOPD newborns had lower GAA activity compared to carrier, pseudodeficiency, and false positive categories, although with a wide range.

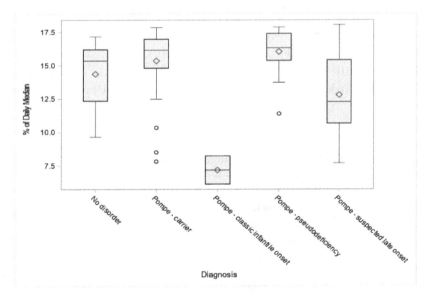

Figure 2. Acid alpha-glucosidase (GAA) activities (% of daily means) by resolution for positive Pompe disease screening.

3.3. GAA Gene Mutations and Allelic Frequency

As shown in Table 3, a total of 120 *GAA* gene variants were reported among the screen-positive cases, including 52 (43.3%) pathogenic variants, 52 (43.3%) pseudodeficiency alleles, and 16 (13.3%) VUS. The c.-32-13T>G variant was the most common pathogenic mutation (34.6% of all pathogenic variants) and was present in 10 of the 16 suspected LOPD cases, followed by c.[752C>T;761C>T]. A homozygous c.1799G>A variant was found in one of the IOPD patients; the c.1979G>A variant and the c.1754+1_1754+12delinsCCA variant were found in the other. The c.[1726G>A;2065G>A] variant was the predominant pseudodeficiency allele (80.8% of all pseudodeficiency variants).

Table 3. Pompe disease variants identified by California newborn screening.

Mutation Name	Count
Pathogenic variant	
c.-32-13T>G	18
c.[752C>T;761C>T] *	8
c.2238G>C, c.1099T>C, c.1799G>A, c.1437+1G>A, c.1548G>A, c.1579delA, c.1754+1_1754+12delinsCCA, c.1856G>A, c.1933G>A, c.1935C>A, c.1979G>A, c.2297A>C *, c.2408_2426del19, c.2560C>T, c.2646+2T>A, c.29delA, c.511del, c.546G>A, c.546G>C, c.573C>A, c.670C>T, c.925G>A	<5
Subtotal	52
Pseudodeficiency allele	
c.[1726G>A;2065G>A]	42
c.2065G>A	5
c.271G>A	5
Subtotal	52
Variant of uncertain significance	
c.1048G>A, c.1019A>G, c.1357G>A, c.1375G>A, c.1392_1393delinsTT, c.1477C>T, c.1757C>T, c.2221G>A, c.2261C>T, c.265C>T, c.266G>A **, c.316C>T, c.546+5G>T, c.726G>A, c.868A>G	<3
Subtotal	16
Total	120

* Noted as presumably non-pathogenic in the updated Pompe variant database: http://pompevariantdatabase.nl. ** Noted as presumably non-pathogenic but pathogenic with a null allele in the updated Pompe variant database: http://pompevariantdatabase.nl.

The overall pathogenic allele frequency was 115 per million (or 1 in 8700) in California's NBS population. Asian and Pacific Islander (API) and African American newborns had relatively higher frequencies (216/1,000,000 and 161/1,000,000, respectively). The overall pseudodeficiency allele frequency was also 115 per million, with API having a significantly higher rate of 432 per million (1 in 2300). Relatively higher frequencies of VUS were found in API and African American as well (Table 4).

Table 4. Allelic frequency by race/ethnicity.

Race/Ethnicity	Pathogenic		Pseudodeficiency Allele		Uncertain Significance	
	Count	Allele Frequency	Count	Allele Frequency	Count	Allele Frequency
African American (*n* = 37,340)	6	161/1,000,000 (1 in 6200)	4	107/1,000,000 (1 in 9300)	3	80/1,000,000 (1 in 12,500)
Asian/Pacific Islander (API, *n* = 69,510)	15	216/1,000,000 (1 in 4600)	30	432/1,000,000 (1 in 2300)	6	86/1,000,000 (1 in 11,600)
Hispanic (*n* = 214,049)	14	66/1,000,000 (1 in 15,300)	7	33/1,000,000 (1 in 30,600)	5	23/1,000,000 (1 in 42,800)
White (*n* = 115,281)	17	148/1,000,000 (1 in 6800)	11	95/1,000,000 (1 in 10,480)	2	17/1,000,000 (1 in 57,600)

3.4. Diagnosed Cases and Case Study of IOPD Patients

Of the 18 infants diagnosed with Pompe disease (IOPD and suspected LOPD), 12 had either a homozygous pathogenic variant or a pair of distinctive pathogenic/likely pathogenic variants (Table 5). The other six had at least one VUS, indicating a less conclusive diagnosis. Three of the 18 diagnosed cases also had a pseudodeficiency allele.

Table 5. Mutation status of diagnosed cases identified by California newborn screening.

Diagnosis	Number of Cases	Mutation Status
Pompe—classic infantile onset	1	Pathogenic, homozygous
	1	Pathogenic & pathogenic
Pompe—suspected late onset	3	Pathogenic, homozygous
	7	Pathogenic & Pathogenic/likely pathogenic
	4	Pathogenic & VUS
	1	VUS, homozygous
	1	VUS & VUS

We examined the testing results and follow-up reports on the two IOPD cases.

Case 1: This is an infant with homozygous pathogenic variant c.1799G>A, a known pathogenic mutation linked to IOPD [33,34]. The GAA confirmatory test showed "markedly reduced" enzyme activity. Further confirmatory testing showed urine glucose tetrasaccharide quantitation (Hex4) was elevated. Hypertrophic cardiomyopathy and arrhythmia were noted on the service report provided by the metabolic specialty care center clinical staff. ERT was started at two months of age.

Case 2: This is an infant with two heterozygous pathogenic variants. The c.1979G>A variant has been associated with both IOPD and LOPD [35,36]; and the c.1754+1_1754+12delinsCCA variant has no reported link to Pompe disease but was deemed as disease-causing in general [37]. Confirmatory tests found reduced GAA enzyme activity and mildly elevated Hex4. Abnormal echocardiogram and electrocardiogram results, as well as hypertrophic cardiomyopathy, were reported at the time of diagnosis. We confirmed that ERT was started but the exact starting age was unclear.

4. Discussion

The present study is one of the first reports on statewide Pompe disease screening outcomes after its placement on the RUSP, especially with a relatively large population base. California GDSP screened almost half a million babies in its first year (2018–2019) and of those referred, indicated a birth prevalence of 1 in 25,200 (IOPD and LOPD combined), which is within the range of previously reported prevalence. However, due to the rare occurrence of the disorder in the general population, only a small number of cases were reported, thus limiting the accuracy of birth prevalence calculation. With only two cases of IOPD, the birth prevalence in California (approximately 1 in 250,000) was lower than in other regions (1 in 138,000 in the Netherlands [38], 1 in 50,000 Taiwan [4,6], or 1 in 4500 in Maroon population of French Guiana [39]). However, the prevalence of potential LOPD (approximately 1 in 37,500) seems to be higher than the previously reported prevalence among the Dutch population (1 in 57,000) [38], but lower than that of Taiwan (approximately 1 in 25,000) [6]. Based on the birth prevalence of diagnosed Pompe disease cases, the calculated carrier frequency using the Hardy-Weinberg principle indicates more than five thousand carriers in our screened population. The number of carriers (34) identified from NBS was significantly fewer than that estimate because the cutoff of GAA activity in NBS aims at identifying Pompe disease cases, which have significantly lower GAA enzyme activity than that of carriers.

Six of the 16 suspected LOPD cases had at least one VUS, and since none of them have exhibited symptoms, some of their diagnoses could be changed to carrier, pseudodeficiency or no disorder based on the future clinical follow-up results. The inherent uncertainty of VUS results leads clinicians to cautiously diagnose a late-onset disorder, but affected children and their families might endure years of anxiety due to the unknown pathogenicity and consequence of the molecular findings [40]. Except when symptoms are clearly identified and a diagnosis has been made by a specialist, our observations are preliminary and incomplete given the short follow-up period of this study.

The diagnosis of Pompe disease identified by NBS is largely based on the results from molecular analysis along with supportive confirmatory testing, especially for patients who have not exhibited any symptoms. The high occurrence of the pathogenic c.-32-13T>G variant in our screen positive samples (40.4% of all pathogenic variants) echoed findings from literature, which reported an allelic frequency from 40% to 70% [41]. For newly screened rare disorders with late-onset phenotypes like Pompe disease, one of the greatest challenges for screening is the VUS category in which cases have an unknown pathogenic molecular profile. Some VUS may eventually be recognized as pathogenic, but barriers to receiving a thorough clinical work-up or ongoing clinical follow-up (such as factors associated with access to care), could play a role in obtaining a more definitive diagnosis later. With a more developed global registry and variant database [32,34] future screening could yield more predictive results.

California has a vastly diverse population. In our study, Pompe disease-positive newborns with Asian and Pacific Islander (API) ancestry had a high occurrence of pseudodeficiency alleles, especially the c.[1726G>A;2065G>A] variant, which represents 80% of all the pseudodeficiency mutations. This finding confirmed the results from other studies with Asian populations [22,42,43]. Unlike these other studies, we did not find any Pompe disease cases (IOPD or LOPD) among nearly 70,000 API newborns, and we only found one c.1935C>A (linked to c.[1726G>A;2065G>A]), which was identified as the most common pathogenic *GAA* variants among Asian countries. African American newborns had a birth prevalence of 54 per million (or 1 in 18,700), which was the highest among all groups. This result may be indicative of a potentially high Pompe disease birth prevalence among African Americans, but more data are needed to be conclusive. Previous research identified c.2560C>T as the most common *GAA* variant among African Americans [34,44]. We did not have a large enough sample size ($n = 7$) of African American infants who had variants to confirm the finding. The only c.2560C>T variant, however, was indeed detected in an African American sample.

In most of the study period (before 21 August 2019), every newborn with GAA activity $\leq$ 18% of the daily median was flagged as an urgent call-out by the laboratory before the results of *GAA* gene sequencing was available. About six months after the Pompe disease newborn screening began, NBS received communications from clinical specialists about the follow-up burden for both patients and providers due to the large number of patients being referred; many of them were either pseudodeficiency or no mutation based on the sequencing findings. Although previous research showed that MS/MS analysis of GAA activity could separate pseudodeficiency and Pompe disease cases [45], our screening test results still showed some overlap in GAA activity for these two groups. GDSP evaluated the available data and modified the protocol in August 2019 to flag only the cases with GAA activity less than 10% of the daily median for urgent call-out (the two IOPD cases identified through the program were well-below this threshold). Newborns with GAA activities between 10% and 18% of the daily median are only referred if the molecular results show pathogenic, likely pathogenic, or VUS mutations. In other words, we wait so that screen-positive newborns with homozygous or heterozygous pseudodeficiency alleles or no mutations are not referred to the specialty care centers for further follow-up. This serves as a good example of how synergy between providers and the newborn screening program minimized the unnecessary referrals and improved screening performance. If we later find infants who have GAA activities between 10% and 18% of the daily median diagnosed with IOPD, we will consider adjusting the cutoff again for urgent call-outs.

More than four years after Pompe disease was added to the RUSP, the adoption and implementation of newborn screening at the state level has been at a moderate pace. In the first year of Pompe disease newborn screening in California, we have gained a better understanding of the disease distribution at the population level, and most importantly, now have experience and evidence to support effective screening. With a robust long-term follow-up component, GDSP values the necessity of monitoring all potential cases, including those with a VUS [46]. The growing knowledge from long-term follow-up will further improve our understanding of the clinical significance of these cases, especially when case management algorithms are still undeveloped for asymptomatic patients [47].

While the two newborns with IOPD were identified while in the NICU, almost all of the newborns with LOPD were identified in the regular nursery. These newborns were asymptomatic and unlikely to be identified as at risk for Pompe disease except by screening. Now that treatment is warranted before symptoms develop, the value of population-based screening is clear: to identify the youngest candidates for treatments that can reduce life-long disability [48].

Author Contributions: Conceptualization, R.S.O., H.T., L.F., and S.S.; methodology, H.T. and S.S.; formal analysis, H.T. and J.M.; resources, T.B.; Data curation, H.T., J.M., and D.M.; writing—original draft preparation, H.T.; writing—review and editing, L.F., S.S., J.M., and D.M.; visualization, H.T., J.M., and S.S.; supervision, L.F. and R.S.O.; project administration, T.B. All authors have read and agreed to the published version of the manuscript.

Acknowledgments: We want to extend our thanks to the staff at the Genetic Disease Laboratory who conduct Pompe disease testing and interpretation of test results as well as to the staff at Perkin-Elmer Life Sciences who conduct the genomic sequencing of screen-positive cases. We also want to thank the staff at the state-contracted California Metabolic Special Care Centers who provide follow-up diagnostic services for referred newborns and the data for our ongoing program evaluation efforts.

References

1. Reuser, A.J.J.; Hirschhorn, R.; Kroos, M.A. Pompe Disease: Glycogen storage disease type II: Acid α-glucosidase (acid maltase) deficiency. In *The Online Metabolic and Molecular Bases of Inherited Disease*; Valle, D., Antonarakis, S., Ballabio, A., Eds.; McGraw-Hill: New York, NY, USA, 2018.

2. Martiniuk, F.; Chen, A.; Mack, A.; Arvanitopoulos, E.; Chen, Y.; Rom, W.N.; Codd, W.J.; Hanna, B.; Alcabes, P.; Raben, N.; et al. Carrier frequency for glycogen storage disease type II in New York and estimates of affected individuals born with the disease. *Am. J. Med. Genet.* **1998**, *79*, 69–72. [CrossRef]

3. Bashan, N.; Potashnik, R.; Barash, V.; Gutman, A.; Moses, S.W. Glycogen storage disease type II in Israel. *Isr. J. Med. Sci.* **1988**, *24*, 224–227.

4. Chiang, S.C.; Hwu, W.L.; Lee, N.C.; Hsu, L.W.; Chien, Y.H. Algorithm for Pompe disease newborn screening: Results from the Taiwan screening program. *Mol. Genet. Metab.* **2012**, *106*, 281–286. [CrossRef]

5. Scott, C.R.; Elliott, S.; Buroker, N.; Thomas, L.I.; Keutzer, J.; Glass, M.; Gelb, M.H.; Turecek, F. Identification of infants at risk for developing Fabry, Pompe, or mucopolysaccharidosis-I from newborn blood spots by tandem mass spectrometry. *J. Pediatr.* **2013**, *163*, 498–503. [CrossRef]

6. Chien, Y.H.; Lee, N.C.; Huang, H.J.; Thurberg, B.L.; Tsai, F.J.; Hwu, W.L. Later-onset Pompe disease: Early detection and early treatment initiation enabled by newborn screening. *J. Pediatr.* **2011**, *158*, 1023–1027. [CrossRef]

7. Dasouki, M.; Jawdat, O.; Almadhoun, O.; Pasnoor, M.; McVey, A.L.; Abuzinadah, A.; Herbelin, L.; Barohn, R.J.; Dimachkie, M.M. Pompe disease: Literature review and case series. *Neurol. Clin.* **2014**, *32*, 751–776. [CrossRef]

8. Van den Hout, H.M.; Hop, W.; van Diggelen, O.P.; Smeitink, J.A.; Smit, G.P.; Poll-The, B.T.; Bakker, H.D.; Loonen, M.C.; de Klerk, J.B.; Reuser, A.J.; et al. The natural course of infantile Pompe's disease: 20 original cases compared with 133 cases from the literature. *Pediatrics* **2003**, *112*, 332–340. [CrossRef]

9. Umapathysivam, K.; Hopwood, J.J.; Meikle, P.J. Correlation of acid alpha-glucosidase and glycogen content in skin fibroblasts with age of onset in Pompe disease. *Clin. Chim. Acta* **2005**, *361*, 191–198. [CrossRef]

10. Chien, Y.H.; Hwu, W.L.; Lee, N.C. Pompe disease: Early diagnosis and early treatment make a difference. *Pediatr. Neonatol.* **2013**, *54*, 219–227. [CrossRef]

11. Lai, C.J.; Hsu, T.R.; Yang, C.F.; Chen, S.J.; Chuang, Y.C.; Niu, D.M. Cognitive development in infantile-Onset Pompe disease under very early enzyme replacement therapy. *J. Child. Neurol.* **2016**, *31*, 1617–1621. [CrossRef]

12. Tarnopolsky, M.; Katzberg, H.; Petrof, B.J.; Sirrs, S.; Sarnat, H.B.; Myers, K.; Dupre, N.; Dodig, D.; Genge, A.; Venance, S.L.; et al. Pompe disease: Diagnosis and management. Evidence-based guidelines from a Canadian expert panel. *Can. J. Neurol. Sci.* **2016**, *43*, 472–485. [CrossRef] [PubMed]

13. Kronn, D.F.; Day-Salvatore, D.; Hwu, W.L.; Jones, S.A.; Nakamura, K.; Okuyama, T.; Swoboda, K.J.; Kishnani, P.S. Pompe Disease Newborn Screening Working Group. Management of confirmed newborn-Screened patients with Pompe disease across the disease spectrum. *Pediatrics* **2017**, *140*, S24–S45.

14. Ortolano, R.; Baronio, F.; Masetti, R.; Prete, A.; Cassio, A.; Pession, A. Letter to the Editors: Concerning "Divergent clinical outcomes of alphaglucosidase enzyme replacement therapy in two siblings with infantile-onset Pompe disease treated in the symptomatic or pre-symptomatic state" by Takashi M et al. *Mol. Genet. Metab. Rep.* **2017**, *11*, 1. [CrossRef] [PubMed]

15. Umapathysivam, K.; Whittle, A.M.; Ranieri, E.; Bindloss, C.; Ravenscroft, E.M.; van Diggelen, O.P.; Hopwood, J.J.; Meikle, P.J. Determination of acid alpha-Glucosidase protein: Evaluation as a screening marker for Pompe disease and other lysosomal storage disorders. *Clin. Chem.* **2000**, *46*, 1318–1325. [CrossRef] [PubMed]

16. Gelb, M.H.; Turecek, F.; Scott, C.R.; Chamoles, N.A. Direct multiplex assay of enzymes in dried blood spots by tandem mass spectrometry for the newborn screening of lysosomal storage disorders. *J. Inherit. Metab. Dis.* **2006**, *29*, 397–404. [CrossRef] [PubMed]

17. Spacil, Z.; Tatipaka, H.; Barcenas, M.; Scott, C.R.; Turecek, F.; Gelb, M.H. High-Throughput assay of 9 lysosomal enzymes for newborn screening. *Clin. Chem.* **2013**, *59*, 502–511. [CrossRef]

18. Gucciardi, A.; Legnini, E.; Di Gangi, I.M.; Corbetta, C.; Tomanin, R.; Scarpa, M.; Giordano, G. A column-Switching HPLC-MS/MS method for mucopolysaccharidosis type I analysis in a multiplex assay for the simultaneous newborn screening of six lysosomal storage disorders. *Biomed. Chromatogr.* **2014**, *28*, 1131–1139. [CrossRef]

19. Tortorelli, S.; Turgeon, C.T.; Gavrilov, D.K.; Oglesbee, D.; Raymond, K.M.; Rinaldo, P.; Matern, D. Simultaneous testing for 6 lysosomal storage disorders and x-Adrenoleukodystrophy in dried blood spots by tandem mass spectrometry. *Clin. Chem.* **2016**, *62*, 1248–1254. [CrossRef]

20. Chien, Y.H.; Chiang, S.C.; Zhang, X.K.; Keutzer, J.; Lee, N.C.; Huang, A.C.; Chen, C.A.; Wu, M.H.; Huang, P.H.; Tsai, F.J.; et al. Early detection of Pompe disease by newborn screening is feasible: Results from the Taiwan screening program. *Pediatrics* **2008**, *122*, e39–e45. [CrossRef]

21. Burton, B.K. Newborn screening for Pompe disease: An update, 2011. *Am. J. Med. Genet. C. Semin. Med. Genet.* **2012**, *160C*, 8–12. [CrossRef]

22. Momosaki, K.; Kido, J.; Yoshida, S.; Sugawara, K.; Miyamoto, T.; Inoue, T.; Okumiya, T.; Matsumoto, S.; Endo, F.; Hirose, S.; et al. Newborn screening for Pompe disease in Japan: Report and literature review of mutations in the GAA gene in Japanese and Asian patients. *J. Hum. Genet.* **2019**, *64*, 741–755. [CrossRef]

23. Wittmann, J.; Karg, E.; Turi, S.; Legnini, E.; Wittmann, G.; Giese, A.K.; Lukas, J.; Golnitz, U.; Klingenhager, M.; Bodamer, O.; et al. Newborn screening for lysosomal storage disorders in hungary. *JIMD Rep.* **2012**, *6*, 117–125. [PubMed]

24. Kemper, A.R. Condition Review Workgroup Evidence Report: Newborn Screening for Pompe Disease. Available online: https://www.hrsa.gov/sites/default/files/hrsa/advisory-committees/heritable-disorders/rusp/previous-nominations/pompe-external-evidence-review-report-2013.pdf (accessed on 14 November 2019).

25. Advisory Committee on Heritable Disorders in Newborns and Children. Recommended Uniform Screening Panel [As of July 2018]. Available online: http://www.hrsa.gov/advisorycommittees/mchbadvisory/heritabledisorders/recommendedpanel (accessed on 14 November 2019).

26. The Newborn Screening Technical Assistance and Evaluation Program (NewSTEPs), Association of Public Health Laboratories. Disorders Screening Status Map: Pompe. Available online: https://www.newsteps.org/resources/newborn-screening-status-all-disorders (accessed on 14 November 2019).

27. California State Legislature. Senate Bill No.1095: Newborn Screening Program. 2016. Available online: https://leginfo.legislature.ca.gov/faces/billTextClient.xhtml?bill_id=201520160SB1095 (accessed on 14 November 2019).

28. Califorina Health and Safety Code, Sections 125001, amended 2016. Available online: https://leginfo.legislature.ca.gov/faces/codes_displayText.xhtml?lawCode=HSC&division=106.&title=&part=5.&chapter=1.&article=2 (accessed on 19 December 2019).

29. Bronstein, M.G.; Pan, R.J.; Dant, M.; Lubin, B. Leveraging evidence-Based public policy and advocacy to advance newborn screening in California. *Pediatrics* **2019**, *143*, e20181886. [CrossRef] [PubMed]

30. The Newborn Screening Technical Assistance and Evaluation Program (NewSTEPs), Association of Public Health Laboratories. NewSTEPs Data Repository Case Definition. Available online: https://www.newsteps.org/case-definitions (accessed on 21 November 2019).

31. Richards, S.; Aziz, N.; Bale, S.; Bick, D.; Das, S.; Gastier-Foster, J.; Grody, W.W.; Hegde, M.; Lyon, E.; Spector, E.; et al. Standards and guidelines for the interpretation of sequence variants: A joint consensus recommendationof the American College of Medical Genetics and Genomics and the Association for Molecular Pathology. *Genet. Med.* **2015**, *17*, 405–424. [CrossRef] [PubMed]

32. Nino, M.Y.; in't Groen, S.L.M.; Bergsma, A.J.; van der Beek, N.A.M.E.; Kroos, M.; Hoogeveen-Westerveld, M.; van der Ploeg, A.T.; Pijnappel, W.W.M.P. Extension of the Pompe mutation database by linking disease-Associated variants to clinical severity. *Hum. Mutat.* **2019**, *40*, 1954–1967. [CrossRef] [PubMed]

33. Reuser, A.J.J.; van der Ploeg, A.T.; Chien, Y.H.; Llerena, J., Jr.; Abbott, M.A.; Clemens, P.R.; Kimonis, V.E.; Leslie, N.; Maruti, S.S.; Sanson, B.J.; et al. GAA variants and phenotypes among 1,079 patients with Pompe disease: Data from the Pompe Registry. *Hum. Mut.* **2019**, *40*, 2146–2164. [CrossRef]

34. Herzog, A.; Hartung, R.; Reuser, A.J.; Hermanns, P.; Runz, H.; Karabul, N.; Gokce, S.; Pohlenz, J.; Kampmann, C.; Lampe, C.; et al. A cross-Sectional single-centre study on the spectrum of Pompe disease, German patients: Molecular analysis of the GAA gene, manifestation and genotype-phenotype correlations. *Orphanet J. Rare Dis.* **2012**, *7*, 35. [CrossRef]

35. Burrow, T.A.; Bailey, L.A.; Kinnett, D.G.; Hopkin, R.J. Acute progression of neuromuscular findings in infantile Pompe disease. *Pediatr. Neurol.* **2010**, *42*, 455–458. [CrossRef]

36. Nazari, F.; Sinaei, F.; Nilipour, Y.; Fatehi, F.; Streubel, B.; Ashrafi, M.R.; Aryani, O.; Nafissi, S. Late-Onset pompe disease in Iran: A clinical and genetic report. *Muscle Nerve* **2017**, *55*, 835–840. [CrossRef]

37. Lek, M.; Karczewski, K.J.; Minikel, E.V.; Samocha, K.E.; Banks, E.; Fennell, T.; O'Donnell-Luria, A.H.; Ware, J.S.; Hill, A.J.; Cummings, B.B.; et al. Analysis of protein-Coding genetic variation in 60,706 humans. *Nature* **2016**, *536*, 285–291. [CrossRef]

38. Ausems, M.G.; Verbiest, J.; Hermans, M.P.; Kroos, M.A.; Beemer, F.A.; Wokke, J.H.; Sandkuijl, L.A.; Reuser, A.J.; van der Ploeg, A.T. Frequency of glycogen storage disease type II in The Netherlands: Implications for diagnosis and genetic counselling. *Eur. J. Hum. Genet.* **1999**, *7*, 713–716. [CrossRef]

39. Elenga, N.; Verloes, A.; Mrsic, Y.; Basurko, C.; Schaub, R.; Cuadro-Alvarez, E.; Kom-Tchameni, R.; Carles, G.; Lambert, V.; Boukhari, R.; et al. Incidence of infantile Pompe disease in the Maroon population of French Guiana. *BMJ Paediatr. Open* **2018**, *2*, e000182. [CrossRef] [PubMed]

40. Pruniski, B.; Lisi, E.; Ali, N. Newborn screening for Pompe disease: Impact on families. *J. Inherit. Metab. Dis.* **2018**, *41*, 1189–1203. [CrossRef] [PubMed]

41. Peruzzo, P.; Pavan, E.; Dardis, A. Molecular genetics of Pompe disease: A comprehensive overview. *Ann. Transl. Med.* **2019**, *7*, 278. [CrossRef] [PubMed]

42. Kroos, M.A.; Mullaart, R.A.; Van Vliet, L.; Pomponio, R.J.; Amartino, H.; Kolodny, E.H.; Pastores, G.M.; Wevers, R.A.; Van der Ploeg, A.T.; Halley, D.J.; et al. p.[G576S.; E689K]: Pathogenic combination or polymorphism in Pompe disease? *Eur. J. Hum. Genet.* **2008**, *16*, 875–879. [CrossRef] [PubMed]

43. Lee, J.H.; Shin, J.H.; Park, H.J.; Kim, S.Z.; Jeon, Y.M.; Kim, H.K.; Kim, D.S.; Choi, Y.C. Targeted population screening of late onset Pompe disease in unspecified myopathy patients for Korean population. *Neuromuscul. Disord.* **2017**, *27*, 550–556. [CrossRef]

44. Becker, J.A.; Vlach, J.; Raben, N.; Nagaraju, K.; Adams, E.M.; Hermans, M.M.; Reuser, A.J.; Brooks, S.S.; Tifft, C.J.; Hirschhorn, R.; et al. The African origin of the common mutatoin in African American patients with glycogen-Storage disease type II. *Am. J. Hum. Genet.* **1998**, *62*, 991–994. [CrossRef]

45. Liao, H.C.; Chan, M.J.; Yang, C.F.; Chiang, C.C.; Niu, D.M.; Huang, C.K.; Gelb, M.H. Mass spectrometry but not fluorimetry distinguisheds affected and pseudodeficiencies in newborn screening for Pompe disease. *Clin. Chem.* **2017**, *63*, 1271–1277. [CrossRef]

46. Feuchtbaum, L.; Yang, J.; Currier, R. Follow-Up status during the first 5 years of life for metabolic disorders on the federal Recommended Uniform Screening Panel. *Genet. Med.* **2018**, *20*, 831–839. [CrossRef]

47. Kemper, A.R.; Boyle, C.A.; Brosco, J.P.; Grosse, S.D. Ensuring the life-Span benefits of newborn screening. *Pediatrics* **2019**, *144*, e20190904. [CrossRef]

48. Yang, C.F.; Yang, C.C.; Liao, H.C.; Huang, L.Y.; Chiang, C.C.; Ho, H.C.; Lai, C.J.; Chu, T.H.; Yang, T.F.; Hsu, T.R.; et al. Very early treatment for infantile-Onset Pompe disease contributes to better outcomes. *J. Pediatr.* **2016**, *169*, 174–180. [CrossRef]

15

Newborn Sickle Cell Disease Screening Using Electrospray Tandem Mass Spectrometry

Yvonne Daniel [1,]* **and Charles Turner** [2]

[1]   Viapath, Guy's & St Thomas Hospital, London SE17EH, UK
[2]   WellChild Laboratory, Evelina London Children's Hospital, London SE17EH, UK;
      Charles.turner@gstt.nhs.uk
*   Correspondence: yvonne.daniel@viapath.co.uk

Abstract: There is a growing demand for newborn sickle cell disease screening globally. Historically techniques have relied on the separation of intact haemoglobin tetramers using electrophoretic or liquid chromatography techniques. These techniques also identify haemoglobin variants of no clinical significance. Specific electrospray ionization-mass spectrometry-mass spectrometry techniques to analyse targeted peptides formed after digestion of the haemoglobin with trypsin were reported in 2005. Since this time the method has been further developed and adopted in several European countries. It is estimated that more than one million babies have been screened with no false-negative cases reported. This review reports on the current use of the technique and reviews the related publications.

Keywords: screening; sickle cell disease; newborn; mass spectrometry

---

1. Introduction

The first report of newborn screening for sickle cell disease (SCD) by mass spectrometry (MS) utilised matrix-assisted laser desorption-time of flight (MALDI-TOF) [1]. Intact haemoglobin chains were initially analysed followed by mass mapping of trypsin-active MS targets to localise the mutation site. This proof of concept had not translated into large-scale trials or prospective screening until recently. Newborn screening using MALDI-TOF is covered in a separate article in this issue and it will not be reviewed further here. The other ionisation mode for MS in common use is electrospray ionisation (ESI). ESI of undigested haemoglobin produces a large number of multiply charged ions, formed in the source when charged droplets are dried in the presence of an inert gas such as nitrogen. The ions formed can then be analysed.

Wild et al. [2] reported the use of ESI-MS to analyse intact globin chains in 147 newborn blood spots. The protocol utilised software to produce a deconvoluted profile spectrum displaying the α, β, and γ globin peaks along with peaks of variant haemoglobins with a mass shift sufficiently different from normal to allow resolution. This allowed detection of sickle globin and other variants with a mass difference of −30 daltons (Da) from normal β chains but did not clearly resolve those clinically significant variants with a mass difference of 1 Da. The method was not specific for Hb S, as there are 5 amino acid substitutions which result in a mass difference of 30 Da. The authors concluded that the technique allowed for detection of sickle cell disease, but samples found to have a positive signal for Hb S would require confirmation by an alternate technique. No large-scale trial of this ESI-MS approach has been published. In 2005, Daniel et al. [3] published the first report of a targeted ESI-MSMS approach, based on tryptic digestion. Developments of this method have been widely adopted into active newborn screening programmes and are the main subject of this review.

2. The MSMS (Tandem Mass Spectrometry) Technique

ESI coupled to tandem mass spectrometry (MSMS), in which ions formed are selected in a first quadrupole (Q1), product ions are produced via collision in Q2 and detected in Q3, is in common use in newborn screening for small molecules such as amino acids and acylcarnitiines. The 2005 paper of Daniel et al. [3] achieved targeted detection of haemoglobin variants including clinically significant variants with 1 Da mass difference from normal using ESI-MSMS with a series of experiments run simultaneously on whole blood samples digested with trypsin. Trypsin cleaves peptide bonds adjacent to arginine and lysine residues producing a predictable and reproduceable series of peptide fragments. As the clinically significant haemoglobin variants have been well characterised, the amino acid sequences are known along with the expected mass differences from normal. The target beta chain haemoglobin variants were Hb S and Hb C, Hb D^{Punjab} and Hb O^{Arab}, and Hb E which occur in tryptic peptides (T) 1, 13, and 3 respectively. Selected reaction monitoring experiments were designed to select the required tryptic peptide in Q1 and a specific fragmentation ion in Q3 generated following collision induced fragmentation in Q2. Experiments were designed for wildtype and the designated haemoglobin variants. Unlike the previous method using intact chains, this method was targeted and highly specific. Additionally, the use of ESI-MSMS allowed rationalisation of equipment and better use of existing resources. The tryptic digestion had been simplified by the demonstration that informative peptides were produced within 30–45 min and that chemical denaturation of the protein or purification of haemoglobin prior to the addition of trypsin was unnecessary. A patent was awarded to the final method in 2006. The method of Daniel et al. [3] was commercialised by SpOtOn Clinical Diagnostics from 2013, and CE-marked reagent kits were made available in 2015. The kits include stable isotope-labeled Hb S peptide and trypsin, and peptide standards for instrument optimization are also available from the company. Dried blood spot samples are punched (3 mm spot), stable isotope and trypsin are added, and the samples incubated at 37 °C for 30 min. Following the addition of mobile phase to stop the reaction and act as diluent, samples are introduced into the MSMS using flow injection (without chromatography). The method utilizes simple acetonitrile/water/formic acid mobile phases as used for newborn screening for amino acids and acyl carnitines. The stable isotope-labeled Hb S allows sample-by-sample assurance of trypsin activity and MSMS performance.

3. Review of Published Results

The initial method was validated in a project funded by the NHS Sickle Cell & Thalassaemia Screening programme, which compared newborn blood spots analysed by the existing isoelectric focussing technique (IEF) in Leeds with the ESI-MSMS technique [4]. Over 40,000 blood spots were tested between August 2007 and August 2008. The results were analysed by reviewing the abundance ratio of the variant peptide to the corresponding wild-type peptide with no discrepant results observed, shown in Table 1.

Subsequently Boemer et al. [5] reported the results of 2082 newborn samples screened using a slightly modified MSMS method with the same principle. Results were compared with IEF and high performance liquid chromatography (HPLC). Only haemoglobins S, C, E, and wild-type β and γ were targeted with multiple experiments for each haemoglobin of interest. No discrepancies were reported. In 2011, the group reported a review of three years' experience presenting the results of 43,736 newborn samples [6]. First-line MSMS analysis identified 444 samples as screen-positive. All were confirmed using molecular techniques. The paper also reported ranges obtained for the amalgamated ratio data of the variant to corresponding wild-type peptides as well as the β to γ peptides used to screen for β thalassaemia disease. These showed clear discrimination between unaffected and affected cases within each of the investigated disease categories, as well as carriers for the haemoglobin variants. The group noted the lack of an experiment to detect Hb Bart's and therefore possible Hb H disease and noted the possibility that Hb S co-inherited with other clinically significant variants not targeted in the experimental protocol would have a result pattern identical to that of a sickle carrier.

Table 1. Results of comparison of blood spots and the isoelectric focussing technique (IEF).

Haemoglobins Detected	Number (*n*)
Total samples tested	40,054
No abnormality detected	39,710
FS	9
FSC	3
FC	1
FAS	187
FAC	38
FAD^{Punjab}	49
FAE	47
FAO^{Arab}	0
Wild-type β absent [#]	4

F = fetal; A = adult/wild type; [#] all subsequently confirmed as β thalassaemia disease.

Moat et al. [7] used the SpOtOn kit method in a study to inform the introduction of newborn screening for sickle cell disease in Wales. The published protocol built on the use of ratios and utilised locked software algorithms to screen for sickle cell and β thalassaemia disease, the latter as a clinically significant by-product. The only parameters available and routinely reviewed by the operator were those required to check for appropriate tryptic sample digestion, prematurity, and transfusion status. The developed algorithms prevented the identification of most sickle cell carriers and all carriers and homozygotes of C, D^{Punjab}, O^{Arab}, and E, as the operator was not alerted to the results of these experiments unless Hb S was detected at levels above the designated ratio action values. Ratio action values were set using the residual blood spots of 2154 normal and 675 known positive cases and were subsequently evaluated using 13,249 blood spots run in parallel with HPLC. The protocol identified some Hb S carriers as ratio action values were set sufficiently low to ensure that all possible cases of coinheritance of Hb S and β plus thalassaemia were detected. Unblinding of the data revealed a further 328 cases of infants who were carriers of either Hb S, C, D^{Punjab}, or E, which had not been identified to the operator using the locked protocol. As the protocol is designed not to identify cases that are carriers of Hb S, it does not permit the detection of rare Hb variants that interact with Hb S. As these rare mutations are not targeted in the protocol, only the sickle mutation will be detected, giving screening results that mimic that of a sickle carrier. Examples include Hb Maputo and Hb North Shore.

An update and three-year review of the Welsh screening programme was published in 2017 [8]. At the time of writing, 100,456 babies had been screened using the protocol. Findings were similar to those of previous studies (10 true-positive sickle cell disease cases and 6 false positives) with no false negatives reported. The latter six cases were sickle cell carriers with results that fell above the action value in the Welsh Programme, which aims to detect only sickle cell disease. Such cases are considered to be false positives. The protocol had been transferred successfully to a second instrument maintaining the set action values, which correlated well with values established by the Public Health England (PHE) Sickle Cell & Thalassaemia screening programme [9]. Work had also been carried out to correlate observed ratios of the γ and β chain ratios to gestational age in premature samples and to age after birth. These ratios were used to guide interpretation of results obtained and to reduce the number of samples referred unnecessarily for second testing.

This work was overlapped by a multi-centre pilot study carried out by the PHE Sickle Cell & Thalassaemia screening programme during 2012 and 2013 [10,11]. The aim of the study was to investigate integration of the SpOtOn Clinical Diagnostics method into routine screening services, determine if common action values could be established for all manufacturers and laboratories, and assess consistency with existing methods. Four laboratories participated in the study; 23,878 samples were analysed using either ABI Sciex AP4000 (2 laboratories) or Waters Micromass (Xevo TQMS (1 laboratory) and Premier (1 laboratory) instruments. The study was unable to recommend the use of the latter instrument in this context, as false-positive rates were unacceptably high due to variable ratios. The need to replicate existing practice and ensure consistency with existing methods (HPLC, capillary electrophoresis (CE), and IEF) required the detection of carriers of the targeted haemoglobin variants as well as beta thalassaemia disease. Common action values were set for all experiments with the exception of Hb C, which has manufacturer-specific values [9].

The programme operates a two-test protocol such that results are only reported following second testing, so conservative action values were set to minimise the likelihood of false-negative results from the first line test. The action values are available online [9] and subject to ongoing review and optimisation with laboratories who have implemented the method. At the time of writing, three English newborn screening laboratories have implemented the protocol with a further three actively assessing the method. Over 150 positive cases have been identified in a cohort of approximately 250,000 babies.

The protocol has also been investigated for use in a German setting with 29,079 newborn samples screened as part of an evaluation project carried out between November 2015 and September 2016 in Berlin [12]. Samples were analysed in parallel with CE, with 100% concordance reported. Samples positive for sickle cell disease ($n = 7$) were also confirmed by molecular techniques. The authors have concluded that MSMS is a suitable technique for newborn screening in Germany, citing the benefits of the existing expertise in MSMS techniques as well as the ability to use software algorithms to only find sickle cell disease cases. This is in keeping with the requirements of their genetic testing act, which prohibits the testing of minors for heterozygous states considered to be not relevant in childhood or adolescence [12].

4. Summary

The development of ESI-MSMS for newborn sickle cell disease screening was driven by the concept that rationalization of resource within newborn screening laboratories would be of benefit in a health care environment where there is increasing pressure on equipment, cost, and workforce skill mix. The protocol uses the same equipment as that used for newborn metabolic screening. Initial set up is more time-consuming when compared to HPLC, and is similar to IEF, however analysis and result interpretation time is significantly reduced, particularly if software algorithms are used to scrutinize the data. This also has the advantage of removing operator-dependent variability. The method is targeted and more specific than existing procedures, whilst the inherent flexibility has enabled users to develop protocols that fit with local practice and requirements. Reported sensitivity for Hb S is 100%, where this data is presented [4,11,12]. Costs vary according to laboratory arrangements but are comparable with other available techniques.

Since the first report of the procedure in 2005 [3], the literature shows that the protocol has been adopted in a number of different settings, and it is estimated that more than one million babies have been screened with no false-negative cases reported. The ability to prevent the operator from identifying the majority of cases of carriers fulfils ethical requirements and is seen as advantageous by some users, although use of the protocol in this way does mean that some rare cases of sickle cell disease will be missed. The rationalization of equipment and skills, along with reduced interpretative requirements, is also advantageous in the current environment. Where screening programmes already exist, it is important to ensure standardization with existing practice, and this has been demonstrated to be possible in the English setting [10]. The current lack of an experiment to detect Hb Bart's may limit uptake in areas where this currently falls into newborn screening requirements. However, strategies to target Hb Bart's are being investigated by the manufacturer. Other areas under development include quality control material.

In conclusion, ESI-MSMS has been shown to be a specific, sensitive, and practical technique for newborn screening for sickle cell disease.

5. Patents

WO2006082389A1, Screening method. WO2008/0135756A1, Peptide Standards.

References

1. Kiernan, U.A.; Black, J.A.; Williams, P.; Nelson, R.W. High-Throughput analysis of haemoglobin from neonates using matrix-assisted laser desorption/ionization time-of-flight mass spectrometry. *Clin. Chem.* **2002**, *48*, 946–949.
2. Wild, B.J.; Green, B.N.; Stephens, A.D. The potential of electrospray ionization mass spectrometry for the diagnosis of hemoglobin variants found in newborn screening. *Blood Cells Mol. Dis.* **2004**, *33*, 308–317. [CrossRef] [PubMed]
3. Daniel, Y.A.; Turner, C.; Haynes, R.M.; Hunt, B.J.; Dalton, R.N. Rapid and specific detection of clinically significant haemoglobinopathies using electrospray mass spectrometry-mass spectrometry. *Br. J. Haem.* **2005**, *130*, 635–643. [CrossRef] [PubMed]
4. Daniel, Y.; Turner, C.; Farrar, L.; Dalton, R.N. A comparison of IEF and MSMS for clinical hemoglobinopathy screening in 40,000 newborns. *Blood* **2008**, *112*, 2387.
5. Boemer, F.; Ketelslegers, O.; Minon, J.-M.; Bours, V.; Schoos, R. Newborn screening for sickle cell disease using tandem mass spectrometry. *Clin. Chem.* **2008**, *54*, 2036–2041. [CrossRef] [PubMed]
6. Boemer, F.; Cornet, Y.; Libioulle, C.; Segers, K.; Bours, V.; Schoos, R. 3-years experience review of neonatal screening for hemoglobin disorders using tandem mass spectrometry. *Clin. Chim. Act.* **2011**, *412*, 1476–1479. [CrossRef] [PubMed]
7. Moat, S.J.; Rees, D.; King, L.; Ifederu, A.; Harvey, K.; Hall, K.; Lloyd, G.; Morell, G.; Hillier, S. Newborn blood spot screening for sickle cell disease by using tandem mass spectrometry: implementation of a protocol to identify only the disease states of sickle cell disease. *Clin. Chem.* **2014**, *60*, 373–380. [CrossRef] [PubMed]
8. Moat, S.J.; Rees, D.; George, R.S.; King, L.; Dodd, A.; Ifederu, A.; Ramgoolam, T.; Hillier, S. Newborn screening for sickle cell disorders using tandem mass spectrometry: Three years' experience of using a protocol to detect only the disease states. *Ann. Clin. Biochem.* **2017**, *54*, 601–611. [PubMed]
9. Daniel, Y.; Henthorn, J. Public Health England. Available online: https://assets.publishing.service.gov.uk/government/uploads/system/uploads/attachment_data/file/664932/Sickle_cell_and_thalassaemia_screening_action_values_for_tandem_mass_spectrometry_screening.pdf (accessed on 23 November 2018).
10. Daniel, Y.; Henthorn, J. Public Health England. Available online: https://assets.publishing.service.gov.uk/government/uploads/system/uploads/attachment_data/file/488858/Tandem_Mass_Spectrometry_for_Sickle_Cell_and_Thalassaemia_Newborn_Screening_Pilot_Study_2015.pdf (accessed on 23 November 2018).
11. Daniel, Y.A.; Henthorn, J. Newborn screening for sickling and other haemoglobin disorders using tandem mass spectrometry: A pilot study of methodology in laboratories in England. *J. Med. Screen.* **2016**, *23*, 175–178. [CrossRef] [PubMed]
12. Lobitz, S.; Klein, J.; Brose, A.; Blankenstein, O.; Frömmel, C. Newborn screening by tandem mass spectromety confirms the high prevalence of sickle cell disease among German newborns. *Ann. Hem.* **2018**. [CrossRef]

16

Critical Congenital Heart Disease Screening Using Pulse Oximetry: Achieving a National Approach to Screening, Education and Implementation in the United States

Lisa A. Wandler * and Gerard R. Martin

Children's National Heart Institute, Washington, DC 20010-2970, USA; gmartin@childrensnational.org
* Correspondence: lhom@childrensnational.org;

Abstract: A national approach to screening for critical congenital heart disease (CCHD) using pulse oximetry was undertaken in the United States. Following the scientific studies that laid the groundwork for the addition of CCHD screening to the U.S. Recommended Uniform Screening Panel (RUSP) and endorsement by professional societies, advocates including physicians, nurses, parents, medical associations, and newborn screening interest groups were able to successfully pass laws requiring the screen on a state by state basis. Public health involvement and screening requirements vary by state. However, a common algorithm, education, and implementation strategies were shared nationally as well as CCHD toolkits to aid in the implementation in hospitals. Health Resources & Services Administration (HRSA) grants to pilot states encouraged the development of a public health infrastructure around screening, data collection, and quality measures. The formation of a CCHD NewSTEPs technical advisory work group provided a systematic way to tackle challenges and share best practices by hosting monthly meetings and webinars. CCHD screening is now required in 48 states, with over 98% of U.S. births being screened for CCHD using pulse oximetry. A standard protocol has been implemented in most states. While the challenges related to screening special populations and quantifying screening outcomes through the creation of a national data repository remain; universal implementation is nearly complete.

Keywords: CCHD screening in the US; newborn screening pulse oximetry; critical congenital heart disease screening

1. Introduction

Critical congenital heart disease (CCHD) screening using pulse oximetry is a point of care newborn screen that relies on the detection of low blood oxygen levels to identify infants who may have CCHD or other life threatening neonatal conditions. Particularly useful for identifying asymptomatic infants with CCHD in well-baby nurseries, the importance of this screen is in its ability to allow for the detection of CCHD prior to when the infant is discharged from the birth hospital. The late detection of CCHD, after hospital discharge, has been shown to increase morbidity and mortality [1].

Congenital heart disease (CHD) is the most common birth defect. In the U.S., approximately 40,000 infants are born with CHD, with 25% of those having CCHD [2–4]. The primary targets for CCHD screening were identified through expert consensus in 2011. The list included those seven lesions most likely to be identified using pulse oximetry: hypoplastic left heart syndrome, pulmonary atresia, tetralogy of Fallot, total anomalous pulmonary venous return, transposition of the great arteries, tricuspid atresia, and truncus arteriosus [5]. This list of core conditions was expanded in 2016, this time by an expert panel convened by the Centers for Disease Control (CDC) and the

American Academy of Pediatrics (AAP) to include coarctation of the aorta, double-outlet right ventricle, Ebstein's anomaly, interrupted aortic arch, single ventricle, and other critical cyanotic lesions not specified. The expert panel also acknowledged the added benefit of identifying secondary targets, including hemoglobinopathy, hypothermia, infection (including sepsis), lung disease, noncritical CHD, persistent pulmonary hypertension, and other hypoxemic conditions as important public health targets of CCHD screening in the U.S. [6].

The goal of this article is to give an overview and insight into how the U.S. was able to achieve systematic implementation of CCHD screening using pulse oximetry including a nationally endorsed screening algorithm, centralized resources coordinated at the state and federal government levels, shared educational strategies, and toolkits; thus, moving within five years from screening in only a few hospitals, mainly associated with research studies with no state requirements, to nearly universal implementation in all but two states.

2. Early Studies and 2009 Scientific Statement

The need for additional methods to identify infants with CCHD early and prior to circulatory collapse was made very clear in one research study that investigated missed diagnosis of CCHD in California. More than 50% of CCHD deaths (up to 30 infants a year) could be attributed to late or missed diagnosis in the neonatal period in the state of California alone [7]. Evidence presented in the Chang study and others [8] demonstrated that additional methods of detection for CCHD, aside from prenatal ultrasound and physical examination of the neonate, were needed. If infants with CCHD could be identified, diagnosed, and receive an intervention (cardiovascular surgery or cardiac catheterization), survival and morbidity outcomes could be improved.

Although the concept of using pulse oximetry as a screening mechanism was explored in research articles both in the U.S. and Europe as early as 1993 [9–12], screening had not yet been implemented in U.S. newborn nurseries or required in any states. In 2005, Mississippi proposed legislation suggesting that pulse oximetry screening be used as a strategy to identify additional instances of newborns with CCHD [13]. Tennessee also considered early pulse oximetry screening legislation, but at that time, cardiologists, concerned about false positive studies, were hesitant to support the concept of CCHD screening as a state mandate [14]. Pulse oximetry screening was gaining significant attention as a potential strategy to improve the timely recognition of CCHD; the scientific community responded by reviewing the state of evidence related to the use of pulse oximetry in newborns to detect CCHD [15].

On behalf of the AAP Section on Cardiology and Cardiac Surgery, and Committee on Fetus and Newborn and the American Heart Association (AHA) Congenital Heart Defects Committee of the Council on Cardiovascular Disease in the Young, Council on Cardiovascular Nursing, and Interdisciplinary Council on Quality of Care and Outcomes Research, an expert writing group was tasked with evaluating the state of evidence on the routine use of pulse oximetry to detect CCHD. In 2009, they released a scientific statement concluding, based on an analysis of papers from 1966 to 2008, the following: CCHD was not being detected in some newborns prior to discharge from their birth hospital, resulting in significant morbidity and occasional mortality; if routine pulse oximetry is performed on asymptomatic newborns after 24 h of life but prior to discharge, additional CCHD could be detected, particularly in hospitals where on-site pediatric cardiologists and pediatric cardiovascular services were available; and that screening could be conducted at very low cost and risk of harm [15]. However, the expert group went on to emphasize that further studies in "larger populations and across a broad range of newborn delivery systems" was required to determine whether pulse oximetry testing should become the standard of care in the routine assessment of neonates [15].

3. Evidence from Europe

While the AHA/AAP expert writing group was performing their review of the evidence and grappling with the need for population level data to validate using pulse oximetry as a CCHD screening tool, researchers in Europe were poised to publish several important studies that would provide the precise evidence needed. Studies from Sweden, the United Kingdom, and Germany demonstrated that screening for CCHD at the population level had the required sensitivity and specificity to meet the criteria for newborn screening.

Perhaps most influential was a study from Sweden by Granelli et al. It was complete but not published in time to be considered in the analysis by the 2009 AAP/AHA writing group. This study analyzed 39,821 newborns who were screened using pulse oximetry and compared the strategy of physical exam alone with pulse oximetry screening alone, and in combination physical exam and pulse oximetry screening. The results were compelling, in addition to having an acceptable sensitivity (82.8% when combined with physical assessment) and specificity (97.8%); many of the false positives of pulse oximetry screening were not CCHD, but true positives for other important pathologies including persistent pulmonary hypertension of the newborn (PPHN), pneumonia, and infections, adding to the value of the screen outside of identifying unknown infants with CCHD. Although not all forms of CCHD can be detected by using pulse oximetry, this study concluded that 92% of ductal dependent cases could be identified if screening was performed in newborn delivery hospitals prior to discharge [16].

An additional study was published in 2010. It involved 34 institutions in Germany in which 42,240 infants were screened (sensitivity 77.78%, specificity 99.90%, and negative predictive value 99.99%). Based on the analysis of those screens, the study team concluded that the addition of pulse oximetry screening could substantially close the postnatal diagnostic gap (those cases of CCHD not identified through prenatal ultrasound or physical assessment) to 4.4% [17].

A meta-analysis conducted by researchers in the United Kingdom, which identified 13 high quality primary studies involving 229,421 infants screened using pulse oximetry, provided additional key support. The calculated sensitivity (76.5%) was similar to the Granelli study and the false positive rate overall was 0.14%. Interestingly, when the data was further broken down, the study found that the false positive rate, if the screening was conducted after 24 h, was significantly lower than if the screening was conducted prior to 24 h of life (false positive rate <24 h 0.5% versus >24 h 0.05%) [18]. This distinction would later factor heavily into the development of the U.S. nationally endorsed protocol. However, it may not have properly acknowledged that additional secondary conditions make up the majority of those false positives.

These studies from Europe provided valuable evidence that would help to inform the development of the U.S. recommended strategies. In fact, two of the U.S. CCHD stakeholder meetings included expert representation from among the authors of the Swedish and UK studies.

4. Call to Action as CCHD Screening Is Added to the RUSP

In October 2010, following the availability of new evidence from Europe and a formal scientific evidence review process, the Secretary's Advisory Committee on Heritable Disorders in Newborns and Children (SACHDNC), whose responsibility it is to identify, evaluate, and make recommendations on which newborn screens should be added to the Recommended Uniform Screening Panel (RUSP), evaluated the research, heard the testimony of experts and families, and agreed that CCHD screening using pulse oximetry be recommended at the national level as part of the standard of care for newborn screening in the US. An additional review to propose a plan of action and to address the evidence gaps by the Interagency Coordinating Committee (ICC) was also completed prior to endorsement by the Secretary of Health and Human Services [19].

A group of experts and stakeholders came together for a two-day meeting sponsored by SACHDNC and hosted by the American College of Cardiology (ACC) at the Heart House in January of 2011. Participants included physicians, nurses, scientists, representatives from Health Resources & Services Administration (HRSA), ACC, AAP, AHA, the American College of Medical Genetics, March of Dimes, the Association of Maternal and Child Health Programs, The Association of Public Health Laboratories (APHL), the National Institutes of Health (NIH), Centers for Disease Control and Prevention (CDC), Food and Drug Administration (FDA), parent advocacy groups, industry partners, state public health program, and healthcare organizations [19]. Initial recommendations and a screening algorithm (see Appendix A) based in large part on the Swedish protocol, specifying that screening be conducted using two limbs (the right hand and either foot) [16] were developed [5]. This algorithm was chosen mainly for its acceptable sensitivity (82.76%) and high specificity (97.88%) when paired with physical assessment. The expert group also recommended screening take place "at or around 24 h or prior to discharge" to maximize sensitivity while minimizing the number of false positives [5].

CCHD screening was added to the RUSP by Secretary Kathleen Sebelius in September of 2011 [20]. This recommendation was a first major step toward systematic implementation and represented buy-in at the federal or national level. The AAP [21], AHA, ACC, and March of Dimes also quickly endorsed CCHD screening.

The need for an additional workgroup and stakeholders meeting arose to address challenges such as the selection of screening equipment, the standards for reporting screening outcomes, the training and education of health care providers and families whose infants were being screened, payment for screening, appropriate follow-up diagnostic testing, public health involvement, and oversight and to identify areas for future research [22]. This additional work group meeting also took place at the Heart House in Washington, D.C. in February, 2012. Importantly, the recommendations from this work group included a minimum data set for both hospital level and state public health level reporting [22].

Secretary Sebelius, as a part of her 2011 adoption of CCHD screening to the RUSP, included a Federal Agency Plan of Action focused on the key areas of (1) research, (2) surveillance, (3) screening standards and infrastructure, and (4) education and training [20]. NIH was tasked with determining the impact of CCHD screening on the health outcomes of infants as well as the development of registries to help address research questions related to screening. The CDC's main area of focus would be surveillance, including the evaluation of cost-effectiveness analysis and the monitoring of CCHD mortality and its link to other health outcomes. The Health Resources and Services Administration (HRSA) was charged with completing a thorough evaluation in collaboration with SACHDNC to evaluate the potential public health impact of universal screening for CCHD and to develop screening standards, and support the development of education tools and the infrastructure required for a public health approach to this point of care screen [20].

HRSA responded by funding six CCHD state demonstration projects over a three year period, specifically to support the validation and dissemination of CCHD screening protocols and for the development of infrastructure around point-of-care screening for CCHD [23]. The state programs chosen were: Michigan, New Jersey, Utah, Virginia, Wisconsin and a consortium of five New England states (Maine, New Hampshire, Vermont, Rhode Island, and Connecticut) [23]. Shortly after the grants to the states were awarded, a third stakeholders meeting took place in Washington, D.C. in September of 2012 to kick-off and coordinate state efforts. Initial lessons learned following the completion of the grant period were published by the grantees in 2017 [23].

The need for building public health infrastructure and sharing best practices and lessons learned with other states was particularly important as CCHD screening was only the second point of care newborn screen to be implemented nationally. The first was newborn hearing screening. HRSA also provided limited funding for another CCHD specific initiative, the Newborn Screening Technical assistance and Evaluation Program (NewSTEPs). NewSTEPs partnered with federal agencies in examining CCHD screening as well as state public health newborn screening programs to provide a central platform for CCHD screening resources. It also brought together a technical assistance CCHD work group and monthly webinars specifically related to implementation, education, and the spread of CCHD best practices [24].

Since the 2011 addition to the RUSP, federal agencies continue to work towards addressing the needs identified in Secretary Sebelius' recommendations. Researchers at the CDC have published studies examining the potential impact of screening implementation on the detection of CCHD and lives saved [25], and cost-effectiveness [26].

5. State-by-State Advocacy

The addition of CCHD screening to the RUSP at the federal level is non-binding on the states. To become required by law, each state would individually need to mandate CCHD screening, which, to date, all of the states, except for three, have done, either by statute, regulation, or executive order. Indiana, New Jersey and Maryland were the first three states to require CCHD screening in 2011, prior to the addition of CCHD screening to the RUSP. Parent groups, nurses, physicians, and professional societies worked together to go state-by-state advocating that CCHD screening be adopted as law. Peak advocacy efforts within the U.S. occurred in 2013 when 25 states adopted CCHD screening [27]. By early 2015, 43 states and the District of Columbia required CCHD screening.

There are nuances in how states selected to implement, with varying levels of public health involvement. Differences in state CCHD screening laws include whether the mandate would be funded, whether all of the infants would be screened or whether exceptions to screening were permissible (special care nurseries, premature infants, out of hospital births, screening at altitude) and whether any aggregate or individual CCHD screening data would be reported. Most states choose to implement the algorithm recommended by the AAP with New Jersey, Tennessee, and Minnesota being among the few exceptions [6]. Data collection, the extent to which education was provided, and the monitoring of implementation by state public health departments also vary greatly.

By the end of 2016, only two states, Idaho and Wyoming, were not screening. One state, Kansas, implemented at all hospital newborn nurseries without a state mandate. As of September 2017, the last two states that do not require screening, Idaho and Wyoming, have proposed regulations pending that would require CCHD screening. Rapid adoption by the states can largely be contributed to the alignment of several key forces, the validation of pulse oximetry as an effective screening method at the federal level, the endorsement of screening by national professional medical societies, and the support in the form of initial financial resources by federal and state public health agencies. Parents and clinical experts also played key roles as advocates [28], testifying at both the state and federal levels in support of CCHD screening and its ability to save lives through early identification.

6. Systematic Implementation

Once required by state law, there was still considerable work to be done to implement CCHD screening in hospitals with newborn nurseries. Several different strategies were employed to ensure an efficient approach. These included the use of CCHD implementation toolkits, the sharing of educational videos for providers and families, a train-the-trainer approach, and the dissemination of resources, best practices, and solutions to common challenges through the aforementioned NewSTEPs webinars.

Systematic implementation was aided by the publication of a feasibility study conducted in Maryland, demonstrating that CCHD screening could be successfully implemented at a community hospital without the need for additional staff members, taking an average of only 3.5 min to screen and with few barriers [29]. Showing that CCHD screening was feasible in a community hospital was important. Prior to this study, most screening implementation was conducted at large, often urban centers and most often associated with research.

In 2013, NewSTEPs, which continues to function as a part of a partnership between the Association of Public Health Laboratories (APHL) and the Colorado School of Public Health, began hosting monthly CCHD technical assistance webinars to assist in the dissemination of best practices and working solutions to commonly identified challenges to screening [23]. Early topics included: educational resources available for parents and screeners, data collection including electronic reporting resources, defining roles and resources from a public health perspective, special populations, and how to address cost/equipment issues [30]. NewSTEPs, in partnership with the Pediatric Congenital Heart Association, also brought together the HRSA grantees and other leaders in CCHD for an in-person meeting in February 2014. The purpose of this meeting was to discuss the current status of CCHD screening in the U.S. and to share ideas and provide guidance for state screening programs involved in all stages of implementation [23].

Toolkits containing materials used to implement in a hospital newborn nursery made it possible to implement screening in a new hospital without having to gather and develop all of the necessary components for implementation each time. These toolkits contained important background evidence on CCHD screening, information on the screening protocol, education for providers, nurses, and parents, as well as competencies and forms to facilitate the documentation of screening results. Children's National Medical Center developed one such CCHD screening implementation toolkit that was shared nationally and adapted to be state specific in Alaska, Missouri, Utah, and Colorado. Other states, including Rhode Island, Texas, and Wisconsin also created and extensively used CCHD screening implementation toolkits within their states.

Educational videos and training modules, incorporating evidence based content, were created and shared to provide those staff tasked with implementing CCHD screening with information on the importance, benefits and limitation of screening, technical assistance in how to perform the screen as well as information for parents on understanding the screens purpose and results [31,32]. Donations from families, federal and state funds all helped support the development of these freely available resources.

7. Lessons Learned

An early concern discussed extensively in stakeholder meetings and prior to the addition to the RUSP was that CCHD screening would result in too many false positives. This initial concern was not valid; early adopters did not find that the number of false positives overwhelmed the care delivery system in the way of unnecessary referrals to specialists or unnecessary echocardiograms [33,34]. Screening with pulse oximetry is not diagnostic for CCHD, it simply identifies an infant for follow-up to determine the cause for hypoxia. Referral and assessment by a pediatric cardiologist and an echocardiogram are required for a diagnosis of CCHD. Other causes of low blood oxygen levels should also be considered, such as assessment and laboratory work for infectious or respiratory causes. This distinction was particularly important in places that were geographically isolated or remote, where an infant would have to be transported over great distances for follow-up to occur. If another cause for a failed screen could be identified first, a referral and echocardiogram may not be required. Initial U.S. recommendations for follow-up stated that a comprehensive evaluation for the causes of hypoxemia be conducted and if the hypoxemia is not explained, a diagnostic echocardiogram with interpretation by a pediatric cardiologist is needed [5]. However, subsequent research from Europe has shown that echocardiography is not always needed if another condition is found to be causing the low blood oxygen saturation, and that only 29% of those that fail the screen require echocardiograms [35]. The number of false positives in the U.S. did not result in a large number of unnecessary echocardiograms once CCHD screening implementation was underway [29,34].

Misinterpretation of the screening algorithm and protocol violations were also reported as early implementation was undertaken. These issues could be addressed or minimized by implementing quality metrics and through the use of electronic decision support tools [33,36]. Best practices are still being developed with regards to screening special populations, particularly home births, births at altitude, and evaluating whether screening of infants in neonatal intensive care units is effective [37]. Colorado requires CCHD screening of infants born at moderate altitude, accepting a higher false positive rate when compared to infants born at sea level [38]. Physicians, midwives, and nurses in Wisconsin and Pennsylvania have tailored the AAP recommended screening protocol for use in out of hospital births [30]. Best practices related to screening these special populations continue to be studied [23,24].

Although a few early adopter states have published data on their initial implementation of CCHD screening [34], states that received grants from HRSA cited the lack of sustained funding for data collection activities to be the most common and important challenge identified [23]. Initial federal and state funds were limited and not renewed. Data collection activities vary greatly by state. In some states, the public health department is not permitted to collect newborn screening data; whereas in others, such as Maryland, Minnesota, Virginia, Florida, and New Jersey results are reported centrally to the state department of health sometimes using electronic birth certificates or rely on the dried blood spot cards as the reporting mechanism. Other states have developed automated systems and have the ability to extract data directly from the pulse oximeter devices and electronically transmit and report results [23]. One survey conducted in 2015 reported that 74% of states collected CCHD screening data or had plans to do so, however, that the amount of data collected varied from aggregate results on whether infants passed or failed, to all individual screening results [27].

The dramatic variation in the amount of CCHD screening data collected and the differences in how the data is collected (electronic, paper, aggregate data vs. individual screening results) has made it difficult to analyze the data to accurately assess and inform the impact that screening has on reducing CCHD morbidity and mortality through early detection and intervention. In particular, the need for an "assessment of the certainty of diagnosis using standardized public health surveillance case definitions" is needed to be able to allow for consistent comparisons across state screening programs and over time [24]. Although a national web-based repository to collect data on CCHD screening outcomes was created through NewSTEPs, without a requirement to collect CCHD screening data, which many of the CCHD screening mandates lack, the data is not available or submitted, to date, for systematic review and analysis nationally.

8. Conclusions

During a follow-up Advisory Committee on Heritable Disorders in Newborns and Children (ACHDNC) meeting in August of 2017, committee members discussed whether CCHD screening may be one of the most successful and impactful additions to the RUSP, particularly in its ability to gain the attention and buy-in of the general public, and publicity in the form of newspaper articles and news coverage. Outcomes analysis to assess the national impact of requiring CCHD screening in the U.S. is currently underway and may rely heavily on administrative data, birth defect and death registry data in the absence of population level CCHD outcomes reporting, since no such robust U.S. clinical dataset currently exists. Data from Europe that was crucial in informing initial recommendations and strategies related to screening may continue to be informative for future U.S. algorithm refinements particularly around the question of ideal timing of the screen [39].

A preliminary report, examining state death registry data from 2007–2013, was presented to ACHDNC in the August 2017 meeting. This report focused on the impact of state policies requiring CCHD screening, and found a 33% reduction in CCHD infant deaths in those states requiring screening and a calculated potential reduction of approximately 120 infant deaths due to CCHD per year in the U.S. as a whole [40]. This reduction in infant deaths is the primary outcome hoped for by the many individuals, government entities, researchers, physicians, nurses, public health staff, industry partners, parents, and others that worked to ensure that CCHD screening using pulse oximetry would be implemented in the U.S. as a national policy. As research studies, federal and state programs continue to focus on CCHD screening, we will learn more about the granular impact of public health involvement and the implementation of screening on decreasing the late identification of infants with CCHD, and the subsequent impact on morbidity and neurodevelopmental outcomes as well as evidence based recommendations for special settings [24].

Acknowledgments: We are grateful to Lindsay Attaway for her graphic designs and editorial assistance.

Author Contributions: Lisa Wandler drafted the initial outline and first draft of the manuscript. Gerard Martin developed the conceptual framework, edited and revised the manuscript.

Appendix A

U.S. Algorithm [5]

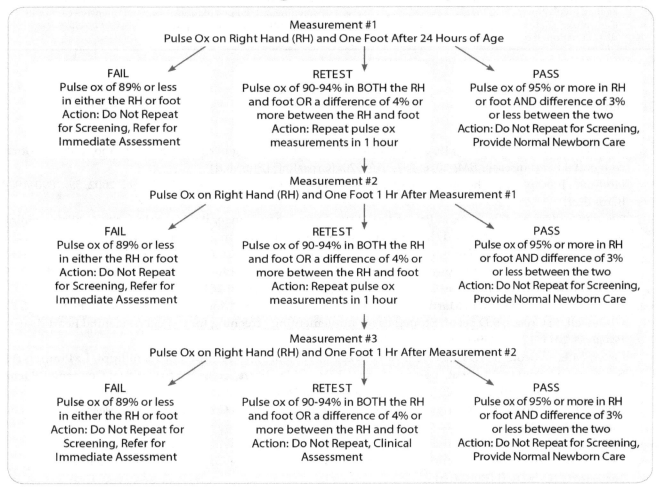

Critical Congenital Heart Disease Screening Program:
Screening Protocol Diagram

Measurement #1
Pulse Ox on Right Hand (RH) and One Foot After 24 Hours of Age

FAIL
Pulse ox of 89% or less in either the RH or foot
Action: Do Not Repeat for Screening, Refer for Immediate Assessment

RETEST
Pulse ox of 90-94% in BOTH the RH and foot OR a difference of 4% or more between the RH and foot
Action: Repeat pulse ox measurements in 1 hour

PASS
Pulse ox of 95% or more in RH or foot AND difference of 3% or less between the two
Action: Do Not Repeat for Screening, Provide Normal Newborn Care

Measurement #2
Pulse Ox on Right Hand (RH) and One Foot 1 Hr After Measurement #1

FAIL
Pulse ox of 89% or less in either the RH or foot
Action: Do Not Repeat for Screening, Refer for Immediate Assessment

RETEST
Pulse ox of 90-94% in BOTH the RH and foot OR a difference of 4% or more between the RH and foot
Action: Repeat pulse ox measurements in 1 hour

PASS
Pulse ox of 95% or more in RH or foot AND difference of 3% or less between the two
Action: Do Not Repeat for Screening, Provide Normal Newborn Care

Measurement #3
Pulse Ox on Right Hand (RH) and One Foot 1 Hr After Measurement #2

FAIL
Pulse ox of 89% or less in either the RH or foot
Action: Do Not Repeat for Screening, Refer for Immediate Assessment

RETEST
Pulse ox of 90-94% in BOTH the RH and foot OR a difference of 4% or more between the RH and foot
Action: Do Not Repeat, Clinical Assessment

PASS
Pulse ox of 95% or more in RH or foot AND difference of 3% or less between the two
Action: Do Not Repeat for Screening, Provide Normal Newborn Care

Appendix B

Timeline of U.S. Implementation

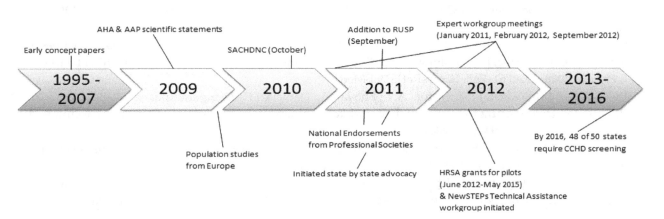

Early concept papers

AHA & AAP scientific statements

SACHDNC (October)

Addition to RUSP (September)

Expert workgroup meetings (January 2011, February 2012, September 2012)

1995 - 2007   **2009**   **2010**   **2011**   **2012**   **2013-2016**

Population studies from Europe

National Endorsements from Professional Societies

Initiated state by state advocacy

HRSA grants for pilots (June 2012-May 2015) & NewSTEPs Technical Assistance workgroup initiated

By 2016, 48 of 50 states require CCHD screening

Table A1. Showing Components for Successful U.S. Implementation & Barriers Addressed.

Components for Successful Implementation	Barriers Addressed and *Solutions*
• Common algorithm/protocol for screening & follow-up • Endorsement by professional societies • Engage parents and clinical stakeholders as advocates • Federal recommendations and agency involvement • Centralized shared educational resources and dissemination of best practices/lessons learned	• Too many false positives—*In most cases, false positives are important secondary conditions* • Unnecessary referrals to pediatric cardiology and echocardiograms—*Found to be reasonable in practice* • Quality control and assurance of protocol adherence and interpretation—*Quality metrics and electronic decision support* • Screening special populations (neonatal intensive care units, at high altitude, out of hospital births)—*Best practices in development*

References

1. Eckersley, L.; Sadler, L.; Parry, E.; Finucane, K.; Gentles, T.L. Timing of diagnosis affects mortality in critical congenital heart disease. *BMJ* **2016**, *101*, 516–520. [CrossRef] [PubMed]

2. Hoffman, J.; Kaplan, S. The incidence of Congenital Heart Disease. *J. Am. Coll. Cardiol.* **2002**, *39*, 1890–1900. [CrossRef]

3. Centers for Disease Control and Prevention. Data & Statistics. Congenital Heart Defects. Available online: https://www.cdc.gov/ncbddd/heartdefects/data.html (accessed on 23 August 2017).

4. American Academy of Pediatrics. Newborn Screening for CCHD. Frequently Asked Questions. Available online: https://www.aap.org/en-us/advocacy-and-policy/aap-health-initiatives/PEHDIC/Pages/Newborn-Screening-for-CCHD.aspx (accessed on 23 August 2017).

5. Kemper, A.R.; Mahle, W.T.; Martin, G.R.; Cooley, W.C.; Kumar, P.; Morrow, W.R.; Kelm, K.; Pearson, G.D.; Glidewell, J.; Grosse, S.D.; et al. Strategies for implementing screening for critical congenital heart disease. *Pediatrics* **2011**, *128*, e1259–e1267. [CrossRef] [PubMed]

6. Oster, M.E.; Aucott, S.W.; Glidewell, J.; Hackell, J.; Kochlias, L.; Martin, G.R.; Phillippi, J.; Pinto, N.M.; Saarinen, A.; Sontag, M.; et al. Lessons Learned From Newborn Screening for Critical Congenital Heart Defects. *Pediatrics* **2016**, *137*, e20154573. [CrossRef] [PubMed]

7. Chang, R.K.; Gurvitz, M.; Rodriguez, S. Missed Diagnosis of Critical Congenital Heart Disease. *Arch. Pediatr. Adolesc. Med.* **2008**, *162*, 969–974. [CrossRef] [PubMed]

8. Mouledoux, J.H.; Walsh, W.F. Evaluating the Diagnostic Gap: Statewide Incidence of Undiagnosed Critical Congenital Heart Disease before Newborn Screening with Pulse Oximetry. *Pediatr. Cardiol.* **2013**, *34*, 1680–1686. [CrossRef] [PubMed]

9. Hoke, T.R.; Druschel, C.M.; Carter, T.; Bawa, P.K.; Mitchell, R.D.; Pathak, A.; Rowe, P.C.; Byrne, B.J. Oxygen saturation as a screening test for critical congenital heart disease: A preliminary study. *Pediatr. Cardiol.* **2002**, *23*, 403–409. [CrossRef] [PubMed]

10. Koppel, R.I.; Druschel, C.M.; Tonia, C.; Barry, E.G.; Prabhu, N.M.; Rohit, T.; Fredrick, Z.B. Effectiveness of Pulse Oximetry Screening for Congenital Heart Disease in Asymptomatic Newborns. *Pediatrics* **2003**, *111*, 45. [CrossRef]

11. Meberg, A.; Brügmann-Pieper, S.; Due, R.; Eskedal, L.; Fagerli, I.; Farstad, T.; Frøisland, D.H.; Sannes, C.H.; Johansen, O.J.; Keljalic, J.; et al. First day of life pulse oximetry screening to detect congenital heart defects. *J. Pediatr.* **2008**, *152*, 761–765. [CrossRef] [PubMed]

12. Ewer, A.K.; Middleton, L.J.; Furmston, A.T.; Bhoyar, A.; Daniels, J.P.; Thangaratinam, S.; Deeks, J.J.; Khan, K.S. Pulse oximetry screening for congenital heart defects in newborn infants (PulseOx): A test accuracy study. *Lancet* **2011**, *378*, 785–794. [CrossRef]

13. Mississippi 2005 Regular Session, House Bill 1052. 2005. Available online: http://billstatus.ls.state.ms.us/documents/2005/pdf/HB/1000-1099/HB1052IN.pdf (accessed on 11 October 2017).

14. Chang, R.K.; Rodriguez, S.; Klitzner, T.S. Screening Newborns for Congenital Heart Disease with Pulse Oximetry: Survey of Pediatric Cardiologists. *Pediatr. Cardiol.* **2009**, *30*, 20–25. [CrossRef] [PubMed]

15. Mahle, W.T.; Newburger, J.W.; Matherne, G.P.; Smith, F.C.; Hoke, T.R.; Koppel, R.; Gidding, S.S.; Beekman, R.H.; Grosse, S.D.; American Heart Association Congenital Heart Defects Committee of the Council on Cardiovascular Disease in the Young, Council on Cardiovascular Nursing, and the Interdisciplinary Council on Quality of Care and Outcomes Research. Role of Pulse Oximetry in Examining Newborns for Congenital Heart Disease: A Scientific Statement from the American Heart Association and American Academy of Pediatrics. *Circulation* **2009**, *120*, 447–458. [CrossRef] [PubMed]

16. Granelli, A.D.; Wennergren, M.; Sandberg, K.; Mellander, M.; Bejlum, C.; Inganäs, L.; Eriksson, M.; Segerdahl, N.; Agren, A.; Ekman-Joelsson, B.M.; et al. Impact of pulse oximetry screening on the detection of duct dependent congenital heart disease: A Swedish prospective screening study in 39821 newborns. *BMJ* **2009**, *338*, a3037. [CrossRef] [PubMed]

17. Riede, F.T.; Worner, C.; Dahnert, I.; Möcke, A.; Kostelka, M.; Schneider, P. Effectiveness of neonatal pulse oximetry screening for detection of critical congenital heart disease in daily clinical routine: results from a prospective multicenter study. *Eur. J. Pediatr.* **2010**, *169*, 975–981. [CrossRef] [PubMed]

18. Thangaratinam, S.; Daniels, J.; Zamora, J.; Khan, K.S.; Ewer, A.K. Pulse oximetry screening for critical congenital heart defects in asymptomatic newborn babies: a systematic review and meta-analysis. *Lancet* **2012**, *379*, 2459–2464. [CrossRef]

19. Bradshaw, E.A.; Martin, G.R. Review: Screening for critical congenital heart disease: advancing detection in the newborn. *Curr. Opin. Pediatr.* **2012**, *24*, 603–608. [CrossRef] [PubMed]

20. Sebelius, K. Secretary of Health and Human Services Recommendation for Pulse Oximetry Screening. 2011. Available online: https://www.hrsa.gov/advisorycommittees/mchbadvisory/heritabledisorders/recommendations/correspondence/cyanoticheartsecre09212011.pdf (accessed on 6 September 2017).

21. Mahle, W.T.; Martin, G.R.; Beekman, R.H.; Morrow, R.; Rosenthal, G.L.; Synder, C.S.; Minich, L.L.; Mital, S.; Towbin, J.A.; Tweddell, J.S. Endorsement of Health and Human Services Recommendation for Pulse Oximetry Screening for Critical Congenital Heart Disease Section on Cardiology and Cardiac Surgery Executive Committee. *Pediatrics* **2012**, *129*, 190–192. [CrossRef] [PubMed]

22. Martin, G.R.; Beekman, R.H.; Mikula, E.B.; Fasules, J.; Garg, L.F.; Kemper, A.R.; Morrow, W.R.; Pearson, G.D.; Mahle, W.T. Implementing Recommended Screening for Critical Congenital Heart Disease. *Pediatrics* **2013**, *132*, e185–e192. [CrossRef] [PubMed]

23. McClain, M.R.; Hokanson, J.S.; Grazel, R.; Van Naarden, B.K.; Garg, L.F.; Morris, M.R.; Moline, K.; Urquhart, K.; Nance, A.; Randall, H.; et al. Critical Congenital Heart Disease Newborn Screening Implementation: Lessons Learned. *Matern. Child. Health J.* **2017**. [CrossRef]

24. Olney, R.S.; Ailes, E.C.; Sontag, M.K. Detection of critical congenital heart defects: Review of contributions from prenatal and newborn screening. *Semin. Perinatol.* **2015**, *39*, 230–237. [CrossRef] [PubMed]

25. Peterson, C.; Ailes, E.; Riehle-Colarusso, T.; Oster, M.E.; Olney, R.S.; Cassell, C.H.; Fixler, D.E.; Carmichael, S.L.; Shaw, G.M.; Gilboa, S.M. Late detection of critical congenital heart disease among US infants: estimation of the potential impact of proposed universal screening using pulse oximetry. *JAMA Pediatr.* **2014**, *168*, 361–370. [CrossRef] [PubMed]

26. Peterson, C.; Grosse, S.D.; Oster, M.E.; Olney, R.S.; Cassell, C.H. Cost- effectiveness of routine screening for critical congenital heart disease in US newborns. *Pediatrics* **2013**, *132*, e595–e603. [CrossRef] [PubMed]

27. CDC. State Legislation, Regulations, and Hospital Guidelines for Newborn Screening for Critical Congenital Heart Defects—United States, 2011–2014. *Morb. Mort. Wkly. Rep.* **2015**, *64*, 625–630.

28. Berger, S.; Health & Science. Saving babies: An inexpensive, easy oxygen test can prevent many deaths. *The Washington Post.* 7 April 2014. Available online: https://www.washingtonpost.com/national/health-science/saving-babies-an-inexpensive-easy-oxygen-test-can-prevent-many-deaths/2014/04/07/3c6c8b2a-9b12-11e3-975d-107dfef7b668_story.html?utm_term=.dde8c8a2d734 (accessed on 23 August 2017).

29. Bradshaw, E.A.; Cuzzi, S.; Kiernan, S.; Nagel, N.; Becker, J.A.; Martin, G.R. Feasibility of implementing pulse oximetry screening for congenital heart disease in a community hospital. *J. Perinatol.* **2012**, *32*, 710–715. [CrossRef] [PubMed]

30. NewSTEPs CCHD Technical Assistance Webinars. Available online: https://newsteps.org/cchd-technical-assistance-webinars (accessed on 24 August 2017).

31. Baby's First Test, Conditions, Critical Congenital Heart Disease. Heart Smart Videos. Available online: http://www.babysfirsttest.org/newborn-screening/conditions/critical-congenital-heart-disease-cchd (accessed on 6 September 2017).

32. Newborn Screening Education. Critical Congenital Heart Disease Course sponsored by the Virginia Department of Health, The University of Virginia School of Medicine and the University of Virginia Children's Hospital. Available online: http://www.newbornscreeningeducation.org/pages/cchd (accessed on 6 September 2017).

33. Kochilas, L.K.; Lohr, J.L.; Bruhn, E.; Borman-Shoap, E.; Gams, B.L.; Pylipow, M.; Saarinen, A.; Gaviglio, A.; Thompson, T.R. Implementation of Critical Congenital Heart Disease Screening in Minnesota. *Pediatrics* **2013**, *132*, e587–e594. [CrossRef] [PubMed]

34. Garg, L.F.; Van Naarden Braun, K.; Knapp, M.M.; Anderson, T.M.; Koppel, R.I.; Hirsch, D.; Beres, L.M.; Sweatlock, J.; Olney, R.S.; Glidewell, J.; et al. Results from the New Jersey statewide critical congenital heart defects screening program. *Pediatrics* **2013**, *132*, e314–e323. [CrossRef] [PubMed]

35. Singh, A.; Rasiah, S.V.; Ewer, A.K. The impact of routine predischarge pulse oximetry screening in a regional neonatal unit. *Arch. Dis. Child. Fetal Neonatal Ed.* **2014**, *99*, F297–F302. [CrossRef] [PubMed]

36. Oster, M.E.; Kuo, K.W.; Mahle, W.T. Quality Improvement in Screening for Critical Congenital Heart Disease. *J. Pediatr.* **2014**, *164*, 67–71. [CrossRef] [PubMed]

37. Van Naarden Braun, K.; Grazel, R.; Koppel, R.; Lakshminrusimha, S.; Lohr, J.; Kumar, P.; Govindaswami, B.; Giuliano, M.; Cohen, M.; Spillane, N.; et al. Evaluation of critical congenital heart defects screening using pulse oximetry in the neonatal intensive care unit. *J. Perinatol.* **2017**, *37*, 1117–1123. [CrossRef] [PubMed]

38. Children's Hospital Colorado. Pulse Oximetry Program: Recommendations for Health Professionals. Available online: https://www.childrenscolorado.org/doctors-and-departments/departments/heart/programs-and-clinics/critical-congenital-heart-disease-screening-program/screening-toolkit-for-health-professionals/program-recommendations/ (accessed on 11 September 2017).

39. Ewer, A.K.; Martin, G.R. Newborn Pulse Oximetry Screening: Which Algorithm Is Best? *Pediatrics* **2016**, *138*, e20161206. [CrossRef] [PubMed]

40. Grosse, S. Reduction in Infant Cardiac Deaths in US States Implementing Policies to Screen Newborns for Critical Congenital Heart Disease. Available online: https://www.hrsa.gov/advisorycommittees/mchbadvisory/heritabledisorders/meetings/2017/0803/8grossecchdscreeningphimpact.pdf (accessed on 14 September 2017).

17

Newborn Screening for Sickle Cell Disease in the Caribbean: An Update of the Present Situation and of the Disease Prevalence

Jennifer Knight-Madden [1], Ketty Lee [2], Gisèle Elana [3], Narcisse Elenga [4],
Beatriz Marcheco-Teruel [5], Ngozi Keshi [6], Maryse Etienne-Julan [7], Lesley King [1],
Monika Asnani [1], Marc Romana [8,9,†] and Marie-Dominique Hardy-Dessources [8,9,10,*,†] on behalf
of the CAREST Network

[1] Caribbean Institute for Health Research—Sickle Cell Unit, The University of the West Indies, Mona, Kingston 7, Jamaica; jennifer.knightmadden@uwimona.edu.jm (J.K.-M.); lesley.king@uwimona.edu.jm (L.K.); monika.parshadasnani@uwimona.edu.jm (M.A.)

[2] Laboratory of Molecular Genetics, Academic Hospital of Guadeloupe, 97159 Pointe-à-Pitre, Guadeloupe; ketty.lee@chu-guadeloupe.fr

[3] Referral Center for Sickle Cell Disease, Department of Pediatrics, Academic Hospital of Martinique, 97261 Fort de France, Martinique, France; gisele.elana@chu-martinique.fr

[4] Referral Center for Sickle Cell Disease, Department of Pediatric Medicine and Surgery, Andrée Rosemon General Hospital, 97306 Cayenne, French Guiana, France; narcisse.elenga@ch-cayenne.fr

[5] National Center of Medical Genetics, 11300 La Habana, Cuba; beatriz@infomed.sld.cu

[6] Paediatric Department, Scarborough General Hospital, 00000 Scarborough, Tobago; nzigokeshi@yahoo.com

[7] Referral Center for Sickle Cell Disease, Sickle Cell Unit, Academic Hospital of Guadeloupe, 97159 Pointe-à-Pitre, Guadeloupe, France; maryse.etienne-julan@chu-guadeloupe.fr

[8] UMR Inserm 1134 Biologie Intégrée du Globule Rouge, Inserm/Université Paris Diderot—Université Sorbonne Paris Cité/INTS/Université des Antilles, Hôpital Ricou, Academic Hospital of Guadeloupe, 97159 Pointe-à-Pitre, Guadeloupe; marc.romana@inserm.fr

[9] Laboratoire d'Excellence du Globule Rouge (Labex GR-Ex), PRES Sorbonne, 75015 Paris, France

[10] CAribbean Network of REsearchers on Sickle Cell Disease and Thalassemia, UMR Inserm 1134, Hôpital Ricou, Academic Hospital of Guadeloupe, 97159 Pointe-à-Pitre, Guadeloupe

* Correspondence: marie-dominique.hardy-dessources@inserm.fr;
† These authors contributed equally to this work.

Abstract: The region surrounding the Caribbean Sea is predominantly composed of island nations for its Eastern part and the American continental coast on its Western part. A large proportion of the population, particularly in the Caribbean islands, traces its ancestry to Africa as a consequence of the Atlantic slave trade during the XVI–XVIII centuries. As a result, sickle cell disease has been largely introduced in the region. Some Caribbean countries and/or territories, such as Jamaica and the French territories, initiated newborn screening (NBS) programs for sickle cell disease more than 20 years ago. They have demonstrated the major beneficial impact on mortality and morbidity resulting from early childhood care. However, similar programs have not been implemented in much of the region. This paper presents an update of the existing NBS programs and the prevalence of sickle cell disease in the Caribbean. It demonstrates the impact of the Caribbean Network of Researchers on Sickle Cell Disease and Thalassemia (CAREST) on the extension of these programs. The presented data illustrate the importance of advocacy in convincing policy makers of the feasibility and benefit of NBS for sickle cell disease when coupled to early care.

Keywords: sickle cell disease; newborn screening; Caribbean

1. Introduction

The Caribbean is defined as the geographical region including the Caribbean Sea, more than 700 islands, and the surrounding coasts. The region is located southeast of the Gulf of Mexico and the North American mainland, East of Central America, and North of South America. A wider definition includes Belize, the Caribbean region of Colombia, the Yucatán Peninsula, and the Guyanas (Guyana, Suriname, French Guiana, the Guyana region in Venezuela, and the state of Amapà in Brazil); these areas have political and cultural ties to the region. The Caribbean islands are organized into 13 sovereign states and 17 overseas territories/departments and dependencies, with 43 million inhabitants and at least five official spoken languages.

The Caribbean countries and territories share some common historical features. Less than two centuries after the arrival of Christopher Columbus in the New World, these territories were all under the rules of the European colonial powers (France, United Kingdom, Spain, Portugal, The Netherlands, and Denmark). The introduction of new crops which needed intensive work, such as tobacco, cotton, and sugarcane, led to the development of the transatlantic slave trade. More than 12 million Africans were deported to the New World [1]. One of the consequences of this massive forced migration was the introduction of sickle cell disease (SCD) into the New World. The migration of Indians as indentured laborers when slavery was abolished led to the introduction of the Arabo-Indian haplotype of the β^S gene and thalassemia alleles.

The Caribbean occupies a unique position in the history of SCD in the modern era. Indeed, the first case ever described in the Western medical literature by Herricks in 1910 was that of a young fellow from Grenada studying dentistry in Chicago (USA) [2]. Additionally, the benefits of newborn screening (NBS) for SCD as a public health tool, including evidence of both the feasibility of the test and its major impact on mortality and morbidity, were first demonstrated in Jamaica [3]. Available data also suggest that the prevalence of SCD in the Caribbean Region is second only to Sub-Saharan Africa [4].

However, prior to 2006, accurate SCD prevalence and epidemiological data were available for only a limited number of these countries and territories. These data were provided from NBS programs implemented in Jamaica [5] and in the French territories [6], as well as from a prenatal diagnosis program in Cuba [7,8]. Collaboration between medical and scientific Caribbean teams began to increase in 2006, leading to the founding in 2011 of the Caribbean Network of Researchers on Sickle Cell Disease and Thalassemia (CAREST) as a not-for-profit organization [9]. Promotion of NBS for the hemoglobinopathies and assistance for the establishment of sickle cell centers were the primary goals of CAREST. CAREST has worked with all regional stakeholders with common goals, including the SickKids Caribbean Initiative. It has included outreach initiatives to clinicians and policy makers to share regional data regarding the status of SCD NBS and the implications for their own countries. As a result, we present an SCD NBS program initiated in Tobago since 2008 and pilot NBS programs conducted in Grenada and Saint Lucia in 2014–2015 and 2015–2017, respectively.

Beyond the presentation and discussion on the experience of CAREST in establishing NBS programs, we also present an update on the prevalence of SCD in the Caribbean.

2. Materials and Methods

2.1. Neonatal Screening for Sickle Cell Disease

Blood samples obtained neonatally are collected on Guthrie cards. As shown in Table 1, cord blood samples are collected in Martinique, Jamaica, and St Lucia, whereas in Guadeloupe, Tobago, Grenada, and French Guiana, heel prick samples are obtained. Heel prick samples were also collected for the Saint Lucia's pilot NBS project funded by the SickKids Caribbean Initiative (2015–2017) and these samples were sent and processed in Jamaica. This project sought to test the feasibility of replacing cord blood sampling and hemoglobin electrophoresis which had been in place since 1992, by heel prick sampling and high-performance liquid chromatography (HPLC); during the pilot, both systems ran concomitantly. Blood samples from Tobago and Grenada are sent by post-mail and analyzed in Guadeloupe (Table 1).

Table 1. Neonatal screening process.

Site	Sample	Screening Center	First Test	Confirmation Test
Guadeloupe Tobago Grenada	Heel prick/Guthrie cards	Guadeloupe	HPLC	IEF
Martinique	Cord blood/Guthrie cards	Martinique	IEF	HPLC
French Guiana	Heel prick/Guthrie cards	France (Lille)	CE	HPLC
Jamaica 1995–2015 Jamaica 2015–2018	Cord blood/Guthrie cards	Jamaica	Citrate agar HPLC	Cellulose acetate IEF
Saint Lucia 1992–2018 [†] Saint Lucia 2015–2017 [††]	Cord blood/Guthrie cards Heel prick/Guthrie cards	Saint-Lucia Jamaica	Citrate agar HPLC	Cellulose acetate IEF

[†] From Alexander et al. [10]; [††] From pilot (results not previously published). HPLC: high-performance liquid chromatography; IEF: isoelectric focusing; CE: capillary electrophoresis.

As indicated in Table 1, the samples are primarily tested in reference laboratories based in Guadeloupe (University Hospital of Guadeloupe), Martinique (University Hospital of Martinique), and Jamaica (Sickle Cell Unit, Caribbean Institute for Health Research, Kingston and Southern Regional Health Authority, Manchester). French Guiana specimens are sent to a reference laboratory based in mainland France (regional center for metabolic disease screening, Lille). Saint Lucian cord blood samples, except for those obtained during the pilot study, are tested locally.

NBS itself now primarily uses three laboratory-based methodologies for detecting Hb variants: isoelectric focusing (IEF), capillary electrophoresis (CE), and high-performance liquid chromatography (HPLC), one is used as the first-line screening method and a second as a confirmatory test. In Saint Lucia, however, hemoglobin cellulose acetate and citrate agar electrophoresis are used locally for cord blood samples. In Guadeloupe, DNA analysis is also secondarily performed as a confirmatory diagnosis of a new sample (peripheral blood on EDTA as anticoagulant) in the following cases: FS phenotype when the two parents cannot be tested in order to distinguish SS, S/beta-thalassemia, or S/HPFH; and the FSX or FCX phenotype in order to formally identify the abnormal hemoglobin (HbX), as well as for ambiguous primary screening results [11,12].

2.2. Prenatal Screening for SCD

In Cuba, the screening for SCD is a prenatal diagnosis based on fetal DNA analysis. This procedure has been established since 1982 for mothers at risk and the screening program is performed on pregnant women at the provincial centers of genetics located all over the country [7,8].

2.3. Initiation of Early Childhood Care for SCD

Children confirmed to have a diagnosis of SCD are enrolled in the different sickle cell centers or clinical structures as soon as possible to initiate clinical management and to provide information to the parents. To shorten delays and promote early medical management of the newly identified SCD children from Tobago, the results are sent by e-mail from the laboratory in Guadeloupe to the appropriate health care provider using secure file transfer systems. Similar communication procedures were also used during the pilot projects in Grenada and Saint Lucia.

2.4. Data Analysis

Allele frequencies were estimated by gene-counting and the prevalence of SCD was calculated from the newborn screening results.

3. Results

Table 2 summarizes the main results of the hemoglobinopathy NBS programs performed in the French territories [6], Jamaica [5], Grenada [13], Tobago [9], and Saint Lucia [10].

Table 2. Results from the newborn screening programs in the Caribbean.

Site	Period	Number of Samples Screened	FAS	FAC	FS	FSC	FC	Other
Jamaica	1995–2006 *	150,803	14,688 9.74% 9.59–9.89%	5420 3.59% 3.50–3.69%	557 0.37% 0.34–0.40%	332 0.22% 0.20–0.25%	115 0.08 0.06–0.09%	972 0.64% 0.61–0.69%
	2016–2017	40,444	4020 9.94% 9.65–10.24	1481 3.66% 3.48–3.85	165 0.41% 0.35–0.47	95 0.23% 0.19–0.29	35 0.09% 0.06–0.12	63 0.16% 0.12–0.20
Guadeloupe	1984–2010	178,428	14,126 7.92% 7.79–8.04%	4375 2.45% 2.38–2.52%	310 0.17% 0.16–0.19%	231 0.13% 0.11–0.15%	39 0.02 0.02–0.03%	248 0.14 0.12–0.16%
Martinique	2009–2015 **	30,171	2134 7.07% 6.79–7.37%	910 3.02% 2.83–3.22%	44 0.15% 0.11–0.20%	29 0.10% 0.07–0.14%	11 0.04% 0.02–0.07%	88 0.29% 0.29–0.36%
French Guiana	1992–2013	115,200	8824 7.66% 7.51–7.81%	2797 2.43% 2.34–2.52%	293 0.25% 0.23–0.29%	186 0.16% 0.14–0.19%	NA	NA
Grenada	2014–2015	1914	183 (9.56%) 8.32–10.96%	63 3.29% 2.58–4.19%	10 0.52% 0.28–0.96%	2 0.10% 0.03–0.38%	1 0.05% 0.01–0.3%	2 0.10% 0.03–0.38%
Tobago	2008–2017	7389	689 9.32% 8.68–10.01%	285 3.86% 3.44–4.32%	28 0.38% 0.26–0.55%	14 0.19% 0.11–0.32%	5 0.07% 0.03–0.16%	21 0.28% 0.19–0.43%
St Lucia	1992–2010 †	36,253	3146 8.68% 8.39–8.97%	NA	180 0.50% 0.43–0.57%	59 0.16% 0.13–0.21%	NA	NA
	2015–2017 ††	2023	238 11.76% 10.43–13.24%	42 2.08% 1.54–2.79%	3 0.15% 0.05–0.44%	5 0.25% 0.11–0.58%	2 0.10% 0.04–3.6%	NA

Number of samples screened with the FAS, FAC, FS, and FSC phenotypes are indicated (first line), as well as the prevalence (%) and (95% confidence interval). Other: samples presenting with an abnormal hemoglobin other than HbS or HbC; NA: Not available; * samples collected under the South–East Regional Jamaican Health Authorities only and tested at the Sickle Cell Unit, Caribbean Institute for Health Research (from King et al. [5]); ** universal screening was initiated in Martinique in 1986 in two different laboratories and in 2009, it was centralized in one single center; reliable data are only available from 2009 onwards; † from Alexander et al. [10]; †† From pilot (results not previously published).

The current coverage of the NBS programs is as follows: Guadeloupe (>98%), Martinique (>99%), Jamaica (>98%), and Tobago (96%). The coverage of the two pilot NBSs in Grenada and Saint Lucia were 79% and 45% respectively. In Cuba, since the beginning of the program until December 2016, 7659 couples at risk have been identified.

The highest frequency of sickle cell trait carriers is observed in Jamaica (9.74–9.94%), Grenada (9.56%), and Tobago (9.32%). In Jamaica, less samples presenting abnormal hemoglobin other than HbS or HbC have been observed during the 2016–2017 period (0.16%) than during the previous screening period (0.64%), probably due to an optimization of the Hb variant detection.

The low screening coverage rate (45%) in Saint-Lucia during the period 2015–2017 could explain the differences in the frequency of phenotypes observed compared to the 1992–2010 period.

Table 3 summarizes the currently available data on β^S and β^C allele frequencies, carrier prevalence, and SCD prevalence in the Caribbean area.

Table 3. SCD birth prevalence in the Caribbean countries and territories.

(A) Neonatal Screening					
Country/Territory	Screening Method	Carrier Prevalence (Hb S and Hb C Trait)	Gene Frequencies	β^S/β^C Ratio	SCD Prevalence
Jamaica	Specific locations (1995–2006) [6]	15%	β^S: 0.055–β^C: 0.019	2.89	0.53%–1/188
	Univ screen (2016–2017)	13.6%	β^S: 0.055–β^C: 0.020	2.75	0.65%–1/153
Guadeloupe	Univ screen	10.5%	β^S: 0.042–β^C: 0.013	3.23	0.33%–1/304
Martinique	Univ screen	10%	β^S: 0.040–β^C: 0.012	3.33	0.31%–1/322
French Guiana	Univ screen	10%	β^S: 0.039–β^C: 0.012	3.25	0.42%–1/235
Tobago	Univ screen	13.2%	β^S: 0.051–β^C: 0.021	2.43	0.57%–1/176
Grenada [7]	Univ screen	12.85%	β^S: 0.054–β^C: 0.018	3.00	0.63%–1/160
Saint Lucia	Univ screen	13.8%	β^S: 0.062–β^C: 0.013	4.77	0.39%–1/253
Haiti [9]	Pilot screen	13.46%	β^S: 0.059–β^C: 0.013	4.54	0.58%–1/173
Saint Vincent & Grenadines [10]	Pilot screen	15.27%	β^S: 0.065–β^C: 0.016	4.06	0.26%–1/382
(B) Prenatal Diagnosis					
Country/Territory	Screening Method	Carrier Prevalence (Hb S and Hb C Trait)	Gene Frequencies	β^S/β^C Ratio	SCD Prevalence
Cuba	Prenatal diagnosis	3.1%	β^S: 0.011–β^C: 0.0036 [a]	3.06	
			β^S: 0.053–β^C: 0.006 [b]	8.83	0.02%–1/5000

Univ screen: universal screening; [a]: Figures for the Western side of Cuba (not including for Havana); [b]: figures for the Southeastern side of Cuba.

Several abnormal genotypes, some of which include hemoglobin variants leading to sickle cell disease when associated with the β^S allele, have also been identified during the course of these NBS programs. Indeed, the second most frequent sickle cell genotype encountered in these populations was the genotype SC, with some differences in the β^S/β^C ratio detected, and the highest was observed in Saint-Lucia and the lowest in Tobago, as indicated in Table 3. The others correspond to S/β-thalassemia compound heterozygosity (including S/E and S/Lepore) and also S/D^{Punjab} [3,6].

Once infants are screened, confirmation and referral for care are ensued. In French speaking territories and in Jamaica, care is provided according to the guidelines of the French Health Authority [14] and the Sickle Cell Unit [15], respectively. The Sickle Cell Unit Clinical Care Guidelines are currently in use in several other Anglophone countries, including Trinidad and Tobago, Saint-Lucia, the Bahamas, and Barbados. The focus is on pneumococcal prevention and general health maintenance (parents' education, counselling) prior to the onset of complications. In Martinique, Guadeloupe, French Guiana, and Jamaica, most of the SCD children identified by the NBS program are followed by Sickle cell centers before the age of three months [5,6]. In Saint-Lucia and Tobago, babies identified are followed up in pediatric outpatient clinics. In Cuba, guidelines for management and treatment have also been developed [8].

4. Discussion

Given the SCD prevalence and the demonstration of the benefit of the NBS program, one might have expected that SCD NBS would be entrenched across the Region. This is clearly not the case and our data suggest several factors which may be at play, with the availability of resources being a major issue [5,6,9].

Caribbean territories which are part of larger states which mandate SCD NBS as part of a larger universal NBS program, have long and well-established programs. These may be the best funded programs in the Region. In the three French territories, Guadeloupe, Martinique, and French Guiana, the cost of the test is borne by the French government. In territories of the United States of America, screening started in Puerto Rico in 1977 and the US Virgin Islands in 1987 [16]. The test mandated by law covers 99% of births, but the hospitals include a charge to the patient for the NBS panel (http://bft.stage.bbox.ly/newborn-screening/states/puerto-rico). Overseas British territories have separate health systems and SCD NBS is not uniformly offered.

Among the independent nations, Cuba has an integrated public health program and SCD prenatal testing for couples at risk and carrier women was mandated by law in 1983 [7,8]. This program seeks to actively prevent the births of children with SCD, and is perhaps the most active in promoting the termination of pregnancies; since termination of pregnancy was requested by 76.5% of at-risk couples.

In the other independent Caribbean nations, screening varies based on factors such as historical context, current champions, and public health commitment. Jamaica has a unique historical context as the site of the Jamaica Sickle Cell Cohort Study. Nevertheless, after the completion of recruitment for the cohort study in 1981, SCD NBS ceased until 1995, when, through the advocacy of the Sickle Cell Support Club of Jamaica (now the Sickle Cell Support Foundation), it was restarted. For a decade, it was limited to three hospitals in the South East Regional Health Authority, providing screening for approximately 43% of all national births. The coverage gradually increased from 2008 to 2015 when essentially universal coverage was achieved. While testing was mandated in the National Strategic Plan for the Prevention and Control of Non-communicable Disease in Jamaica 2012–2018, there is no legislative mandate and the integration of the program into the fabric of the public health system remains incomplete. Thus, the sustainability of the program depends on the support of incumbent policy makers.

The Saint Lucia Sickle Cell Association (SSCA), a local non-governmental organization, has been strong for many years. It was influential in the introduction of universal SCD NBS in 1992 and its integration into the Ministry of Health's Community Child Health Service (CCHS) [10]. The program uses hemoglobin electrophoresis to test cord blood samples. A pilot program funded by the SickKids Caribbean Initiative using HPLC testing of heel prick samples had a disappointing uptake and the initial approach continues. The pilot in Tobago has also been successful; it has been continuous for a decade. It is funded by the Regional Health Authority of Tobago, which has made the diagnosis and treatment of SCD a priority. Screening of the immediate family of babies identified with the trait or the disease is done by electrophoresis in the hospital laboratory, thus a greater percentage of the population now know their genotype and there is a greater awareness through education. The initiation of SCD NBS at a major obstetric hospital in Trinidad in 2018 is further evidence of the acceptance of this program.

Pilot screening projects in Grenada [13], St Vincent and the Grenadines [17], and Haiti [18], funded by CAREST, the Medical University of South Carolina (Charleston, SC, USA), and University Hospitals Medical Center (Cleveland, OH, USA), respectively, were not sustained once project funding ended. Local policy makers were not able to identify funding and human resources for continued screening. A pilot posited in Barbados was not undertaken [19]. Instead, screening of pregnant women and testing postnatally of at risk children was the approach chosen.

Currently, champions in Antigua and Guyana are pressing to start pilots and perhaps sustainable programs. These outcomes again indicate the importance of advocacy in convincing policy makers of the feasibility and benefit of SCD NBS. In both Jamaica and Saint Lucia, advocacy groups have been critical to convincing public health officials to initiate and maintain screening. CAREST has a role in supporting their advocacy efforts to secure governmental support and sustainable funding, even as screening begins. In this framework, CAREST has recently obtained funding from the European Regional Development Fund. This funding dedicated to the development of cooperation between the French Departments of the Americas and the other countries/territories of the Caribbean Basin will allow the screening of Grenada to be re-launched, initiate a pilot study for Antigua, and evaluate strategies to ensure the sustainability of this NBS.

The Saint-Lucia and Tobago experience clearly demonstrate that the model of using a few regional laboratories to increase efficiencies of scale, decreasing per cost tests, can be used. Actually, given the high cost of equipment and requisite disposables, and the relatively small populations in the Region, the use of two regional laboratories (Jamaica and Guadeloupe) proved to be a cost-effective approach, once reasonably costed transportation of samples and secure data flows are available. However, it is worthwhile to notice that a significant proportion of the Caribbean populations do not have access to screening program, such as Haiti, which accounts for more than 90% the Francophone inhabitants of the Caribbean, and the Dominican Republic, with approximately 40% of Spanish-speakers. Up to now, only a little more than 50% of the English and Spanish speaking infants are screened.

The cost of national SCD NBS programmes may decrease significantly if efficient, accurate, and inexpensive point-of-care (POC) devices become available; a number of such POC testing devices have recently been developed [20]. These low-cost devices, which must have high specificity to detect HbS and HbC in the presence of HbF and the capacity to distinguish the trait (HbAS) from samples with SCD, must also be easy to use. Two of them, relying on lateral flow immunoassays, the SickleSCAN [21] and the HemoTypeSC tests [22], could be viable screening tools for the early diagnosis of SCD conducted by health workers with little expertise. Preliminary data using the HemoTypeSC test on a small series of children and adults in Martinique, in comparison with a larger series in Ghana and the USA, showed the good specificity and sensitivity of the test [23]. We plan to conduct larger studies to evaluate the performance and implementation feasibility of these POC testing devices as screening tools in Caribbean territories where the reference "gold-standard" tests, IEF, and HPLC are not available. This approach may also reduce the number of samples to be screened by the reference laboratories and the delay between the blood sampling and the transmission of the result and ultimately reduce the age of inclusion of the newly identified children. Mothers would get immediate feedback if their children's tests are normal, and be advised of the need to do confirmatory tests in cases consistent with traits or SCD. This promising strategy is expected to promote the extension of screening programs, and lead to the clarification of the prevalence and to a better management of SCD in the Caribbean. Audits of important outcomes, such as time to enrollment in clinic, initiation of splenic palpation, and Pneumococcal prophylaxis, as well as continued ongoing ascertainment of survival in countries and territories with SCD NBS, will help to determine what implementation models are most successful and guide the subsequent initiation of programs in other settings.

Differences of SCD prevalence in the Caribbean islands could be observed, with the highest being detected in Jamaica and Grenada and the lowest in Cuba. Various factors may explain these variations, such as the selective introduction of crop production requiring a greater or lesser need for slaves, the settlement policy of the colonial powers with France and the United Kingdom importing few of their own population compared to Spain, for example, as well as the significance of migrations after the end of slavery (ranging from 1804 in Haiti to 1888 in Brazil). In addition, various β^S/β^C ratios have been detected in the studied populations. Since the distribution of the β^C allele is more restricted than that of the β^S allele in Africa, this data could be related to differences in the African origins of the deported slaves in these territories. These differences in the β^S/β^C ratio could also result from sampling effects; a relatively small number of newborns were screened in some populations. Few epidemiological data from continental countries of the Western coast of the Caribbean Sea coast have been produced so far. An NBS pilot study was conducted in Costa Rica with a total of 70,943 samples and led to the identification of five SS and one SC children [24]. In addition, several clinical reports or genetic studies indicating the presence of SCD in Panama [25], Colombia [26], and Venezuela [27] have been published, but none of these countries have implemented an NBS program on SCD and no accurate data of the prevalence of the disease are available so far, to the best of our knowledge.

In summary, SCD is a perfect example of a disease which fulfils all requirements for doing NBS. Parents are usually asymptomatic and may not know of their risk. Tests done on an asymptomatic baby can allow them to access interventions that decrease morbidity and preventable mortality. CAREST will continue to advocate and work towards universal SCD NBS across the Caribbean Region, regardless of language, per capita income, or political system.

Author Contributions: Conceptualization: M.R., M.-D.H.-D., B.M.-T., and J.K.-M.; Methodology: M.R., L.K., K.L., N.E., G.E., M.E.-J., B.M.-T., M.-D.H.-D., and J.K.-M.; Resources: L.K., K.L., N.E., G.E., M.E.-J., B.M.-T., M.A., and N.K.; Writing-Original Draft Preparation: M.R., J.K.-M., B.M.-T., and M.-D.H.-D.; Writing-Review & Editing: M.R., M.-D.H.-D., L.K., K.L., J.K.-M., B.M.-T., M.A., N.E., G.E., and N.K.; Project administration: M.-D.H.-D., and J.K.-M.

Acknowledgments: The authors wish to acknowledge the contribution of the team of the diagnostic laboratory of hemoglobinopathies of the University Hospital of Guadeloupe for its implication in the NBS of Tobago and Grenada.

References

1. Curtin, P.D. Distribution in space: The colonies of the North Europeans. In *The Atlantic Slave Trade: A Census*; University of Wisconsin Press: Madison, WI, USA, 1969; pp. 51–94.
2. Herrick, J.B. Peculiar elongated and sickle-shaped red blood cell corpuscules in a case of severe anemia. *Arch. Intern. Med.* **1910**, *6*, 517–521. [CrossRef]
3. Serjeant, G.; Serjeant, B.E.; Forbes, M.; Hayes, R.J.; Higgs, D.R.; Lehmann, H. Haemoglobin gene frequencies in the Jamaican population: A study in 100,000 newborns. *Br. J. Haematol.* **1986**, *64*, 253–262. [CrossRef] [PubMed]
4. Kato, G.J.; Piel, F.B.; Reid, C.D.; Gaston, M.H.; Ohene-Frempong, K.; Krishnamurti, L.; Smith, W.R.; Panepinto, J.A.; Weatherall, D.J.; Costa, F.F.; et al. Sickle cell disease. *Nat. Rev. Dis. Primers* **2018**, *4*, 18010. [CrossRef] [PubMed]
5. King, L.; Fraser, R.; Forbes, M.; Grindley, M.; Ali, S.; Reid, M. Newborn sickle cell disease screening: The Jamaican experience (1995–2006). *J. Med. Screen.* **2007**, *14*, 117–122. [CrossRef] [PubMed]
6. Saint-Martin, C.; Romana, M.; Bibrac, A.; Brudey, K.; Tarer, V.; Divialle-Doumdo, L.; Petras, M.; Keclard-Christophe, L.; Lamothe, S.; Broquere, C.; et al. Universal newborn screening for haemoglobinopathies in Guadeloupe (French West Indies): A 27-year experience. *J. Med. Screen.* **2013**, *20*, 177–182. [CrossRef]
7. Heredero-Baute, L. Community-based program for the diagnosis and prevention of genetic disorders in Cuba. Twenty years of experience. *Community Genet.* **2004**, *7*, 130–136. [CrossRef]
8. Svarch, E.; Machín García, S.; Marcheco Teruel, B.; Triana, R.M.; González Otero, A.; Menéndez Veitía, A. Program for comprehensive sickle cell disease care in Cuba. *Revista Cubana de Hematología, Inmunología y Hemoterapia* **2017**, *33*, 1–2.
9. Knight-Madden, J.; Romana, M.; Villaescusa, R.; Reid, M.; Etienne-Julan, M.; Boutin, L.; Elana, G.; Elenga, N.; Wheeler, G.; Lee, K.; et al. CAREST—Multilingual Regional Integration for Health Promotion and Research on Sickle Cell Disease and Thalassemia. *Am. J. Public Health* **2016**, *106*, 851–853. [CrossRef]
10. Alexander, S.; Belmar-George, S.; Eugene, A.; Elias, V. Knowledge of an attitudes toward heel prick screening for sickle cell disease in Saint Lucia. *Rev. Panam. Salud Publica* **2017**, *41*, e70.
11. Kéclard, L.; Romana, M.; Lavocat, E.; Saint-Martin, C.; Berchel, C.; Mérault, G. Sickle cell disorder, beta-globin gene cluster haplotypes and alpha-thalassemia in neonates and adults from Guadeloupe. *Am. J. Hematol.* **1997**, *55*, 24–27. [CrossRef]
12. Romana, M.; Kéclard, L.; Froger, A.; Lavocat, E.; Saint-Martin, C.; Berchel, C.; Mérault, G. Diverse genetic mechanisms operate to generate atypical betaS haplotypes in the population of Guadeloupe. *Hemoglobin* **2000**, *24*, 77–87. [CrossRef] [PubMed]
13. Antoine, M.; Lee, K.; Donald, T.; Belfon, Y.; Drigo, A.; Polson, S.; Martin, F.; Mitchell, G.; Etienne-Julan, M.; Hardy-Dessources, M.D. Prevalence of sickle cell disease among Grenadian newborns. *J. Med. Screen.* **2018**, *25*, 49–50. [CrossRef] [PubMed]
14. Available online: https://www.has-sante.fr/portail/upload/.../ald_10_pnds_drepano_enfant_web.pdf (accessed on 2 April 2010).
15. Aldred, K.; Asnani, M.; Beckford, M.; Bhatt-Poulose, K.; Bortolusso Ali, S.; Chin, N.; Daley, C.; Grindley, M.; Hammond-Gabbadon, C.; Harris, J.; et al. *Sickle Cell Disease: The Clinical Care Guidelines of the Sickle Cell Unit*; Bortolusi-Ali, S., Ed.; Sickle Cell Unit, Tropical Medicine Research Institute, University of the West Indies: Kingston, Jamaica, 2016.

16. Morales, A.; Wierenga, A.; Cuthbert, C.; Sacharow, S.; Jayakar, P.; Velazquez, D.; Loring, J.; Barbouth, D. Expanded newborn screening in Puerto Rico and the US Virgin Islands: Education and barriers assessment. *Genet. Med.* **2009**, *11*, 169–175. [CrossRef] [PubMed]

17. Williams, S.A.; Browne-Ferdinand, B.; Smart, Y.; Morella, K.; Reed, S.G.; Kanter, J. Newborn Screening for Sickle Cell Disease in St. Vincent and the Grenadines: Results of a Pilot Newborn Screening Program. *Glob. Pediatr. Health* **2017**, *4*. [CrossRef]

18. Rotz, S.; Arty, G.; Dall'Amico, R.; De Zen, L.; Zanolli, F.; Bodas, P. Prevalence of sickle cell disease, hemoglobin S, and hemoglobin C among Haitian newborns. *Am. J. Hematol.* **2013**, *88*, 827–828. [CrossRef] [PubMed]

19. Quimby, K.R.; Moe, S.; Sealy, I.; Nicholls, C.; Hambleton, I.R.; Landis, R.C. Clinical findings associated with homozygous sickle cell disease in the Barbadian population–do we need a national SCD registry? *BMC Res. Notes* **2014**, *7*, 102. [CrossRef] [PubMed]

20. McGann, P.T.; Hoppe, C. The pressing need for point-of-care diagnostics for sickle cell disease: A review of current and future technologies. *Blood Cells Mol. Dis.* **2017**, *67*, 104–113. [CrossRef]

21. Nwegbu, M.M.; Isa, H.A.; Nwankwo, B.B.; Okeke, C.C.; Edet-Offong, U.J.; Akinola, N.O.; Adekile, A.D.; Aneke, J.C.; Okocha, E.C.; Ulasi, T.; et al. Preliminary Evaluation of a Point-of-Care Testing Device (SickleSCAN™) in Screening for Sickle Cell Disease. *Hemoglobin* **2017**, *41*, 77–82. [CrossRef]

22. Quinn, C.T.; Paniagua, M.C.; DiNello, R.K.; Panchal, A.; Geisberg, M. A rapid, inexpensive and disposable point-of-care blood test for sickle cell disease using novel, highly specific monoclonal antibodies. *Br. J. Haematol.* **2016**, *175*, 724–732. [CrossRef]

23. Steele, C.; Sinski, A.; Asibey, J.; Hardy-Dessources, M.D.; Elana, G.; Brennan, C.; Odame, I.; Hoppe, C.; Geisberg, M.; Serrao, E.; et al. Point-of-care screening for sickle cell disease in low-resource settings: A multi-center evaluation of HemoTypeSC, a novel rapid test. *Am. J. Hematol.* **2018**. [CrossRef]

24. Abarca, G.; Navarrete, M.; Trejos, R.; de Céspedes, C.; Saborío, M. Abnormal haemoglobins in the newborn human population of Costa Rica. *Rev. Biol. Trop.* **2008**, *56*, 995–1001. [PubMed]

25. Rusanova, I.; Cossio, G.; Moreno, B.; Javier Perea, F.; De Borace, R.G.; Perea, M.; Escames, G.; Acuña-Castroviejo, D. β-globin gene cluster haplotypes in sickle cell patients from Panamá. *Am. J. Hum. Biol.* **2011**, *23*, 377–380. [CrossRef] [PubMed]

26. Fong, C.; Lizarralde-Iragorri, M.A.; Rojas-Gallardo, D.; Barreto, G. Frequency and origin of haplotypes associated with the beta-globin gene cluster in individuals with trait and sickle cell anemia in the Atlantic and Pacific coastal regions of Colombia. *Genet. Mol. Biol.* **2013**, *36*, 494–497. [CrossRef] [PubMed]

27. Arends, A.; Alvarez, M.; Velázquez, D.; Bravo, M.; Salazar, R.; Guevara, J.M.; Castillo, O. Determination of beta-globin gene cluster haplotypes and prevalence of alpha-thalassemia in sickle cell anemia patients in Venezuela. *Am. J. Hematol.* **2000**, *64*, 87–90. [CrossRef]

18

Inconclusive Diagnosis after Newborn Screening for Cystic Fibrosis

Anne Munck

Hopital Necker Enfants-Malades, AP-HP, CF centre, Université Paris Descartes, 75015 Paris, France; anne.munck1@gmail.com;

Abstract: An unintended consequence of newborn screening for cystic fibrosis (CF) is the identification of infants with a positive screening test but an inconclusive diagnostic testing. These infants are designated as CF transmembrane conductance regulator-related metabolic syndrome (CRMS) in the US and CF screen-positive, inconclusive diagnosis (CFSPID) in Europe. Recently, experts agreed on a unified international definition of CRMS/CFSPID which will improve our knowledge on the epidemiology and outcomes of these infants and optimize comparisons between cohorts. Many of these children will remain free of symptoms, but a number may develop clinical features suggestive of CFTR-related disorder (CFTR-RD) or CF later in life. Clinicians should to be prepared to identify these infants and communicate with parents about this challenging and stressful situation for both healthcare professionals and families. In this review, we present the recent publications on infants designated as CRMS/CFSPID, including the definition, the incidence across Europe, the assessment of the CFTR protein function, the outcomes with the rates of conversion to a final diagnosis of CF and their management.

Keywords: cystic fibrosis; CF transmembrane conductance regulator-related metabolic syndrome; CF screen positive; inconclusive diagnosis; newborn screening

1. Introduction

Newborn screening (NBS) for cystic fibrosis (CF), when combined with very early multidisciplinary care at CF centers (CFC), is acknowledged as the optimal approach to CF diagnosis, as it maximizes the long-term prognosis and survival of these children [1–3]. However, beyond the goal of NBS and irrespective of the screening protocol used, there is the detection of infants with a positive NBS test and an inconclusive designation [4]. The terminology used for these infants is CF transmembrane conductance regulator-related metabolic syndrome (CRMS) in the US [5] and CF screen-positive, inconclusive diagnosis (CFSPID) in Europe [6]. Many of these children will remain asymptomatic, but later in life, a number of them may develop symptoms suggestive or CFTR-related disorder (CFTR-RD) or CF [7]. The approach to these infants is evolving as clinical experience grows; nevertheless, uncertainty remains challenging for families and caregivers

2. Inconclusive Diagnosis after Newborn Screening

2.1. Definition of CRMS/CFSPID

For infants with a positive NBS test but an inconclusive diagnosis, a definition has been created using the terminology CRMS in the US since 2009 [5] that is included in the International Statistical Classification of Diseases and Related Health Problems, Ninth Revision medical code (277.9), which is mandatory in the US for healthcare delivery. Recently, in Europe, a Delphi process conducted by the European CF Society (ECFS) Neonatal Screening Working Group (NN WG) identified the need for a designation, and the terminology CFSPID was introduced in 2015 [6]. The differences between these two definitions were minor. To optimize comparisons between cohorts and thus improve our knowledge on the epidemiology and outcomes, experts from around the world gathered at a Diagnosis Consensus Conference held in the US, in 2015, and agreed on a unified definition (Table 1) of CRMS/CFSPID [8], with a recently published algorithm for this definition in Figure 1 [9]. This definition incorporates the knowledge on *CFTR* variants characteristics as "CF causing", "non-CF causing", "varying clinical consequences" or "unknown significance" [10] in the CFTR2 database, which is regularly updated and searchable on the website https://cftr2.org. However, an international survey conducted in 2018 by ECFS NN WG, with support of the Cystic Fibrosis Foundation (CFF) NBS Quality Improvement Group, showed significant confusion in regard to the correct designation of inconclusive diagnosis in six scenarios of infants screening positive. In one-third to half of the respondents, who were either CF doctors or pediatric pulmonologists [9], the diagnosis option was incorrect, thus identifying the need for improved education and communication.

Table 1. Definitions for CF transmembrane conductance regulator-related metabolic syndrome (CRMS) and CF screen-positive, inconclusive diagnosis (CFSPID) and the harmonized definition CRMS/CFSPID.

	Positive NBS	And	Or
CRMS [5] US	Asymptomatic infants with hypertrypsinemia at birth	Persistently intermediate sweat chloride levels [1] and fewer than 2 CF-causing CFTR mutations	Sweat chloride concentration <30 mmol/L and 2 CFTR mutations with 0 or 1 known to be CF-causing
CFSPID [6] Europe	Asymptomatic infants with hypertrypsinemia at birth	0 or 1 CFTR mutation, plus intermediate sweat chloride (30–59 mmol/L)	2 CFTR mutations, at least 1 of which has unclear phenotypic consequences, plus a normal sweat chloride (<30 mmol/L)
CRMS/CFSPID [8]	Infants with positive newborn screening test	Sweat chloride <30 mmol/L and 2 CFTR mutations with 0 or 1 CF-causing CFTR mutation	Sweat chloride 30–59 mmol/L and 0 or 1 CF-causing CFTR mutation

[1] Sweat chloride levels: 30–59 mmol/L if age < 6 months or 40–59 mmol/L if age ≥6 months.

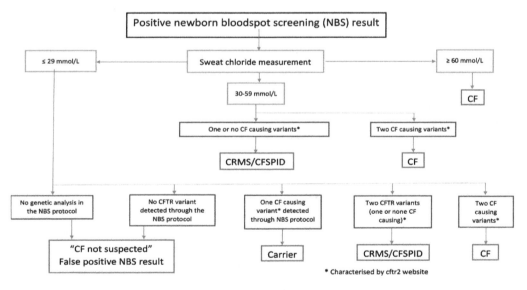

Figure 1. An algorithm for the designation of infants, following the positive newborn screening (NBS) result [9]. CF: Cystic fibrosis, CFTR: CF transmembrane conductance regulator (gene), CFMS: CFTR-related metabolic syndrome, CFSPID: CF screen-positive, inconclusive diagnosis.

2.2. Incidence of CRMS/CFSPID across Europe

Within the two past decades, there has been a huge increase in NBS programs for CF worldwide, including in Europe. A recent European survey [4] reported data from 16 out of the 17 national

NBS protocols with centralized data collection. Since then, national programs have been developed in Portugal (2015), Germany (2016), Denmark (2016), Macedonia (2018) and Belgium (2020); and Spain and Italy have regional programs that provide extensive coverage of the population. Strategies of NBS protocols and structure of programs vary widely, like the proportion of cases designated CRMS/CFSPID, reflecting the different approaches. This survey collected data during the year 2014, when the definition of CFSPID was not yet available, and therefore the recognition of infants may possibly be underestimated. The ratio of infants with CF compared to CFSPID ranged from 1.2:1 (Poland) to 32:1 (Ireland), and protocols, including larger panels of DNA mutations, were more likely to identify those infants. Minimizing the number of cases with CRMS/CFSPID remains an important consideration in NBS programs, as referring and following these infants create a burden for their families and healthcare professionals, and the benefits remain unclear.

2.3. Assessment of CFTR Protein Function

In cases where repeated sweat tests' levels remain within the intermediate range, functional analyses measuring CFTR activity may help clarify the diagnosis. The assessment of the level of CFTR function is based on in vivo pharmacological studies, such as nasal potential difference (NPD) [11] or ex vivo intestinal current measurement (ICM) performed on rectal biopsies perfused in Ussing chambers [12], and on some occasion in combination with intestinal organoids analysis [13]. These evaluations of the CFTR function are performed exclusively in highly specialized CF centers and are not currently used in clinical practice. A diagnosis of CF can be ruled out when these functional analyses are within the normal range. The level of CFTR function further defines the likelihood of developing CF, as there is a continuum of CFTR dysfunction, and the paradigm of CF can be defined in terms of risk, depending on the severity of the dysfunction.

3. Monitoring Infants Designated CRMS/CFSPID

3.1. Outcomes and Conversion to a Final Diagnosis of CF in Infants Designated CRMS/CFSPID

Infants designated CRMS/CFSPID may later develop a diagnosis of CFTR-RD, and a number may have symptoms suggestive of CF and convert to a final diagnosis of CF (a less classical form in most cases). The range of conversion to CF varied widely in retrospective or registry database studies [14–18], from 6% [14] to 48% [15] (Table 2). Neither the definition of cases with an inconclusive diagnosis nor the diagnosis criteria for conversion to CF was consistent among these studies, as well as the duration of follow-up, thus providing an explanation in this wide range of conversion to CF. Reclassification to CF should be based either on subsequent positive sweat test and/or two *CFTR* variants as CF causing *in trans* according to new knowledge acquired in CFTR2. Conversion to CF is also more likely related to individual CFTR variants [19–21] and to infants with an initial intermediate sweat chloride (SC) value compared to normal SC [16]. In two recent prospective studies, the conversion rate varied from 11% [19] to 44% [21]. The first prospective study was set up by Ooi et al. [19] in eight CF centers in Canada and Italy. Eighty-two positive NBS infants with an inconclusive diagnosis of CF, born 2007–2013, were matched 1:1 with a cohort diagnosed with CF through NBS ($n = 80$) and were evaluated at a median age of 2.2 years. Those with a CRMS/CFSPID designation at baseline had significantly lower median IRT (77 µg/L vs. 144 µg/L, $p < 0.0001$) and SC values (27.3 mmol/L vs. 83.2 mmol/L, $p < 0.0001$) compared to those diagnosed with CF. During follow-up, compared to those with CF, they all had sustained exocrine pancreatic sufficiency and less respiratory symptoms as well as identification of *Pseudomonas aeruginosa* (12% vs. 31%) and *Staphylococcus aureus* (40% vs. 70%). Among the 82 cases with a CRMS/CFSPID diagnosis, nine (11%) children converted to a delayed CF diagnosis based on positive SC value ($n = 2$), with the identification of two CF-causing mutations *in trans* in the CFTR2 database at the time of data analysis ($n = 4$) or both in three cases. Serial repeated sweat testing showed a mean age of 21.3 months at the time of conversion in those diagnosed with CF with a positive SC value. Those who converted to CF had higher initial SC values, no clinical or anthropometric differences and a trend toward more *Pseudomonas aeruginosa* identification compared to those who did not convert to CF. Authors shed light on the limited duration of follow-up with a caution in interpretation, as manifestations suggestive of CF may not develop until adolescence or adulthood. The same team [22] analyzed a larger cohort with CRMS/CFSPID and found a difference in initial NBS IRT median values in those with delayed CF ($n = 14$) compared to those who remained CRMS/CFSPID ($n = 83$), respectively with a median [Q1-Q3] of 108.9 (72.3–126.8) vs. 73.7 (60.0–96.0); $p = 0.02$, suggesting IRT initial value and trajectory over time as a potential tool to stratify young infants into high-risk or low-risk groups of developing CF. Munck et al. [21] reported a prospective multicenter study in France. Sixty-three positive NBS infants with an inconclusive diagnosis of CF, born 2002–2009, were matched 1:1 with a cohort diagnosed CF through NBS ($n = 63$) and evaluated at a mean age of 7.4 years. Those with a CRMS/CFSPID designation at baseline had a significantly lower median IRT (97 µg/L vs. 166 µg/L, $p < 0.0001$) and SC values (40 mmol/L vs. 110 mmol/L, $p < 0.0001$) compared to those diagnosed CF. During follow-up, compared to those with CF, they all had sustained exocrine pancreatic sufficiency, less respiratory symptoms and identification of *Pseudomonas aeruginosa* (24% vs. 82%) and *Staphylococcus aureus* (68% vs. 90%). Among the 63 cases with a CRMS/CFSPID diagnosis, 28 (44%) children converted to a delayed CF diagnosis based on a positive SC value ($n = 8$), with the identification of two CF-causing mutations *in trans* in the CFTR2 database at the time of data analysis ($n = 12$) or both in eight cases. All but six presented during follow-up respiratory symptoms suggestive of CF (productive cough, pathogens, antibiotic courses), although not specific to CF. Those who converted to CF had similar initial SC values, no clinical, anthropometric, respiratory pathogens, radiological or spirometry differences at final assessment compared to those who did not convert to CF. Infants recruited in these two studies reflected children currently diagnosed as CRMS/CFSPID, and the conversion to CF was defined by the above strict criteria. Explanations for the discrepancy in CF conversion rates among studies may be a time lag in infants' birth dates with differences in updated CFTR2 knowledge at the time of data analysis, as well as variations in the duration of follow-up.

3.2. Management of Infants with CRMS/CFSPID Designation

Whether screening newborns for CRMS/CFSPID is of clinical benefit has yet to be established, as most of these infants seem unlikely to develop any phenotype. Those designated CRMS/CFSPID have no clinical feature suggestive of CF at initial evaluation. It is important to provide accurate information to parents who feel psychologically distressed with the delivery of an initial positive NBS result and an inconclusive designation [23]. For an appropriate follow-up, most CF physicians agree that a balance is needed to avoid both overmedicalization and undertreatment, which can be a missed opportunity to prevent manifestations later in life. Nevertheless, there is no evidence that early proactive treatment leads to better long-term outcomes. Considering the US guidelines [5] published in 2009 and European recommendations [21,24] published in 2009 and updated in 2015 on early management, they are in agreement on care issues and on regular follow-up by a physician with an interest in CF encouraging clinical assessment rather than unnecessary explorations and including regular sweat testing. Clear information should be provided to the family and the primary care physician over time. Ooi et al. [19] considered his study as an interim one according to the short duration of monitoring and that CF-like manifestations may not develop until adolescence or adulthood. Data of Munck et al. [21], with a longer monitoring period and a more comprehensive respiratory status assessment, support a less intensive approach in the management of these infants compared to those with CF. They consider a possible discharge from the CF center after six years of age if the child has not converted to CF with the primary care physician remaining vigilant, especially for unexplained chronic lung disease. The best practice for monitoring these children is still an unanswered issue. Both prospective studies shed light on the need of further long-term prospective studies. In parallel, the ECFS NN WG is now working on a consensual document for monitoring these individuals from initial assessment to six years of age, with a diagnostic testing section, a care management section, including respiratory phenotype, and a review of evidence from a year-six assessment, with shared a decision on future care plans with the family.

Table 2. Summary of recent studies of CRMS/CFSPID.

	Kharrazi et al. [14]	Groves et al. [15]	Ren et al. [16]	Levy et al. [17]	Terlizzi et al. [18]	Ooi et al. [19]	Munck et al. [21]
Study design	Retrospective	Retrospective case control	CFF registry	Cross sectional	Retrospective	Prospective case control	Prospective case control
Country	USA California	Australia	US	US Wisconsin	Italy Tuscany	Canada, Italy	France
Birth period	2007–2012	1996–2010	2010–2012	1994–2012	2011–2016	2007–2013	2002–2009
Follow up duration (y)	Mean 4.5	10	1	8	Median 0.6	Median 2.2	Mean 7.4
Number CF	345	225	1540	300	32	80	63
Number CRMS/CFSPID	533	29 [2]	309	57	50	82	63 [2]
CF:CRMS/CFSPID	0.65:1	7.8:1	5:1	5.2:1	0.64:1	1.8:1 [6]	6.3:1 [6]
Conversion to CF, N (%)	20 (5.8)	14/29 (48) matched to CF	NA [4]	NA [4]	5 (10)	9 (11)	28(44)
Increased SCC ≥60 mmol/L	17	2 [3]			5	2	8
2 CF causing mutations	0	0			0	4	12
Both criteria	0	0			0	3	8
Other criteria	3	12			0	0	0
Age at conversion (y)	Mean 2.5 ± 1.4				Median 2 (0.2–4)	Mean 1.8 ± 1.2	Unk [1]
Pseudomonas aeruginosa, N (%)	Unk [1]	78.6	10.7	39	25 [5]	12	24
Pancreatic insufficiency, N (%)	3/15 (15)	4/29 (14)	14/309 (4.5)	0	0	0	0
F508del/R117H, N (%)	Unk [1]	4/14 (29)	80/309 (26)	37/57 (63)	0	16/82 (19.5)	27/63 (43)

[1] Unk: unknown; [2] definition slightly different from CRMS/CFSPID; [3] only 8/14 had a repeated sweat test; [4] NA: non-applicable; [5] only 8/50 had swab culture. CF: CF; [6] CF:CRMS/CFSPID ratio from the algorithm. Cystic fibrosis, CFTR: CF transmembrane conductance regulator (gene), CFMS: CFTR-related metabolic syndrome, CFSPID: CF screen-positive, inconclusive diagnosis, SCC: sweat chloride concentration

4. CRMS/CFSPID Registry Database

Analysis of the 2010–2012 CFF Patient Registry database by Ren et al. [15] showed a high rate of misclassification of NBS-positive infants. On one hand, 11% of infants with CRMS had to be reclassified as CF after expansion of the number of CF-causing mutations and/or subsequent positive SC; and on the other hand, 41% of infants with CRMS were assigned as CF, despite not fulfilling the criteria. Now with the unified definition for infants designated CRMS/CFSPID, we can speculate that registry databases monitoring long-term outcomes will provide an accurate assessment of the risk of moving through adolescence or adulthood to CFTR-RD and CF diagnosis and will contribute to better define the modalities of monitoring. The ECFS NN WG is now working with the ECFS Registry team to prepare a European survey for infants with a designation of CRMS/CFSPID, aimed at recording the current situation of existing national or regional registries or databases, or plans and timelines to develop them.

Acknowledgments: The author would like to thank K.W. Southern, Liverpool, UK, for his agreement to publish in the review Figure 1 and D. Delmas for her technical support.

References

1. Dijk, F.N.; Fitzgerald, D.A. The impact of newborn screening and earlier intervention on the clinical course of cystic fibrosis. *Paediatr. Respir. Rev.* **2012**, *13*, 220–225. [CrossRef] [PubMed]
2. Yen, E.H.; Quinton, H.; Borowitz, D. Better nutritional status in early childhood is associated with improved clinical outcomes and survival in patients with cystic fibrosis. *J. Pediatr.* **2013**, *162*, 530–535. [CrossRef] [PubMed]
3. Tridello, G.; Castellani, C.; Meneghelli, I.; Tamanini, A.; Assael, B.M. Early diagnosis from newborn screening maximises survival in severe cystic fibrosis. *ERJ Open Res.* **2018**, *4*, 00109–2017. [CrossRef] [PubMed]
4. Barben, J.; Castellani, C.; Dankert-Roelse, J.; Gartner, S.; Kashirskaya, N.; Linnane, B.; Mayell, S.; Munck, A.; Sands, D.; Sommerburg, O.; et al. The expansion and performance of national newborn screening programmes for cystic fibrosis in Europe. *J. Cyst. Fibros.* **2017**, *16*, 207–213. [CrossRef]
5. Borowitz, D.; Parad, R.B.; Sharp, J.K.; Sabadosa, K.A.; Robinson, K.A.; Rock, M.J.; Farrell, P.M.; Sontag, M.K.; Rosenfeld, M.; Davis, S.D.; et al. Cystic Fibrosis Foundation practice guidelines for the management of infants with cystic fibrosis transmembrane conductance regulator-related metabolic syndrome during the first two years of life and beyond. *J. Pediatr.* **2009**, *155* (Suppl. S6), S106–S116. [CrossRef]
6. Munck, A.; Mayell, S.J.; Winters, V.; Shawcross, A.; Derichs, N.; Parad, R.; Barben, J.; Southern, K.W. ECFS Neonatal Screening Working Group. Cystic Fibrosis Screen Positive, Inconclusive Diagnosis (CFSPID): A new designation and management recommendations for infants with an inconclusive diagnosis following newborn screening. *J. Cyst. Fibros.* **2015**, *14*, 706–713. [CrossRef]
7. Ren, C.L.; Borowitz, D.S.; Gonska, T.; Howenstine, M.S.; Levy, H.; Massie, J.; Milla, C.; Munck, A.; Southern, K.W. Cystic Fibrosis Transmembrane Conductance Regulator-Related Metabolic Syndrome and Cystic Fibrosis Screen Positive, Inconclusive Diagnosis. *J. Pediatr.* **2017**, *181*, S45–S51. [CrossRef]
8. Farrell, P.M.; White, T.B.; Ren, C.L.; Hempstead, S.E.; Accurso, F.; Derichs, N.; Howenstine, M.; McColley, S.A.; Rock, M.; Rosenfeld, M.; et al. Diagnosis of Cystic Fibrosis: Consensus Guidelines from the Cystic Fibrosis Foundation. *J. Pediatr.* **2017**, *181*, S4–S15. [CrossRef]
9. Southern, K.W.; Barben, J.; Gartner, S.; Munck, A.; Castellani, C.; Mayell, S.J.; Davies, J.C.; Winters, V.; Murphy, J.; Salinas, D.; et al. Inconclusive diagnosis after a positive newborn bloodspot screening result for cystic fibrosis; clarification of the harmonised international definition. *J. Cyst. Fibros.* **2019**, *18*, 778–780. [CrossRef]
10. Sosnay, P.R.; Salinas, D.B.; White, T.B.; Ren, C.L.; Farrell, P.M.; Raraigh, K.S.; Girodon, E.; Castellani, C. Applying Cystic Fibrosis Transmembrane Conductance Regulator Genetics and CFTR2 Data to Facilitate Diagnoses. *J. Pediatr.* **2017**, *181*, S27–S32. [CrossRef]

11. Sermet-Gaudelus, I.; Girodon, E.; Roussel, D.; Deneuville, E.; Bui, S.; Huet, F.; Guillot, M.; Aboutaam, R.; Renouil, M.; Munck, A.; et al. Measurement of nasal potential difference in young children with an equivocal sweat test following newborn screening for cystic fibrosis. *Thorax* **2010**, *65*, 539–544. [CrossRef]

12. Derichs, N.; Sanz, J.; Von Kanel, T.; Stolpe, C.; Zapf, A.; Tümmler, B.; Gallati, S.; Ballmann, M. Intestinal current measurement for diagnostic classification of patients with questionable cystic fibrosis: Validation and reference data. *Thorax* **2010**, *65*, 594–599. [CrossRef] [PubMed]

13. De Winter-de Groot, K.M.; Berkers, G.; Marck-van der Wilt, R.E.P.; van der Meer, R.; Vonk, A.; Dekkers, J.F.; Geerdink, M.; Michel, S.; Kruisselbrink, E.; Vries, R.; et al. Forskolin-induced swelling of intestinal organoids correlates with disease severity in adults with cystic fibrosis and homozygous F508del mutations. *J. Cyst. Fibros.* **2019**, in press. [CrossRef] [PubMed]

14. Kharrazi, M.; Yang, J.; Bishop, T.; Lessing, S.; Young, S.; Graham, S.; Pearl, M.; Chow, H.; Ho, T.; Currier, R.; et al. California Cystic Fibrosis Newborn Screening Consortium. Newborn Screening for Cystic Fibrosis in California. *Pediatrics* **2015**, *136*, 1062–1072. [CrossRef] [PubMed]

15. Groves, T.; Robinson, P.; Wiley, V.; Fitzgerald, D.A. Long-term outcomes of children with intermediate sweat chloride values in infancy. *J. Pediatr.* **2015**, *166*, 1469–1474. [CrossRef]

16. Ren, C.L.; Fink, A.K.; Petren, K.; Borowitz, D.S.; McColley, S.A.; Sanders, D.B.; Rosenfeld, M.; Marshall, B.C. Outcomes of infants with indeterminate diagnosis detected by cystic fibrosis newborn screening. *Pediatrics* **2015**, *135*, e1386–e1392. [CrossRef]

17. Levy, H.; Nugent, M.; Schneck, K.; Stachiw-Hietpas, D.; Laxova, A.; Lakser, O.; Rock, M.; Dahmer, M.K.; Biller, J.; Nasr, S.Z.; et al. Refining the continuum of CFTR-associated disorders in the era of newborn screening. *Clin. Genet.* **2016**, *89*, 539–549. [CrossRef]

18. Terlizzi, V.; Mergni, G.; Buzzetti, R.; Centrone, C.; Zavataro, L.; Braggion, C. Cystic fibrosis screen positive inconclusive diagnosis (CFSPID): Experience in Tuscany, Italy. *J. Cyst. Fibros.* **2019**, *18*, 484–490. [CrossRef]

19. Ooi, C.Y.; Castellani, C.; Keenan, K.; Avolio, J.; Volpi, S.; Boland, M.; Kovesi, T.; Bjornson, C.; Chilvers, M.A.; Morgan, L.; et al. Inconclusive diagnosis of cystic fibrosis after newborn screening. *Pediatrics* **2015**, *135*, e1377–e1385. [CrossRef]

20. Salinas, D.B.; Azen, C.; Young, S.; Keens, T.G.; Kharrazi, M.; Parad, R.B. Phenotypes of California CF Newborn Screen-Positive Children with CFTR 5T Allele by TG Repeat Length. *Genet. Test. Mol. Biomark.* **2016**, *20*, 496–503. [CrossRef]

21. Munck, A.; Bourmaud, A.; Bellon, G.; Picq, P.; Farrell, P.M.; DPAM Study Group. Phenotype of children with inconclusive cystic fibrosis diagnosis after newborn screening. *Pediatr. Pulmonol.* **2016**, *20*, 496–503. [CrossRef] [PubMed]

22. Ooi, C.Y.; Sutherland, R.; Castellani, C.; Keenan, K.; Boland, M.; Reisman, J.; Bjornson, C.; Chilvers, M.A.; van Wylick, R.; Kent, S.; et al. Immunoreactive trypsinogen levels in newborn screened infants with an inconclusive diagnosis of cystic fibrosis. *BMC Pediatr.* **2019**, *19*, 369. [CrossRef] [PubMed]

23. Hayeems, R.Z.; Miller, F.A.; Barg, C.J.; Bombard, Y.; Carroll, J.C.; Tam, K.; Kerr, E.; Chakraborty, P.; Potter, B.K.; Patton, S. Psychosocial Response to Uncertain Newborn Screening Results for Cystic Fibrosis. *J. Pediatr.* **2017**, *184*, 165–171. [CrossRef] [PubMed]

24. Mayell, S.J.; Munck, A.; Craig, J.V.; Sermet, I.; Brownlee, K.G.; Schwarz, M.J.; Castellani, C.; Southern, K.W. European Cystic Fibrosis Society Neonatal Screening Working Group. A European consensus for the evaluation and management of infants with an equivocal diagnosis following newborn screening for cystic fibrosis. *J. Cyst. Fibros.* **2009**, *8*, 71–78. [CrossRef]

19

Newborn Screening for Sickle Cell Disease: Indian Experience

Roshan B. Colah, Pallavi Mehta and Malay B. Mukherjee *

ICMR-National Institute of Immunohaematology, KEM Hospital Campus, Mumbai 400012, India;
colahrb@gmail.com (R.B.C.); sarthi710@gmail.com (P.M.)
* Correspondence: malaybmukherjee@gmail.com

Abstract: Sickle cell disease (SCD) is a major public health problem in India with the highest prevalence amongst the tribal and some non-tribal ethnic groups. The clinical manifestations are extremely variable ranging from a severe to mild or asymptomatic condition. Early diagnosis and providing care is critical in SCD because of the possibility of lethal complications in early infancy in pre-symptomatic children. Since 2010, neonatal screening programs for SCD have been initiated in a few states of India. A total of 18,003 babies have been screened by automated HPLC using either cord blood samples or heel prick dried blood spots and 2944 and 300 babies were diagnosed as sickle cell carriers and SCD respectively. A follow up of the SCD babies showed considerable variation in the clinical presentation in different population groups, the disease being more severe among non-tribal babies. Around 30% of babies developed serious complications within the first 2 to 2.6 years of life. These pilot studies have demonstrated the feasibility of undertaking newborn screening programs for SCD even in rural areas. A longer follow up of these babies is required and it is important to establish a national newborn screening program for SCD in all of the states where the frequency of the sickle cell gene is very high followed by the development of comprehensive care centers along with counselling and treatment facilities. This comprehensive data will ultimately help us to understand the natural history of SCD in India and also help the Government to formulate strategies for the management and prevention of sickle cell disease in India.

Keywords: newborn screening; sickle cell disease; India; tribal; non-tribal; Guthrie spots; cord blood; automated HPLC

1. Introduction

Hemoglobinopathies are the most common monogenic disorders in India posing a significant health burden. Sickle cell disease (SCD) was the first molecular disease to be described where a single point mutation (A→T) resulted in the substitution of the 6th aminoacid in the β globin chain from glutamic acid to valine leading to an altered electrophoretic mobility of the hemoglobin molecule. SCD includes a variety of conditions, the primary hemoglobin disorder being sickle cell anemia (SCA) due to homozygosity for hemoglobin S (HbS) as well as the compound heterozygous conditions, HbS-β thalassemia, HbSD disease, HbSE disease, HbSC disease and HbS-O Arab disease [1].

2. Geographic Distribution of HbS in India

HbS is widespread in African, Mediterranean, Middle Eastern, Indian, Caribbean and South and Central American populations [1]. In India, SCA is prevalent among tribal populations who are considered to be the original inhabitants in south Gujarat, Maharashtra, Madhya Pradesh, Chhattisgarh, and western Odisha with a smaller focus in the southern region in Andhra Pradesh, Karnataka, northern Tamil Nadu and Kerala. They often reside in remote regions away from the mainstream populations. Sickle cell anemia is also prevalent in some of the scheduled castes and other backward classes (non-tribal populations) mainly in central India, in particular, among the Mahar, Kunbi and Teli castes but is rare in other castes where it may be seen due to admixture. These are economically and socially disadvantaged populations living largely in rural areas. Carrier frequencies ranging from 1 to 35% have been described in these groups and their distribution in different states of the country has been mapped earlier [2–4]. Many of these populations also harbor the β thalassemia gene but screening for β thalassemia had not been extensively carried out among them earlier. A recent report from Akola district in central India showed that 36 out of 91 pediatric SCD patients (39.6%) had sickle-β thalassemia [5].

3. Sickle Haplotypes in India

In the eastern province of Saudi Arabia and in India, the sickle gene is linked to the Arab Indian or Asian haplotype, which is associated with higher fetal hemoglobin (HbF) levels and a milder clinical presentation than the Benin haplotype seen in west and north Africa and the Bantu haplotype seen in east and central Africa [6]. There are limited studies on haplotype analysis from different regions in India, however, all of them have shown that around 90% of sickle genes have the Asian haplotype while few other atypical haplotypes including the BantuA2 and the Senegal haplotype have been associated with around 10% of sickle genes [7]. Yet, recent studies have indicated more severe clinical manifestations even among the Asian haplotype.

4. Clinical Manifestations of Sickle Cell Disease in India

Initial studies on sickle cell disease patients from western Odisha demonstrated a mild clinical course with higher hemoglobin levels, lower reticulocyte counts, persistence of splenomegaly, infrequent leg ulcers and priapism compared to patients with the disease of African origin [8]. Subsequently, in western and central India it was found that the disease was milder among tribal populations in Valsad in south Gujarat compared to non-tribal populations in Nagpur in Maharashtra. Apart from higher HbF levels, a significant ameliorating factor was the presence of associated α thalassemia, which was very common in tribal populations in Gujarat [9]. Since then, reports of more severe features, particularly from central India have raised the question of geographic variations in the manifestations of SCD within India. In a retrospective study, where 316 children with sickle cell anemia were followed up for a period of 5.8 ± 5.7 years in Nagpur, there were 1725 hospitalizations among 282 patients and 96 children had severe disease with severe vaso occlusive crises, severe anemia, splenic sequestration, stroke and hypersplenism being reported and 10 babies died during this period [10]. Another retrospective analysis of 110 adult patients with sickle cell disease who attended out-patient clinics or were admitted to the hospital showed that 75.4% of them had a severe disease in spite of all the sickle genes being linked to the Asian haplotype and the presence of associated α thalassemia [11]. Thus, sickle cell disease has an extremely variable clinical presentation in Indian patients.

5. Providing Comprehensive Care in Rural Regions

As a large majority of sickle cell disease cases are born in rural India, it is necessary to provide adequate care for these patients, which can be challenging in remote areas. However, few studies from different regions have demonstrated that this is possible with the involvement of Government and Non-Government Organizations as well as representatives from the local population. It was shown in a study from the Bardoli district in Gujarat that giving basic health care training to a local villager to regularly visit households and monitor sickle cell disease cases and identify those with significant complications and refer them to the coordinating hospital would have a significant impact on tribal communities with a high prevalence of SCD [12]. In another study undertaken in a remote tribal village in Gudalur in south India, it was shown that 71% of 111 patients with sickle cell disease were able to have at least one annual comprehensive care visit. Premature deaths were seen in 19 patients at a median age of 23 years due to acute chest syndrome, sepsis, severe anemia, stroke or sudden unexplained deaths [13]. A comprehensive care model at Sewa Rural in Gujarat was successfully implemented, which included screening, both out-patient and in-patient care of SCD patients as well as health education. A one year follow up of 164 SCD patients in this rural region was possible and pain crises were seen in 72 patients (43.9%); 59 patients (35.9%) required hospitalization, 43 patients (26.2%) required blood transfusions and three patients (1.6%) died during this short follow up [14].

6. Benefits of Newborn Screening and Comprehensive Care

Newborn screening (NBS) enables the identification of babies with sickle cell disease at birth or soon after, within the first few days of their life before they present with any symptoms or complications. These babies can then be regularly followed up with the provision of comprehensive care and timely management to reduce morbidity and mortality. It has been demonstrated in several countries that early diagnosis and providing care is critical in SCD because of the possibility of lethal complications in the first few years of life in pre-symptomatic children. Young children with SCD have an increased susceptibility to bacteremia due to *Streptococcus pneumonia*, which can be fatal in many cases. Acute splenic sequestration crisis is another cause for mortality in infancy. Many studies done globally have shown that early prophylactic penicillin can significantly reduce the morbidity and mortality due to pneumococcal sepsis and they have also shown the importance of pneumococcal vaccines for the prevention of pneumococcal sepsis, thus justifying the need for implementing newborn screening programs for SCD [15,16].

7. Newborn Screening Initiatives in India

It has been estimated that three countries, Nigeria, D R Congo and India are most affected by SCD and widespread newborn screening and follow up care could save the lives of almost 10 million children by 2050. It is also estimated that 15% of the world's neonates with sickle cell anemia are born in India [17]. Thus, newborn screening has a great relevance in this country. There is no National neonatal screening program for SCD as yet and affected children are generally identified when they become symptomatic. However, few newborn screening programs have been initiated in some regions in the last 5 to 6 years. Figure 1 shows the location of the different centers involved in newborn screening programs in India. Table 1 summarizes the programs undertaken in a few states in this vast country.

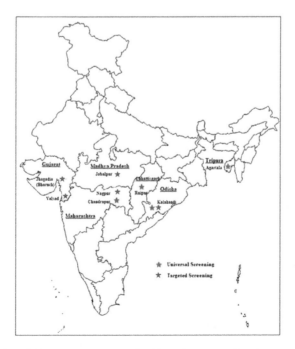

Figure 1. Location of the different centers in India where newborn screening was undertaken.

Table 1. Summary of newborn screening programs initiated in India.

State	District	Target Population	Sample	Technology for Screening	No. Screened	No(%)AS	No(%)SCD	Follow Up	Reference
South Gujarat Phase 1	Valsad	All Tribal babies	Heel prick-Dried blood spot	HPLC-Variant NBS machine	5467	687 (12.5%)	46 (0.8%)	5-6 years	Italia et al., 2015 [18]
South Gujarat Phase 2	Valsad, Bharuch	All Tribal babies	Heel prick-Dried blood spot	HPLC-Variant NBS machine	2944	649 (22.0%)	76 (2.6%)	2 years	Unpublished
Maharashtra	Nagpur	Largely non-tribal, babies of AS mothers	Cord blood, heel prick	HPLC-Variant Hb Testing System	2134	978 (45.8%)	113 (5.3%)	4-5 years	Upadhye et al., 2016 [19]
Madhya Pradesh	Jabalpur	Tribal, babies of AS mothers	Cord blood, heel prick	HPLC-Variant Hb Testing System	461	36 (7.8%)	6 (1.3%)	1 year	Unpublished
Chhattisgarh	Raipur	Tribal and non-tribal babies	Heel prick-Dried blood spot	HPLC-Variant NBS machine	1158	61 (5.3%)	6 (0.5%)	No follow up reported	Panigrahi et al., 2012 [20]
Odisha	Kalahandi	Tribal and non-triba babies	Heel prick-Dried blood spot	HPLC-Variant Hb Testing System	1668	293 (17.6%)	34 (2.0%)	No follow up reported	Mohanty et al., 2010 [21]
Odisha	Kalahandi	Tribal babies	Cord blood	HPLC-Variant Hb Testing System	761	112 (14.7%)	13 (1.7%)	No follow up reported	Dixit et al., 2015 [22]
Tripura	Agartala	Tribal & non tribal babies	Cord blood	HPLC-Variant Hb Testing System	2400	15 (0.6%)	0 (0.0%)	Not done	Upadhye et al., 2018 [23]
Maharashtra	Chandrapur	Tribal and non-tribal babies	Cord blood, heel prick	HPLC-Variant Hb Testing System	1010	85 (8.4%)	4 (0.4%)	Not done	Unpublished

Most of the above were pilot studies undertaken in different states, which showed that it was feasible to undertake newborn screening for SCD even in rural regions and register affected babies for follow up and comprehensive care although the outcome of the follow up was not reported in all these studies.

8. Technologies Used for Newborn Screening in India

Globally, isoelectric focusing (IEF) using eluates from dried blood spots was initially used for screening of newborn babies for sickle cell disease but at many centers this had been replaced by high-performance liquid chromatography (HPLC) analysis [24,25]. In all of the Indian reports on newborn screening for SCD, HPLC analysis has been used. This was mainly due to two reasons. Automated HPLC machines were already in use at these centers for other programs, hence, no additional cost for infrastructure was required. Secondly, it was felt that these machines would be easier to operate and maintain even in rural areas. The Variant NBS machine (BioRad laboratories, Hercules, CA, USA) has been used for hemoglobin analysis from dried blood spots or the Variant Hemoglobin Testing System (BioRad laboratories) for cord blood samples using either the sickle cell short or the β thal short programs. The β thal short program had the advantage of picking up other hemoglobin abnormalities including some rare non-deletional α chain variants like Hb Fontainebleau, Hb O Indonesia and Hb Koya Dora [26]. More recently, several point-of-care devices have been developed for screening, which are either paper-based screening protocols or antibody-based rapid diagnostic devices based on lateral flow immunoassay technologies. They are simple to use and relatively inexpensive as they do not require any specific equipment or even electricity, which is often not always available in remote rural regions. These commercial devices are still being validated for newborn screening for SCD [27,28]. Presently, we are also undertaking a multicenter validation of one of these newborn screening kits to evaluate its suitability for use in newborn screening programs in India in the future.

9. Follow up of Birth Cohorts of Sickle Cell Disease in India

A systematic follow up of SCD babies for around 4 to 5 years had been possible in at least two newborn screening programs in the country in Valsad in south Gujarat and Nagpur in Maharashtra [18,19]. The program in Gujarat targeted mainly tribal newborn babies from four districts. These babies were largely from nine different tribes, the highest numbers being from the Dhodia Patel, Kukna and Halpita tribes. It involved 13 centers (government district hospitals to community health centers) for neonatal sample collection on filter paper. These dried blood spots were sent for processing on the NBS variant machine to the centralized laboratory in Valsad. Of the 5467 babies screened, 687 were identified as sickle cell trait and 46 babies had sickle cell disease (SS-33, S-β-thal-13). After confirmation of the diagnosis, the SCD babies were registered for comprehensive care. Follow up from 1.5 to 5 years was possible only in 32 (69%) of these babies. Pneumococcal vaccination and folic acid supplementation were given to all of the babies. In this cohort, 18 babies (SS-11, S-β thal-7) had no clinical complications till the last follow-up. The majority of the babies who became symptomatic presented after 2 years of age. Seven babies (SS-6, S-β thal-1) had severe complications, which included severe infections, vasoocclusive crises, severe anemia and acute chest syndrome. Few others had mild febrile episodes and mild splenomegaly and hepatomegaly were seen in some babies. One baby died at the age of 4 years during the follow up period. Although haplotyping was not done in all of the SS babies, the Xmn1 polymorphism in 24 SS babies, where this was determined, was Xmn1 (+/+) in all of them. The HbF levels varied from 12.5 to 30.2% among those SS babies who were between 2.4 and 5 years of age. The prevalence of α thalassemia was 92% in this population, the most common α genotype being $-\alpha^{3.7}/-\alpha^{3.7}$ [18]. In the second phase of this program, mobile phones were given to the parents of affected babies to improve compliance for follow ups and this had a significant impact.

In Nagpur in Maharashtra, newborn screening was done at a single government medical college where only babies born to sickle heterozygous mothers were screened making the program more cost-effective. The population here was largely non-tribal, the majority being from the Mahar community. A total of 2134 babies of mothers having a positive solubility test were screened by the collection of cord blood at birth or a heel prick sample subsequently and analyzed by HPLC on the Variant Hemoglobin Testing System. There were 978 babies with sickle cell trait and 113 babies with sickle cell disease (SS-104, S-βthal-7, SD-2). In this cohort too, 73% of the babies could be followed up for 3 to 5 years. Penicillin prophylaxis was given to the babies who could be followed up. Here several babies presented much earlier than the cohort in Gujarat and 45% of the SCD babies required hospitalization between 3 months and 2 years. Infections, severe anemia and painful events were the common presenting features. Eight sickle homozygous babies had sepsis. Six SCD babies died during the follow up period. Haplotyping was done in 75 SS babies and 141 of the 150 SS chromosomes (94%) were linked to the Asian haplotype. Six SS chromosomes were linked to the Bantu A2 haplotype and three to an atypical haplotype. The mean HbF level in the SS cohort was 21.4 ± 5.4%. The prevalence of α thalassemia in this cohort was 28%, the $-\alpha^{3.7}/\alpha\alpha$ genotype being the commonest defect.

Newborn screening for hemoglobinopathies was also undertaken in the malaria endemic northeastern region in Agartala in Tripura where Hb E is widely prevalent but Hb S is also seen among the tea garden workers who are migrant laborers from other states [23]. Only 15 newborn babies with sickle cell trait were identified but 9.3% of babies had HbE trait, 3.3% were Hb E homozygous and one baby had HbE-β thalassemia. Screening for G6PD deficiency was also done and few babies with Hb abnormalities were also G6PD deficient.

The clinical presentation among sickle cell disease babies was quite variable in the two cohorts which could be followed up for at least 4 to 5 years. As mentioned in a recent editorial, the question remains whether the intervention programs developed for African disease could be applied to Indian patients with the Asian haplotype [29]. Newborn cohort studies in different regions in India will be able to answer these questions once they have been systematically undertaken and the affected babies followed up for a longer duration.

10. Lessons Learnt from Pilot Studies on Newborn Screening for Sickle Cell Disease in India

The feasibility of establishing newborn screening programs in tribal areas in rural regions has been shown. Follow up of birth cohorts in the studies where this was done showed that the clinical presentation was very variable in different regions. Further efforts and motivation are needed to ensure that the maximum number of babies can be enrolled and continue to receive comprehensive care and the follow up of babies can be done for a longer duration. Newborn screening programs must be extended to other states where the sickle gene is prevalent. Guidelines for a National Hemoglobinopathy Program have been recently laid down by the Ministry of Health and Family Welfare which also includes newborn screening for SCD and these will be followed for understanding the natural history of sickle cell disease in India [30].

Author Contributions: Conceptualization, R.B.C. and M.B.M.; Data Compilation, R.B.C., P.M. and M.B.M.; Writing—Review and Editing, R.B.C. and M.B.M.

Acknowledgments: We thank all the investigators associated with these studies.

References

1.   Serjeant, G.R.; Serjeant, B.E. (Eds.) *Sickle Cell Disease*; Oxford Medical Publications: New York, NY, USA, 2001.
2.   Urade, B.P. Incidence of sickle cell anemia and thalassemia in Central India. *Open J. Blood Dis.* **2012**, *2*, 71–80. [CrossRef]
3.   Colah, R.; Mukherjee, M.; Ghosh, K. Sickle cell disease in India. *Curr. Opin. Hematol.* **2014**, *21*, 215–223. [CrossRef] [PubMed]

4. Colah, R.B.; Mukherjee, M.B.; Martin, S.; Ghosh, K. Sickle cell disease in tribal populations in India. *Indian J. Med. Res.* **2015**, *141*, 509–515. [PubMed]

5. Jain, D.; Warthe, V.; Dayama, P.; Sarate, D.; Colah, R.; Mehta, P.; Serjeant, G. Sickle Cell Disease in Central India: A Potentially Severe Syndrome. *Indian J. Pediatr.* **2016**, *83*, 1071–1076. [CrossRef] [PubMed]

6. Pagnier, J.; Mears, J.G.; Dunda-Belkhodja, O.; Schaefer-Rego, K.E.; Beldjord, C.; Nagel, R.L.; Labie, D. Evidence for the multicentric origin of the sickle cell hemoglobin gene in Africa. *Proc. Natl. Acad. Sci. USA* **1984**, *81*, 1771–1773. [CrossRef] [PubMed]

7. Mukherjee, M.B.; Surve, R.R.; Gangakhedkar, R.R.; Ghosh, K.; Colah, R.B.; Mohanty, D. β-globin gene cluster haplotypes linked to the βS gene in western India. *Hemoglobin* **2004**, *28*, 157–161. [CrossRef] [PubMed]

8. Kar, B.C.; Satapathy, R.K.; Kulozik, A.E.; Kulozik, M.; Sirr, S.; Serjeant, B.E.; Serjeant, G.R. Sickle cell disease in Orissa State, India. *Lancet* **1986**, *2*, 1198–1201. [CrossRef]

9. Mukherjee, M.B.; Lu, C.Y.; Ducrocq, R.; Gangakhedkar, R.R.; Colah, R.B.; Kadam, M.D.; Mohanty, D.; Nagel, R.L.; Krishnamoorthy, R. The effect of alpha thalassemia on sickle cell anemia linked to the Arab-Indian haplotype among a tribal and non-tribal population in India. *Am. J. Hematol.* **1997**, *55*, 104–109. [CrossRef]

10. Jain, D.; Italia, K.; Sarathi, V.; Ghosh, K.; Colah, R. Sickle cell anemia from central India: A retrospective analysis. *Indian Pediatr.* **2012**, *49*, 911–913. [CrossRef] [PubMed]

11. Italia, K.; Kangne, H.; Shanmukaiah, C.; Nadkarni, A.H.; Ghosh, K.; Colah, R.B. Variable phenotypes of sickle cell disease in India with the Arab-Indian haplotype. *Br. J. Haematol.* **2015**, *168*, 156–159. [CrossRef] [PubMed]

12. Patel, J.; Patel, B.; Gamit, M.; Serjeant, G.R. Screening for the sickle cell gene in Gujarat, India; a village based model. *J. Community Genet.* **2013**, *4*, 43–47. [CrossRef] [PubMed]

13. Nimgaonkar, V.; Krishnamurti, L.; Prabhakar, H.; Menon, N. Comprehensive integrated care of patients with sickle cell disease in a remote aboriginal tribal population in southern India. *Pediatr. Blood Cancer* **2014**, *61*, 702–705. [CrossRef] [PubMed]

14. Desai, G.; Dave, K.P.; Bannerjee, S.; Barbaria, P.; Gupta, R. Initial outcomes of a comprehensive care model for sickle cell disease among a tribal population in rural western India. *Int. J. Community Med. Public Health* **2016**, *3*, 1282–1287. [CrossRef]

15. Gaston, M.H.; Verter, J.I.; Woods, G.; Pegelow, C.; Kelleher, J.; Presbury, G.; Zarkowsky, H.; Vichinsky, E.; Iyer, R.; Lobel, J.S.; et al. Prophylaxis with oral penicillin in children with sickle cell anemia: A randomized trial. *N. Engl. J. Med.* **1986**, *314*, 1593–1599. [CrossRef] [PubMed]

16. Adamkiewicz, T.V.; Sarnaik, S.; Buchanan, G.R.; Iyer, R.V.; Miller, S.T.; Pegelow, C.H.; Rogers, Z.R.; Vichinsky, E.; Elliott, J.; Facklam, R.R.; et al. Invasive pneumococcal infections in children with sickle cell disease in the era of penicillin prophylaxis, antibiotic resistance, and 23-valent pneumococcal polysaccharide vaccination. *J. Pediatr.* **2003**, *143*, 438–444. [CrossRef]

17. Piel, F.B.; Hay, S.I.; Gupta, S.; Weatherall, D.J.; Williams, T.N. Global burden of sickle cell anaemia in children under five, 2010–2050: Modelling based on demographics, excess mortality, and interventions. *PLoS Med.* **2013**, *10*, e1001484. [CrossRef] [PubMed]

18. Italia, Y.; Krishnamurti, L.; Mehta, V.; Raicha, B.; Italia, K.; Mehta, P.; Ghosh, K.; Colah, R. Feasibility of a Newborn Screening and Follow-up Programme for Sickle Cell Disease among South Gujarat (India) Tribal Populations. *J. Med. Screen.* **2015**, *22*, 1–7. [CrossRef] [PubMed]

19. Upadhye, D.S.; Jain, D.L.; Trivedi, Y.L.; Nadkarni, A.H.; Ghosh, K.; Colah, R.B. Neonatal screening and the clinical outcome in children with sickle cell disease in central India. *PLoS ONE* **2016**, *11*, e0147081. [CrossRef] [PubMed]

20. Panigrahi, S.; Patra, P.K.; Khodiar, P.K. Neonatal screening of sickle cell anemia: A preliminary report. *Indian J. Pediatr.* **2012**, *79*, 747–750. [CrossRef] [PubMed]

21. Mohanty, D.; Das, K.; Mishra, K. Newborn screening for sickle cell disease and congenital hypothyroidism in western Orissa. In Proceedings of the 4th International Congress on Sickle Cell Disease, Raipur, India, 22–27 November 2010; pp. 29–30.

22. Dixit, S.; Sahu, P.; Kar, S.K.; Negi, S. Identification of the hot spot areas for sickle cell disease using cord blood screening at a district hospital: An Indian perspective. *J. Community Genet.* **2015**, *6*, 383–387. [CrossRef] [PubMed]

23. Upadhye, D.; Das, R.; Ray, J.; Acharjee, S.; Ghosh, K.; Colah, R.; Mukherjee, M. Newborn screening for hemoglobinopathies and red cell enzymopathies in Tripura state: A malaria endemic state in Northeast India. *Hemoglobin* **2018**, *42*, 43–46. [CrossRef] [PubMed]

24. Consensus Development Summaries. *Newborn Screening for Sickle Cell Disease and Other Hemoglobinophathies*; Connecticut Medicine; National Institutes of Health: Bethesda, MD, USA, 1987; Volume 51, pp. 459–463.

25. Michlitsch, J.; Azimi, M.; Hoppe, C.; Walters, M.C.; Lubin, B.; Lorey, F.; Vichinsky, E. Newborn screening for hemoglobinopathies in California. *Pediatr. Blood Cancer* **2009**, *52*, 486–490. [CrossRef] [PubMed]

26. Upadhye, D.S.; Jain, D.; Nair, S.B.; Nadkarni, A.H.; Ghosh, K.; Colah, R.B. First case of Hb Fontainebleau with sickle haemoglobin and other non-deletional α gene variants identified in neonates during newborn screening for sickle cell disorders. *J. Clin. Pathol.* **2012**, *65*, 654–659. [CrossRef] [PubMed]

27. Piety, N.Z.; George, A.; Serrano, A.; Lanzi, M.R.; Patel, P.R.; Note, M.P.; Kahan, S.; Nirenburg, D.; Camanda, J.F.; Airewale, G.; et al. A paper based test for screening newborns for sickle cell disease. *Sci. Rep.* **2017**, *7*, 45488. [CrossRef] [PubMed]

28. Quinn, C.T.; Paniagua, M.C.; DiNello, R.K.; Panchal, A.; Geisberg, M. A rapid inexpensive and disposable point-of-care blood test for sickle cell disease using novel, highly specific monoclonal antibodies. *Br. J. Haematol.* **2016**, *175*, 724–732. [CrossRef] [PubMed]

29. Serjeant, G.R. Evolving locally appropriate models of care for Indian sickle cell disease. *Indian J. Med. Res.* **2016**, *143*, 405–413. [CrossRef] [PubMed]

30. *National Health Mission Guidelines on Hemoglobinopathies in India*; Ministry of Health and Family Welfare, Government of India: New Delhi, India, 2016.

20

Utilising the 'Getting to Outcomes®' Framework in Community Engagement for Development and Implementation of Sickle Cell Disease Newborn Screening in Kaduna State, Nigeria

Baba P.D. Inusa [1,*], Kofi A. Anie [2], Andrea Lamont [3], Livingstone G. Dogara [4], Bola Ojo [5], Ifeoma Ijei [4], Wale Atoyebi [6], Larai Gwani [7], Esther Gani [8] and Lewis Hsu [9]

[1] Department Evelina Children's Hospital, Guy's and St Thomas' NHS Foundation Trust, London SE1 7EH, UK
[2] Department of Haematology and Sickle Cell Centre, London North West University Healthcare NHS Trust and Imperial College, London NW10 7NS, UK; kofi.anie@nhs.net
[3] Department of Implementation Science, University of South Carolina, Columbia, SC 29208, USA; alamont082@gmail.com
[4] Department of Haematology, School of Medicine , Kaduna State University, Barau Dikko Teaching Hospital, Kaduna 800212, Nigeria; dogaralivingstone@gmail.com (L.G.D.); ijeiip@yahoo.com (I.I.)
[5] Sickle Cell Cohort Research Foundation, WUSE Zone II, Abuja 70032, Nigeria; bolaibilola@yahoo.co.uk
[6] Department of Haematology, Oxford University Hospitals NHS Foundation Trust, Oxford OX3 9DU, UK; Wale.Atoyebi@ouh.nhs.uk
[7] Kaduna State Assembly Office, Kaduna 800212, Nigeria; laraigwani@gmail.com
[8] Library Department, Kaduna State University, Kaduna 800241, Nigeria; ganiestty@gmail.com
[9] Department of Pediatric Hematology-Oncology, University of Illinois at Chicago, Chicago, IL 60612, USA; LewHsu@UIC.EDU
* Correspondence: baba.inusa@nhs.net;

Abstract: Background: Sickle Cell Disease (SCD) has been designated by WHO as a public health problem in sub-Saharan Africa, and the development of newborn screening (NBS) is crucial to the reduction of high SCD morbidity and mortality. Strategies from the field of implementation science can be useful for supporting the translation of NBS evidence from high income countries to the unique cultural context of sub-Saharan Africa. One such strategy is community engagement at all levels of the healthcare system, and a widely-used implementation science framework, "Getting to Outcomes®" (GTO), which incorporates continuous multilevel evaluation by stakeholders about the quality of the implementation. Objectives: (1) to obtain critical information on potential barriers to NBS in the disparate ethnic groups and settings (rural and urban) in the healthcare system of Kaduna State in Nigeria; and, (2) to assist in the readiness assessment of Kaduna in the implementation of a sustainable NBS programme for SCD. Methods: Needs assessment was conducted with stakeholder focus groups for two days in Kaduna state, Nigeria, in November 2017. Results: The two-day focus group workshop had a total of 52 participants. Asking and answering the 10 GTO accountability questions provided a structured format to understand strengths and weaknesses in implementation. For example, we found a major communication gap between policy-makers and user groups. Conclusion: In a two-day community engagement workshop, stakeholders worked successfully together to address SCD issues, to engage with each other, to share knowledge, and to prepare to build NBS for SCD in the existing healthcare system.

Keywords: Sickle Cell Disease; 'Getting to Outcomes'; newborn screening); sub-Saharan Africa; Nigeria; Kaduna State; implementation science; public health engagement

1. Introduction

Sickle Cell Disease (SCD) has been designated by the World Health Organisation (WHO) as a public health problem in sub-Saharan Africa [1–3]. It is projected that, unless specific action is taken, the burden of disease will continue to increase into 2050, especially in Nigeria and Democratic Republic of Congo, where this increase is estimated to be more than 100% [4]. The number of annual births with SCD is estimated to be 100,000 to 150,000 in Nigeria. Our pilot Newborn screening (NBS) study of infants up to six months old in an area within Kaduna State, Nigeria, reported an incidence of 1.7% [4,5], which suggests that over 4000 babies with SCD are born every year (based on 240,000 annual overall births per state). Consistent with WHO's call to action, national and regional policies for the management and control of SCD are required, especially in the view of limited resources across most of sub-Saharan Africa. SCD represents an urgent health burden, both in terms of mortality and morbidity. It is estimated that it accounts for 8–16% of under-five mortality in sub-Saharan Africa [6]. Mortality among children with SCD in Africa is estimated at 50% to 90% by 10 years of age, mostly from preventable infections [2].

Effective management of SCD should incorporate NBS with the prevention of infections (including pneumococcal septicaemia and malaria), parental education, and support at all levels of healthcare provision to enable the timely recognition of SCD complications and health maintenance. The development of NBS programmes in sub-Saharan Africa is crucial to the reduction of high infant mortality. These programmes must be guided by empirical evidence, often accumulated in high income countries, such as United States of America (USA) and United Kingdom (UK), and simultaneously fit within the unique cultural context of sub-Saharan Africa (which is very distinct from the setting of the original clinical trial). This often poses a challenge in implementation where the original trial does not fit with the local context. Strategies from the field of implementation science, defined as the "scientific study of methods to promote the systematic uptake of research findings and other evidence-based practices into routine practice, and, hence, to improve the quality and effectiveness of health services and care" [7] can be useful for supporting the translation of evidence from clinical trials to implementation in contexts vastly different from that originally employed in the clinical trial, such as Kaduna State in Africa. One such strategy is community engagement at all levels of the healthcare system [8].

Kaduna State in northern Nigeria was the country's old colonial capital, it is a microcosm of the entire country, and has a population of over eight million made up of over 60 different ethnic groups, with 23 local governments, three geopolitical (senatorial) zones, with over 30 health care facilities for secondary care, two academic institutions (tertiary care and undergraduate training), and five teaching hospitals (tertiary care) hospitals. The academic institutions are Ahmadu Bello University Teaching Hospital and Barau Dikko Teaching Hospital, Kaduna State University, and the other four tertiary care level hospitals are National Eye Centre, National Ear Care Centre, Federal Neuro-Psychiatric Hospital, and 44 Nigerian Armed Forces Reference Hospital. The State offers free healthcare for pregnant women and children up to five years of age. Kaduna State Primary Health Care Agency is led by an Executive Secretary to oversee primary care centres and clinics in conjunction with the local governments.

We embarked on community engagement as the initial step to informing the development and implementation of an NBS programme for SCD in Kaduna State. Community engagement has been broadly defined as involving communities in information giving, consultation, decision-making, planning, co-design, governance, and delivery of services [9]. This was an early phase of sustained engagement with a broad range of community representatives to be inclusive and aimed for equal partnership. Furthermore, the application of implementation science within health systems is of benefit to the development and implementation of health interventions. Despite favourable evidence in clinical trials, programmes often fail to reach their desired outcomes in the real world due to limitations outside the trial environment and challenges with implementation.

Implementation science provides strategies to help guide implementation, therefore improving access to evidence-based services that fit with the culture of the population in need. The first phase usually consists of descriptive, formative research to better understand the major implementation challenges and to design potential strategies to overcome these [10]. We employed a widely-used implementation science framework, "Getting to Outcomes®" (GTO), which incorporates continuous multilevel evaluation by stakeholders about the quality of the implementation [11–13]. GTO is a 10-step system of accountability that guides the user through the process of planning, monitoring, and evaluating programmes. The continuous evaluation facilitates adaptation of the programme to local capacity and motivation for change, which maximizes the chances of programme success.

The objectives of the community engagement were two-fold. First, to obtain critical information pertaining to disparate ethnic groups and settings (rural and urban), including potential barriers to a successful NBS with the Kaduna State healthcare system and subsequent policy implementation. Second, to assist in the readiness assessment of Kaduna State in the implementation of a sustainable NBS programme for SCD.

2. Methods

Qualitative research methodology was employed in a two-day focus group workshop with an identical format over the two days in Kaduna. A representative group of participants were invited for each of the two focus group sessions. These comprised parents of children with SCD, adults with SCD, representatives of patient association and support groups, community leaders, health professionals, and policy-makers from the three health zones in Kaduna state, including nurses and midwives. Community health extensions workers from primary healthcare centres, doctors, and nurses from general and teaching hospitals were among the participants. In addition, five participants from the neighbouring Niger State were invited to the first focus group session to highlight the anticipated differences between states.

Focus group discussions were facilitated by a faculty of five international and local experts in SCD from the UK and Nigeria, including paediatricians, haematologists, a psychologist, and a professional in community engagement. The focus group format included brief introductory lectures on SCD and NBS. This was followed by a series of 10 questions based on the ten-point GTO framework for discussion. Each participant was given the opportunity and was encouraged to be candid with their responses and discussions in a relaxed and open atmosphere and speak in any language of their preference. Proceedings were transcribed by a professional scribe and audio-recorded. Subsequently, transcripts were produced from the audio recordings by two professionals that were experienced in transcribing (LG) and qualitative research (EG). Their combined report was reviewed by the facilitators of focus groups for accuracy and consistency (KAA, BO, and BI).

3. Results

There was a total of 52 participants for the two-day focus group workshop (Table 1). Discussions based on the GTO questions and additional issues are summarised by themes generated below.

Table 1. Participants of the Two-Day Community Engagement Focus Group Sessions.

Institution or Participant	Number
Adult with Sickle Cell Disease	2
Ahmadu Bello University Teaching Hospital–Zaria	4
Ahmadu Bello University Teaching Hospital School of Nursing–Zaria	1
Barau Dikko Teaching Hospital–Kaduna	8
Fantsuam Foundation–Kafanchan	3
Gambo Sawaba Memorial Hospital–Zaria	1
Federal Ministry of Finance–Abuja (Independent Participant)	1
Kaduna State Primary Healthcare Development Agency	2
Media Representatives	2
Mil-Goma Community Leaders–Zazzau Emirate	2
Niger State Government–(Jumai Babangida Aliyu Maternal and Neonatal Hospital) Minna, Niger State	5
Panaf Schools–Kaduna	2

Table 1. *Cont.*

Institution or Participant	Number
Parent of a Child/Children with Sickle Cell Disease	3
Rahma Integrated Sickle Cell Research Centre–Kaduna	1
Safiya Sickle Cell Foundation Zaria–Kaduna and Abuja	3
Samira Sanusi Sickle Cell Foundation–Kaduna	4
Sickle Cell Health Promotion Centre–Kaduna	2
Sir Patrick Ibrahim Yakowa Hospital–Kafanchan	4
Kaduna State House of Assembly	1
Kaduna State Ministry of Health and Human Services	1

3.1. Objectives of a SCD Programme

- Early detection and reduction of SCD in our communities
- To offer subsidised testing and treatment
- To minimize the cost of treatment and maintenance
- Reduce psychological and emotional trauma amongst family members
- To reduce the financial drain on the families of SCD patients
- Increase awareness of SCD most especially in the rural areas
- Improve the health status of SCD patients
- Eradicate stigma
- Healthy communities to function better
- Accurate data to inform policy makers in improved planning
- Give hope to patients with SCD to live normal fulfilled lives
- Improve standard of diagnosis to rule out confusion
- Increase the life expectancy of patients and eradication of SCD
- Reduce morbidity and mortality

3.2. Perceptions about NBS

- Early diagnosis and administering Penicillin improve on the patient's life expectancy
- Strong perception about SCD not having a cure affects the minds of families
- Poverty and financial constraint hinder families from accessing NBS
- Myths and traditional beliefs about SCD being associated with witchcraft creates an obstacle to NBS
- Most SCD babies not tested at birth end up dying from malaria even before SCD is detected

3.3. Implementation of NBS

- The early diagnosis should be at primary, secondary and tertiary health care centres
- Parents of affected children should be confidentially informed of the implication of SCD and how to prepare for the child's welfare
- World Sickle Cell Day should be emphasised with adequate publicity
- Screening, diagnosis, counselling and service delivery should be inter faced
- Blood samples should be taken at birth and in post-natal clinics
- Incentivising the process by giving out souvenirs
- NBS should be free and patients be given free or subsidized medication
- The Government should give SCD a priority

3.4. Why We Need a NBS Programme

- To create the opportunity for effective management of SCD

- To inform the community on the importance of screening
- To inform parents on how to prepare for the child's welfare
- Early detection will make the government have up to date data on SCD for adequate planning
- To increase the chances of controlling the disease
- To help in reducing stigma and disabuse the perception of the community
- To properly manage patients and parents

3.5. Best Practices to Adopt

- Community based approach by involving Volunteer Community Mobilisers (VCMs) and Traditional Birth Attendants (TBAs)
- Facility based approach
- Utilising media to disseminate information through drama on radio and television
- Incorporate the importance of NBS during antenatal health talks
- Involve community and religious organizations for sensitization campaigns like in the case of the "child spacing" campaigns
- Development partners, NGOs and media collaboration to expand
- More Sickle cell centres should be made available, accessible and affordable
- Social networks should be utilized for campaigns of SCD
- Train existing staff and employ additional qualified staff to run the centres
- Compulsory routine testing at birth
- Build linkages between the community and health care facilities

3.6. Resources and Capacity Building Needed

- Train TBAs to use simple testing for NBS
- Train Village Community Mobilisers
- Train existing staff and employ additional qualified professionals
- Existing health facilities should be equipped
- Build on existing HIV infrastructure
- Technical and financial support from development partners, and charitable organizations
- Continuous advocacy for dissemination of the facts about SCD
- Newborn testing should be available, accessible and affordable

3.7. How to Evaluate the Success of the Programme

- Using existing data to plan
- Correct and appropriate documentation is essential for evaluation
- Continuous monitoring of the programme
- Training and re-training of personnel

In addition, core themes identified within the GTO framework and categorised by the type of participant or institution are presented in Table 2.

Table 2. Ten Steps of the "Getting to Outcomes®" Framework for Sickle Cell Disease New Born Screening and Key Messages from Participants.

	Parent of Sickle Cell Disease (SCD) Child	Community Health Worker	Health Centre Doctor	Health System Hospital Administrator	Laboratory Technician	Patient Organisation Representative
Step 1: Needs & Resources	Early diagnosis & pre-marital counselling	Early awareness of SCD status	Early diagnosis & lack of treatment facilities	Innovative utilisation of resources	Equipment, reagents & quality assurance	Use of media for public awareness
Step 2: Goals & Objectives	Knowledge of diagnosis and access to treatment	Address ignorance, stigma & beliefs	Early detection of SCD and provision of medical care	Equity on service provision for SCD similar to HIV	To eliminate errors in diagnosis	Public perception about SCD
Step 3: Best Practices	Immunisation programme which is accessible	Strong educational elements of family planning campaign	HIV/AIDS programme structure & funding	Low cost intervention that is affordable	Reduce false positives & false negatives results	SCD education for families & general public
Step 4: Programme Fit for NBS	Testing during other clinics such as immunisation	Community worker leadership important	Primary health care system to reach local communities	Combine with other dried blood sample testing	Staff trained for IEF [a] & would like skills in HPLC [b] in addition	Encourage community participation
Step 5: Capacity for NBS	Staff must be competent	Partnership with community	Shortages of staff, medicines & development of skills	Limited resources, 3 tiers of government & community participation	Reagents supply, storage & inventory	Public engagement and sensitisation
Step 6: NBS Implementation Plan	Provide medicines & access to staff	Counselling, treatment for patients & families	Health status, treatment, tracking & follow up	Need to know SCD burden, resource implication	Clear standard operating procedures	Address myths & stigma
Step 7: Evaluation for NBS	Is my baby growing well?	Reporting outcome of babies visiting the SCD centre, verbal autopsies	Diagnosed babies receiving penicillin & attending SCD clinic	Infant & childhood mortality, immunisation coverage	Monthly & quarterly arranged Quality Assurance	Parliamentary oversight & reports to constituents.
Step 8: NBS Outcome Evaluation	Knowledgeable staff & a Sickle Cell Centre	Number of patients accessing counselling services	Percentage of diagnosed babies with SCD, penicillin prophylaxis	Survival for SCD children at 1, 5 &10 years of age	Accurate & timeliness of laboratory results	A sickle cell centre for Kaduna state
Step 9: Continuous Quality Improvement	Parent support & input in care	Education & step-down training	Teleconference discussion on NBS programme results & troubleshooting	Continuous assessment & Peer Review Systems	Weekly quality reports on results, timeliness & errors	Sensitise general public, religious & community leaders
Step 10: Sustainability of NBS Programme	Not limited to a state governor's term in office	Involve all sectors of health care	Multidisciplinary team, government support	Involvement of all parties	Train personnel for additional laboratory procedures	Educate to accept responsibility of both men & women

[a] Isoelectric Focusing (IEF). [b] High Performance Liquid Chromatography (HPLC).

4. Discussion

Readiness is part of GTO, but what we did in this focus group was broader than readiness alone. We organized the findings by GTO steps, which served to (1) understand differences in perspectives across the different levels (this is important for addressing potential barriers) and (2) to remain accountable for implementation. From an implementation standpoint, one of the challenges faced in health care settings is the transport of interventions from a research trial to naturalistic setting. There are many factors that get in the way of successful implementation in naturalistic settings, especially in complex settings, like the multilevel healthcare structure in Kaduna. Differences in the vision, needs, resources, and goals of different levels of the health system may get in the way of successful implementation. This complexity is compounded by differences in contextual factors between the setting of the original clinical trial of the intervention and the local context where the intervention is being implemented. Most likely adaptations are needed to achieve the similar outcomes of a well-funded clinical trial in a developing country. In order to identify which adaptations are needed, and at which level these adaptations are needed, community engagement at each healthcare level is needed.

SCD poses a major public health problem in Nigeria. Community engagement as a first step to developing and implementing a sustainable NBS programme was carried out by SCD experts from UK, USA, and Nigeria, working with a charity in Nigeria called the Sickle Cell Cohort Research (SCORE) Foundation. Focus group discussions employing an implementation science approach with patients, parents, community leaders, doctors, nurses, and community health workers allowed active participation and important information to be gathered about the difficulties and solutions for testing newborn babies in these communities, including cultural and religious beliefs.

This study employed a well-known implementation framework to guide community engagement. Through focus groups, we uncovered certain areas where potential barriers to implementation may exist and where certain adaptations may be needed to improve the chances of achieving programmatic success. For example, we found a major communication gap between policy-makers and user groups. There is an absence of patient-users consultation within the state policy framework and therefore the lack of opportunity to incorporate their views in service planning and implementation. Asking and answering the 10 GTO accountability questions provided a structured format to understand the strengths and weaknesses in the implementation setting. This led nicely to the development of plans that support quality implementation. In this way, the hospitals will be more prepared for implementation and increase their chances of programmatic success.

The goals and objectives were addressed. Outcomes include the opportunity for participants working together to address SCD issues, to network, and engage with each other. Shared knowledge by participants, greater awareness of what is in place albeit on a small scale. Some myths and misinformation were addressed. There is no doubt that the importance of NBS for SCD programme development and implementation in Kaduna State, Niger State and the entire country cannot be over emphasised. To ensure the sustainability of the programme, the government has to be fully committed to it by providing the legal framework, policies, and adequate funding. It is also important to note that issues such as lack of public awareness and concerns could be barriers to a successful programme. Therefore, it is necessary to educate the general public through media campaigns, and advocate in partnership with the support of religious and traditional leaders within.

5. Summary and Conclusions

The two-day workshop successfully set the stage for the development and implementation plan of the NBS programme for SCD communities. Recommendations for the next steps to developing a Kaduna State NBS for SCD programme were made to the State's Commissioner of Health, and subsequently an initial four-day training workshop was organised prior to step by step implementation: (i) Procurement of reagents (ii) collection of blood spots from one local government area (1/23) of the state to test robustness of specimen collection, transportation to the laboratory, analysis turnaround time; result disclosure to families, (iii) counselling to families; and, (iv) referral to treatment clinic. A number of key themes from this 'Getting To Outcomes' (10 steps) assessment process require urgent implementation by Kaduna State through the setting up of steering committee to address the issues that were raised regarding the Objectives of a SCD programme, Perceptions, and Implementation of NBS. For the State to adopt Community based approach by involving Volunteer Community Mobilisers (VCMs) and Traditional Birth Attendants (TBAs) for maximum benefit and to ensure that a robust monitoring and evaluation process is in place.

Author Contributions: Conceptualization, K.A.A., L.H., A.L., B.P.D.I. and B.O.; Methodology, K.A.A., L.H., A.L., B.P.D I. and B.O.; Formal Analysis, L.G., E.G. and K.A.A.; Resources, B.P.D., L.G.D. and I.I.; Data Curation, L.G., E.G., K.A.A. and B.O.; Writing-Original Draft Preparation, K.A.A., B.P.D.I, L.H., A.L., L.G.D., B.O., I.I., W.A.; Writing-Review & Editing, B.P.DI., K.A.A., L.H., A.L., L.G.D., B.O., I.I., W.A.

Acknowledgments: We are sincerely indebted to the invaluable leadership and support of Paul Dogo, Commissioner of Health—Kaduna State, regarding the development and implementation of Newborn Screening in Kaduna State. We acknowledge Amina Abubakar Bello, wife of Niger state Governor for facilitating her state's involvement in the Focus group activity in Kaduna. We are very grateful to all the participants of the two day focus group workshops, and Barau Dikko Teaching Hospital, Kaduna.

References

1. Secretariat FNWHA. Sickle Cell Anaemia. 2006. Available online: http://apps.who.int/gb/ebwha/pdf_files/WHA59-REC3/WHA59_REC3-en.pdf (accessed on 30 August 2018).
2. Williams, T.N. Sickle Cell Disease in Sub-Saharan Africa. *Hematol. Oncol. Clin. N. Am.* **2016**, *30*, 343–358. [CrossRef] [PubMed]
3. World Health Organisation. Sickle-Cell Anaemia Report by the Secretariat. Fifty Ninth World Health Assembly 2006. Available online: http://apps.who.int/gb/ebwha/pdf_files/WHA59/A59_9-en.pdf (accessed on 30 August 2018).
4. Piel, F.B.; Patil, A.P.; Howes, R.E.; Nyangiri, O.A.; Gething, P.W.; Dewi, M.; Temperley, W.H.; Williams, T.N.; Weatherall, D.J.; Hay, S.I. Global epidemiology of Sickle haemoglobin in neonates: A contemporary geostatistical model-based map and population estimates. *Lancet* **2013**, *381*, 142–151. [CrossRef]
5. Inusa, B.P.; Juliana Olufunke, Y.D.; John Dada, L. Sickle Cell Disease Screening in Northern Nigeria: The Co-Existence of Thalassemia Inheritance. *Pediatr. Ther.* **2015**, *5*, 3–6. [CrossRef]
6. Makani, J.; Cox, S.E.; Soka, D.; Komba, A.N.; Oruo, J.; Mwamtemi, H.; Magesa, P.; Rwezaula, S.; Meda, E.; Mgaya, J.; et al. Mortality in sickle cell anemia in Africa: A prospective cohort study in Tanzania. *PLoS ONE* **2012**, *6*, e14699. [CrossRef] [PubMed]
7. Eccles, M.P.; Mittman, B.S. Welcome to implementation science. *Implement. Sci.* **2006**. [CrossRef]
8. Anie, K.A.; Treadwell, M.J.; Grant, A.M.; Dennis-Aantwi, J.A.; Asafo, M.K.; Lamptey, M.E.; Ojodu, J.; Yusuf, C.; Otaigbe, A.; Ohene-Frempong, K. Community engagement to inform the development of a sickle cell counselor training and certification program in Ghana. *J. Community Genet.* **2016**, *7*, 195–202. [CrossRef] [PubMed]
9. Swainston, K.; Summerbell, C. *The Effectiveness of Community Engagement Approaches and Methods for Health Promotion Interventions*; University of Teeside: Teeside, UK, 2008.
10. CDI Study Group. Community-directed interventions for priority health problems in Africa: Results of a multicountry study. *Bull. World Health Organ.* **2010**, *88*, 509–518. [CrossRef] [PubMed]
11. Chinman, M.; Hunter, S.B.; Ebener, P.; Paddock, S.M.; Stillman, L.; Imm, P.; Wandersman, A. The getting to outcomes demonstration and evaluation: An illustration of the prevention support system. *Am. J. Community Psychol.* **2008**, *41*, 206–224. [CrossRef] [PubMed]

12. Meyers, D.C.; Durlak, J.A.; Wandersman, A. The quality implementation framework: A synthesis of critical steps in the implementation process. *Am. J. Community Psychol.* **2012**, *50*, 462–480. [CrossRef] [PubMed]

13. Wandersman, A.; Alia, K.; Cook, B.S.; Hsu, L.L.; Ramaswamy, R. Evidence-Based interventions Are Necessary but Not Sufficient for Achieving Outcomes in Each Setting in a Complex World: Empowerment Evaluation, Getting to Outcomes, and Demonstrating Accountability. *Am. J. Eval.* **2016**, *37*, 544–561. [CrossRef]

21

The Timely Needs for Infantile Onset Pompe Disease Newborn Screening

Shu-Chuan Chiang [1], **Yin-Hsiu Chien** [1,2,*], **Kai-Ling Chang** [1], **Ni-Chung Lee** [1,2] and **Wuh-Liang Hwu** [1,2]

[1]   Department of Medical Genetics, National Taiwan University Hospital, Taipei 100, Taiwan
[2]   Department of Pediatrics, National Taiwan University Hospital, Taipei 100, Taiwan
*   Correspondence: chienyh@ntu.edu.tw;

Abstract: Pompe disease Newborn screening (NBS) aims at diagnosing patients with infantile-onset Pompe disease (IOPD) early enough so a timely treatment can be instituted. Since 2015, the National Taiwan University NBS Center has changed the method for Pompe disease NBS from fluorometric assay to tandem mass assay. From 2016 to 2019, 14 newborns were reported as high-risk for Pompe disease at a median age of 9 days (range 6–13), and 18 were with a borderline risk at a median age of 13 days (9–28). None of the borderline risks were IOPD patients. Among the 14 at a high-risk of Pompe disease, four were found to have cardiomyopathy, and six were classified as potential late-onset Pompe disease. The four classic IOPD newborns, three of the four having at least one allele of the cross-reactive immunologic material (CRIM)-positive variant, started enzyme replacement therapy (ERT) at a median age of 9 days (8–14). Western Blot analysis and whole gene sequencing confirmed the CRIM-positive status in all cases. Here, we focus on the patient without the known CRIM-positive variant. Doing ERT before knowing the CRIM status created a dilemma in the decision and was discussed in detail. Our Pompe disease screening and diagnostic program successfully detected and treated patients with IOPD in time. However, the timely exclusion of a CRIM-negative status, which is rare in the Chinese population, is still a challenging task.

Keywords: infantile-onset Pompe disease; GAA sequencing; immune modulation therapy; enzyme replacement therapy; cross-reactive immunologic material

1. Introduction

Pompe disease, a genetic disorder caused by variants of the glucosidase alpha acid (*GAA*) gene, leads from acid alpha-glucosidase (GAA) deficiency. The phenotypes of Pompe disease vary widely, ranging from the most severe classic infantile-onset Pompe disease (IOPD) to the later-onset Pompe disease (LOPD). Currently, enzyme replacement therapy (ERT) with recombinant human GAA (rhGAA) is the only approved therapy. We have performed newborn screening (NBS) for Pompe disease [1] since 2005, and our results demonstrate that the early initiation of treatment improves the prognosis IOPD patients [2], thus confirming the value of newborn screening for Pompe disease.

However, there are still challenges when an infant receives a positive screening result. First, the phenotype cannot be predicted by GAA activity [3,4]. Mutation analysis of the *GAA* gene can predict the phenotype in a portion of patients [5]. But more precisely, newborns with classic IOPD should have presented with cardiomyopathy and muscle weakness at birth clinically [2,6]. Second, ERT with rhGAA may trigger an immune response with neutralizing antibodies, especially in patients negative for the cross-reactive immunologic material (CRIM) [7]. Prophylactic immunologic modulation therapy may overcome the problem, but the CRIM status needs to be defined before initiating ERT [8]. Nowadays, some GAA variants are associated with a known CRIM status [9].

The National Taiwan University Hospital (NTUH) Newborn Screening Center, established since 1985, is responsible for the screening of more than one-third of all newborns in Taiwan [10]. In 2005, we were the first to implement Pompe disease newborn screening [1]. Initially, dried blood spot (DBS) GAA activities were measured using fluorogenic (4-methylumbelliferone) substrates [4]. Since 2015, we have been using tandem mass assay (MS/MS) substrates in order to accommodate multiplexing ability [11]. The medical genetics department in the NTUH is also the referral center for Pompe disease detected by the NTUH. The hospital staff work closely with the screening center in order to make a timely management of IOPD. Here, we describe our practice in the past seven years.

2. Methods

NBS for inborn errors of metabolism in Taiwan was established in 1985, and, currently, the National Taiwan University Hospital (NTUH) holds one of the three screening centers in Taiwan. There are more than 300 birthing facilities that collect newborn dried bloodspots (DBS) and ship them promptly to the NBS labs. DBS sampling is usually performed 48–72 h after the birth of the babies, and shipping by priority mail typically takes less than two days. The NBS labs are requested to report high-risk results within 72 h after receiving the samples [10]. Although NBS is not mandatory in Taiwan, close to 100% of newborns acquired NBS. In 2008, Pompe disease newborn screening was added by the NTUH NBS Center and also by the other two screening centers [12], but written consent from the parent(s) is required. More than 95% of parents receiving service of NTUH NBS center provide consents for having Pompe disease newborn screening. The methods of Pompe disease NBS has been described previously [1,11,13]. Initially, GAA activity in DBS elute is measured using fluorogenic substrates, but the method was changed to the tandem mass spectrometry (MS/MS) at the end of 2015. From the first DBS, we set two cutoffs of the GAA activity measurements. Values exceeding the critical cutoff imply a high risk of having Pompe disease and that emergent confirmatory diagnostic testing is necessary. Values exceeding the borderline cutoff, mostly due to pseudodeficiency, will trigger a second-tier test, generating the value of % inhibition, before the final assignment [4]. If the second-tier test is positive, the baby will be suggested to have the confirmatory diagnostic testing. Since 2013, we employed the second-tier test to avoid requesting a second sample to prevent delay in the initiation of treatment. DBS DNA genotyping [14] may be applied to categorise the newborns. For confirmatory diagnostic testing, a whole blood sample was used for the measurement of GAA activity, genotyping, and CRIM test [10]. The CRIM test was performed by Western Blot analysis, using anti-GAA and anti-alpha-tubulin antibodies. For GAA protein detection, 15 μL of sonicated lymphocytes protein from patients was loaded in each lane (only 2 μL was used for normal control) and the X-ray film was exposed overnight. For alpha-tubulin (the control protein), 10 μL of sonicated protein was loaded in each lane and the X-ray film was exposed for 15 min. The Taiwanese common variant, p.D645E (p.Asp645Glu) [6,15], was rapidly screened by polymerase chain reaction-restriction fragment length polymorphism analysis (RFLP) using the *Bsa*HI restriction enzyme. Since p.D645E is a CRIM-positive variant [16], patients with this variant should be CRIM-positive. Enzyme replacement therapy (ERT) is scheduled for the next day after the heart involvement is confirmed, unless immunomodulation therapy to prevent anti-GAA antibodies production is planned. For babies without heart involvement at birth, a follow-up plan was initiated, including the development milestone, motor function, and biomarkers as described [10], and ERT was initiated until abnormalities appeared in the follow-up period.

3. Results

3.1. Performance of Screening and Diagnostic Testing

From 2016 to 2019, Pompe disease NBS was performed by the MS/MS method. The timeliness of the performance of other screening conditions (glucose-6-phosphate dehydrogenase deficiency, congenital hypothyroidism, galactosemia, congenital adrenal hyperplasia, and MS/MS acylcarnitine profile) during this period was similar to the previous three years (2013–2015); i.e., the compliance rates of reporting NBS results by 8 days of age were between 98.66% to 99.01%, compared to 98.85%–99.14% in the previous 3 years. With the MS/MS platform, 14 newborns were reported as high-risk for Pompe disease at a median age of 9 days (range 6–13). For newborns with a borderline risk for Pompe disease, 18 were reported at a median age of 13 days (9–28), but none of them were IOPD. During the previous 3 years (2013–2015), when Pompe disease NBS was performed using the 4MU platform, there were no Pompe disease high-risk newborns and 44 were reported as a borderline risk reported at a median age of 12 days (7–41), but none were IOPD.

Among the 14 newborns at a high risk of Pompe disease, four were found to have cardiomyopathy, as shown by electrocardiography, chest X-ray, echocardiography, and an elevation of serum creatine kinase (CK) and pro-brain natriuretic peptide (pro-BNP). Six [11,13] were found to have GAA deficiency and biallelic GAA variants but normal CK and no cardiomegaly and therefore were classified as potential LOPDs. The remaining four of the total 14 newborns were not affected. As for the 18 infants with the borderline risk, only 2 infants [11] were classified as potential LOPDs, while the rest were not affected. The four classic IOPD newborns were treated starting from a median of 9 days (8–14 days). *GAA* gene sequencing confirmed all pathogenic variants in these patients. Three of the four had at least one allele of the p.D645E variant. CRIM status (all CRIM positive (denoted as CRIM +)) was approved by Western Blot analysis in all four patients, including the one who did not have the p.D645E variation. The newborn who did not have the p.D645E variant did create a dilemma in the decision, and the history is described below.

3.2. Case Description

A 7-days-old female newborn was requested to visit our hospital due to an abnormal Pompe disease screening result [13]. She was born at full-term to a G1P1 mother with a birth bodyweight of 4380 gm. The parents denied poor feeding, poor activity, nor weak crying in this baby. NBS included Pompe disease, and other conditions were performed on her third day of life. On Day 4, our NBS laboratory received her sample. On Day 6, a high risk of Pompe disease was reported (GAA activity 0.18 uM/h (critical cutoff < 0.5); ratio 42.87 (critical cutoff acid β-glucosidase (ABG)/GAA ≥ 20) so an urgent visit to our hospital was arranged on Day 7. When we saw her, she had normal muscle power, normal reflex, no macroglossia, but her facial folds decrease slightly. Laboratory examination revealed an elevation of pro-BNP (8738 pg/mL), CK (722 U/L), and alanine aminotransferase (ALT) (112 U/L). A chest X-ray revealed mild cardiomegaly (Figure 1). Echocardiography revealed moderate left ventricle (LV) and right ventricle (RV) hypertrophy, with a LV mass index (LVMI, measured by 2-D method) of 115.7 g/m^2 (normal range < 65 g/m^2). A whole blood sampling at Day 7 revealed deficient lymphocyte GAA activity (1.33 nmol/g pro/h, normal mean 66.7) and thus confirmed the diagnosis of IOPD. However, she did not have the common CRIM-positive Taiwan Pompe disease p.D645E variant, tested using DNA extracted from the first DBS. Although her CRIM status was unknown, her parents refused prophylactic immune modulation therapy. Western Blot analysis using the white blood cells as the material soon revealed the 110 kDa precursor GAA band (Figure 2), suggesting a CRIM-positive status. She received her first dose of rhGAA (20 mg/kg) at the age of 8 days. Mutation analysis showed heterozygous c.2024_2026del (p.N675del) and c.2040+1G>T variants *in trans*, compatible with IOPD. There were no CRIM status predictions about these two variants [9].

The study was approved by the ethical committee of National Taiwan University Hospital, Taipei, Taiwan (201906053RINB, 1st approved date 2019/08/05). The clinical information was gathered from the hospital medical records retrospectively, and no individual's consent was required.

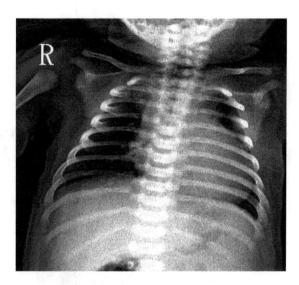

Figure 1. CXR at D7 in a newborn with a positive Pompe newborn screening result. Mild cardiomegaly was noted.

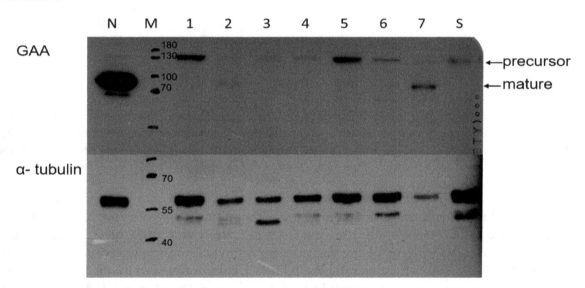

Figure 2. Blood glucosidase alpha acid (GAA) Western Blotting of this case (S), indicating a cross-reactive immunologic material (CRIM)-positive status. The lymphocytes were sonicated and then blotted with antibodies to detect human GAA and α-tubulin protein presence. M: marker; N: normal newborn; No. 1 and No. 3 were from infantile-onset Pompe disease (IOPD) patients with the CRIM(+) GAA variant; No. 2, No. 4–7 were from newborns with low GAA activity. N: normal control sample; M: marker. Precursor: 110 kDa GAA. Mature: 70/76 kDa GAA.

4. Discussion

Pompe newborn screening was included in Taiwan's newborn screening system as well as in the Recommended Uniform Screening Panel (RUSP) in the USA. Therefore, the timeliness requirements of newborn screening, i.e., the efficient collection, transportation, testing, and reporting of the results, also benefit Pompe newborn screening. In Taiwan, the recommended timelines for the high-risk babies is to report and communicate the results to the newborn's healthcare provider/parent(s) within 6–8 days of life, regardless of the location of newborns, which maybe 300 km away from the screening centers/treatment centers (Figure 3). The compliance rate for reporting by age 8 days in our center was over 99%. In the present case, we informed the result by D6 and made the diagnosis by D7, demonstrating the discrimination power of applying the critical cutoffs and the well-established newborn screening system in Taiwan.

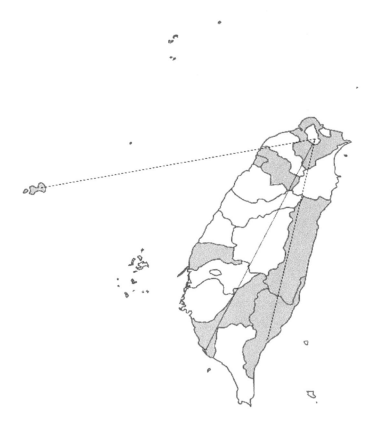

Figure 3. The coverage map of the National Taiwan University Hospital Newborn Screening Center. The samples ship from the gray areas to our screening center, designated by the government, including the three far areas indicated by the lines. The distances from the birthplaces to the screening center were around 300 km.

The more challenging part of this case was the preparation of ERT, starting after the confirmation of cardiomegaly and muscle damage. In this case, the decision for ERT was tentatively made at D7 and the ERT was initiated at D8, after reconfirming the GAA deficiency and confirming the CRIM status. In such classic IOPD newborns waiting for the decision of prophylaxis immunomodulation, we routinely check the predicted CRIM status by screening the p.D645E, commonly seen in our Pompe patients [6], using RFLP so that we could have the result in half day. Since p.D645E is related to CRIM-positive status [16], patients with at least one p.D645E allele will be CRIM-positive, and doing prophylaxis immunomodulation on such cases may not achieve benefit-risk balance. On the other hand, we plan to apply prophylactic immune modulation therapy for IOPD infants if a CRIM-negative status is confirmed. Therefore, in this case, we performed the blood Western Blotting assay as described [17] to determine the CRIM status since the GAA sequencing result took more time, and the CRIM status for a novel variant may not be predicable, especially for the splicing mutation [9] presented in this case. Rapid sequencing, or screening for several common variants, may replace the blood CRIM status measurement in such a situation.

In conclusion, we demonstrate here the performance of the NBS system in Taiwan and the decision steps for positive Pompe NBS. Knowing the genotype/CRIM status was necessary for the ERT initiation but it made for very intensive work. Depending on the different geographic regions and various resources available, each team needs to prepare themselves with a standardized and comprehensive algorithm for the confirmation and treatment of classic IOPD patients. With the timeliness of screening and diagnosis, we were able to start the treatment as early as possible to achieve the best treatment outcome.

Author Contributions: Data curation, S.-C.C. and K.-L.C.; Formal analysis, Y.-H.C. and N.-C.L.; Methodology, S.-C.C., W.-L.H. All authors have read and agreed to the published version of the manuscript.

References

1. Chien, Y.H.; Chiang, S.C.; Zhang, X.K.; Keutzer, J.; Lee, N.C.; Huang, A.C.; Chen, C.A.; Wu, M.H.; Huang, P.H.; Tsai, F.J.; et al. Early detection of Pompe disease by newborn screening is feasible: Results from the Taiwan screening program. *Pediatrics* **2008**, *122*, e39–e45. [CrossRef] [PubMed]

2. Chien, Y.H.; Lee, N.C.; Thurberg, B.L.; Chiang, S.C.; Zhang, X.K.; Keutzer, J.; Huang, A.C.; Wu, M.H.; Huang, P.H.; Tsai, F.J.; et al. Pompe disease in infants: Improving the prognosis by newborn screening and early treatment. *Pediatrics* **2009**, *124*, e1116–e1125. [CrossRef] [PubMed]

3. Chien, Y.H.; Lee, N.C.; Huang, H.J.; Thurberg, B.L.; Tsai, F.J.; Hwu, W.L. Later-onset Pompe disease: Early detection and early treatment initiation enabled by newborn screening. *J. Pediatr.* **2011**, *158*, 1023–1027.e1. [CrossRef] [PubMed]

4. Chiang, S.C.; Hwu, W.L.; Lee, N.C.; Hsu, L.W.; Chien, Y.H. Algorithm for Pompe disease newborn screening: Results from the Taiwan screening program. *Mol. Genet. Metab.* **2012**, *106*, 281–286. [CrossRef] [PubMed]

5. Reuser, A.J.J.; van der Ploeg, A.T.; Chien, Y.H.; Llerena, J., Jr.; Abbott, M.A.; Clemens, P.R.; Kimonis, V.E.; Leslie, N.; Maruti, S.S.; Sanson, B.J.; et al. GAA variants and phenotypes among 1,079 patients with Pompe disease: Data from the Pompe Registry. *Hum. Mutat.* **2019**, *40*, 2146–2164. [CrossRef] [PubMed]

6. Chien, Y.H.; Lee, N.C.; Chen, C.A.; Tsai, F.J.; Tsai, W.H.; Shieh, J.Y.; Huang, H.J.; Hsu, W.C.; Tsai, T.H.; Hwu, W.L. Long-term prognosis of patients with infantile-onset Pompe disease diagnosed by newborn screening and treated since birth. *J. Pediatr.* **2015**, *166*, 985–991. [CrossRef] [PubMed]

7. Banugaria, S.G.; Patel, T.T.; Mackey, J.; Das, S.; Amalfitano, A.; Rosenberg, A.S.; Charrow, J.; Chen, Y.T.; Kishnani, P.S. Persistence of high sustained antibodies to enzyme replacement therapy despite extensive immunomodulatory therapy in an infant with Pompe disease: Need for agents to target antibody-secreting plasma cells. *Mol. Genet. Metab.* **2012**, *105*, 677–680. [CrossRef] [PubMed]

8. Messinger, Y.H.; Mendelsohn, N.J.; Rhead, W.; Dimmock, D.; Hershkovitz, E.; Champion, M.; Jones, S.A.; Olson, R.; White, A.; Wells, C.; et al. Successful immune tolerance induction to enzyme replacement therapy in CRIM-negative infantile Pompe disease. *Genet. Med.* **2012**, *14*, 135–142. [CrossRef] [PubMed]

9. Bali, D.S.; Goldstein, J.L.; Banugaria, S.; Dai, J.; Mackey, J.; Rehder, C.; Kishnani, P.S. Predicting cross-reactive immunological material (CRIM) status in Pompe disease using GAA mutations: Lessons learned from 10 years of clinical laboratory testing experience. *Am. J. Med. Genet. C Semin. Med. Genet.* **2012**, *160*, 40–49. [CrossRef] [PubMed]

10. Chien, Y.H.; Hwu, W.L.; Lee, N.C. Newborn screening: Taiwanese experience. *Ann. Transl. Med.* **2019**, *7*, 281. [CrossRef] [PubMed]

11. Chiang, S.-C.; Chen, P.-W.; Hwu, W.-L.; Lee, A.-J.; Chen, L.-C.; Lee, N.-C.; Chiou, L.-Y.; Chien, Y.-H. Performance of the Four-Plex Tandem Mass Spectrometry Lysosomal Storage Disease Newborn Screening Test: The Necessity of Adding a 2nd Tier Test for Pompe Disease. *Int. J. Neonatal Screen.* **2018**, *4*, 41. [CrossRef]

12. Yang, C.F.; Liu, H.C.; Hsu, T.R.; Tsai, F.C.; Chiang, S.F.; Chiang, C.C.; Ho, H.C.; Lai, C.J.; Yang, T.F.; Chuang, S.Y.; et al. A large-scale nationwide newborn screening program for Pompe disease in Taiwan: Towards effective diagnosis and treatment. *Am. J. Med. Genet. A* **2014**, *164A*, 54–61. [CrossRef] [PubMed]

13. Chien, Y.H.; Lee, N.C.; Chen, P.W.; Yeh, H.Y.; Gelb, M.H.; Chiu, P.C.; Chu, S.Y.; Lee, C.H.; Lee, A.R.; Hwu, W.L. Newborn screening for Morquio disease and other lysosomal storage diseases: Results from the 8-plex assay for 70,000 newborns. *Orphanet J. Rare Dis.* **2020**. [CrossRef] [PubMed]

14. Chien, Y.H.; Chiang, S.C.; Chang, K.L.; Yu, H.H.; Lee, W.I.; Tsai, L.P.; Hsu, L.W.; Hu, M.H.; Hwu, W.L. Incidence of severe combined immunodeficiency through newborn screening in a Chinese population. *J. Formos. Med. Assoc.* **2015**, *114*, 12–16. [CrossRef] [PubMed]

15. Labrousse, P.; Chien, Y.H.; Pomponio, R.J.; Keutzer, J.; Lee, N.C.; Akmaev, V.R.; Scholl, T.; Hwu, W.L. Genetic heterozygosity and pseudodeficiency in the Pompe disease newborn screening pilot program. *Mol. Genet. Metab.* **2010**, *99*, 379–383. [CrossRef] [PubMed]

16. Chien, Y.H.; Hwu, W.L.; Lee, N.C. Pompe disease: Early diagnosis and early treatment make a difference. *Pediatr. Neonatol.* **2013**, *54*, 219–227. [CrossRef] [PubMed]

17. Wang, Z.; Okamoto, P.; Keutzer, J. A new assay for fast, reliable CRIM status determination in infantile-onset Pompe disease. *Mol. Genet. Metab.* **2014**, *111*, 92–100. [CrossRef] [PubMed]

22

Early Detection with Pulse Oximetry of Hypoxemic Neonatal Conditions: Development of the IX Clinical Consensus Statement of the Ibero-American Society of Neonatology (SIBEN)

Augusto Sola [1] **and Sergio G. Golombek** [2,3,*]

[1] Professor of Pediatrics and Neonatology, Medical Executive Director of SIBEN, Wellington, FL 33414, USA; augusto.sola@siben.net

[2] President of SIBEN, Professor of Pediatrics and Clinical Public Health, New York Medical College, 40 Sunshine Cottage RD, Valhalla, NY 10595, USA

[3] Attending Neonatologist, Maria Fareri Children's Hospital at Westchester Medical Center, 100 Woods Road, Valhalla, NY 10595, USA

*   Correspondence: sergio_golombek@nymc.edu

Abstract: This article reviews the development of the Ninth Clinical Consensus Statement by SIBEN (the Ibero-American of Neonatology) on "Early Detection with Pulse Oximetry (SpO$_2$) of Hypoxemic Neonatal Conditions". It describes the process of the consensus, and the conclusions and recommendations for screening newborns with pulse oximetry.

Keywords: pulse oximetry; hypoxia; newborn; screening

---

1. Introduction and Methodology

For many years, the education, training, and advances in neonatology in Spanish and Portuguese speaking countries have been inconsistent—although this is also probably true for many countries. In 2004, the Ibero-American Society of Neonatology (SIBEN) was created, with the principal objective of contributing to the improvement of the quality of life for newborn infants and their families in the Ibero-American population. SIBEN is a new society, with members from 29 different countries that focuses on neonatology facilitating education, communication, and professional advancement that contributes to the welfare and well-being of newborns and their families, in order to improve neonatal outcomes in the region. Over the past years, it has been demonstrated that the process of medical consensus could be a way of increasing professional collaboration, as well as improving uniformity in the care given to newborn infants. In 2007, SIBEN began annual meetings of a Clinical Consensus Group, where we—under the guidance of an expert or opinion leader in the topic—organized several subgroups of neonatal professionals in the Ibero-American region. Each subgroup critically reviews all the available literature in order to find the answers to several questions that had been posed to them. SIBEN's consensus process is the first of its kind in the region. It has led to active and collaborative participation of Ibero-American neonatologists of 19 countries and has significantly improved education of all participants. At SIBEN, we believe that the critical review and summary of available clinical data as well as the recommendations made by the SIBEN consensus contribute to consistent best practice for newborn care and develops a useful foundation and valuable model to reduce the gaps in knowledge and the clinical care every newborn baby receives in in this region, thus decreasing the disparity in the care provided and improving short and long-term outcomes. Several important neonatal topics, all relevant to neonatal clinical practice, have been covered so far by SIBEN's clinical consensus including patent ductus arteriosus (PDA), hemodynamic management, bronchopulmonary dysplasia (BPD), hematology, nutrition, persistent pulmonary hypertension of the newborn (PPHN), and hypoxic ischemic encephalopathy, which have been published in consensus statements and peer reviewed journals. This paper is a summary of SIBEN's consensus statement on newborn screening with pulse oximetry.

2. Background on Screening for Congenital Heart Disease

The prevalence, epidemiology, and impact of delay in the diagnosis of CHD have been described in several publications [1–8]. Critical congenital heart defects (CCHD) affect approximately 2 out of every 1000 live births; it is estimated that about 40,000 babies are born with CCHD per year in the US, and 1.35 million worldwide, including ductus-dependent lesions. CCHD represent about 40% of deaths due to congenital malformations and the majority of deaths from cardiovascular disease occurring in the first year of life. It is known that more than 30% of CCHD deaths have been attributed to errors in diagnosis or late diagnosis [9]. For example, in UK it was estimated that 25% of congenital heart disease defects are not diagnosed until after discharge from hospital, and newborns may become seriously ill or die. It is now understood that prenatal or postnatal examination is inadequate for the early detection of these potentially lethal and treatable conditions. Delay in the diagnosis of CCHD may increase the risk of death or permanent injury in newborn babies [10,11].

In 2009, de-Wahl Granelli et al. [12] published a cohort study in which 39,821 children had oxygen saturation measured by pulse oximetry (SpO$_2$) in the upper and lower extremities and demonstrated acceptable test accuracy for the detection of CCHD. Ewer et al. [13], in a similar study in 20,055 asymptomatic newborns, reported similar findings and Zhao and colleagues [14] in China studied 100,000 newborns and demonstrated the same.

In 2011, the US Advisory Committee on Heritable Disorders in Newborns and Children Advisory Committee on Hereditary Diseases [15–17] found that there was sufficient evidence to recommend screening with pulse oximetry [1–64]. The heart defects that can be detected early are mainly the following specific lesions: hypoplastic left heart syndrome, pulmonary atresia, tetralogy of Fallot, anomalous pulmonary venous return, transposition of large vessels, tricuspid atresia, and truncus arteriosus. Screening can also detect: interrupted aortic arch, critical aortic stenosis, aortic valve stenosis, pulmonary valve stenosis. In addition, pulse oximetry screening is useful for the early detection of other conditions with neonatal hypoxemia, such as respiratory disorders (e.g., congenital pneumonia, meconium aspiration, pneumothorax, transient tachypnea of the newborn), neonatal sepsis, and pulmonary hypertension. These findings and others were summarized in a meta-analysis and systematic review by Thangaratinam and colleagues [18].

3. SIBEN's Consensus on Screening with Pulse Oximetry: An Overview

Based on the issues described above, we proceeded to organize the Ninth Clinical SIBEN Consensus on "Early Detection with Pulse Oximetry (SpO$_2$) of Neonatal Hypoxemic Conditions". The concern about the late diagnosis of CCHD led to the investigation of early detection with SpO$_2$ screening. These screening programs have detected other conditions that also present with hypoxemia in addition to CCHD that would have been diagnosed later if not for the evaluation with SpO$_2$ [19]. In order to make recommendations for the Ibero-American region to implement programs pulse oximetry screening, 39 neonatologists and 4 neonatal nurses from 18 Ibero-American countries were invited to participate and to collaborate. They worked for several months with an intense and collaborative methodology, and met in person at San José de Costa Rica, in September 2015, during the Annual SIBEN Conference. Professor Andrew Ewer from the UK was the leader and expert opinion for this ninth SIBEN's Consensus. Neonatal hypoxemia, such as it occurs in critical congenital heart disease (CCHD) and other conditions, is an abnormal situation, potentially fatal if not diagnosed or if diagnosed late, PO screening allows earlier detection and thus the opportunity to optimize their management and improve outcomes.

Several questions of clinical significance were developed on the early detection with SpO_2 of diseases that present with neonatal hypoxemia. They included:

1. Cyanosis and related concepts.
2. What is hypoxemia?
3. What is hypoxia?
4. What is pulse oximetry, and what are the normal values in a healthy term newborn?
5. What is the hemoglobin dissociation curve?
6. How does altitude influence on the SpO_2?
7. Which are the lesions that can be detected early?
8. How should you do the screening?
9. What are normal and abnormal results?
10. What are false positive and false negative results?
11. How should you interpret the pre- and post-ductal SpO_2 difference?
12. What should we do with an apparently healthy newborn that fails the screening?
13. How should we take care of the family of a newborn that has either a positive or negative screening?
14. Is this program cost-effective?
15. When should we order an echocardiogram?
16. Importance of the information and participation of the healthcare team—what data should you record?
17. Who should do the screening?
18. What limitations does pulse oximetry have?
19. What role can the Perfusion Index (PI) have during the screening?

The subgroups were tasked with answering 2–4 of the above questions. They methodically searched and reviewed the available literature, then interacted and worked together as a whole group to find consensus for the answers to all the questions. This SIBEN Clinical Consensus Group concluded that pulse oximetry is a non-invasive method that allows the rapid measurement of saturation of hemoglobin in arterial blood that can detect hypoxemia in asymptomatic and apparently healthy newborns who suffer from severe health conditions such as critical congenital heart disease. In addition to CCHD, the following conditions can be diagnosed early with SpO_2 screening:

- Early sepsis
- Congenital pneumonia
- Pulmonary hypertension
- Meconium aspiration
- Transient tachypnea
- Pneumothorax
- Other various less frequent neonatal conditions

The early use of pulse oximetry in apparently healthy babies is simple, very easy to perform, fast, non-invasive, cost effective [20,21], and provides a significant improvement in quality and safety in neonatal healthcare. Thus, SIBEN recommended that programs of early detection or screening with SpO_2 are implemented in all places where neonatal care is delivered in Latin America. In summary, the early evaluation of all the newborns with SpO_2 is a complementary, non-invasive, easy-to-perform, and low cost test that is performed between 12–48 h of life and is of great clinical utility to detect potentially serious diseases in asymptomatic and apparently healthy newborn infants. The universal implementation of this evaluation in clinical practice leads to a narrowing of the diagnostic gap for newborns to increase patient safety and to reduce the morbidity, sequelae, and mortality of these babies.

4. SIBEN's Consensus on Screening with Pulse Oximetry: A Summary

We summarize answers to some of the specific questions and recommendations below.

4.1. Evaluation with SpO₂ Monitors and Sampling Sites

Neonatal screening for the detection of pathologies associated with hypoxemia has been introduced in clinical practice in the USA since 2011. Since then, studies and meta-analysis [18] show that it meets the criteria for population screening test, as well as being a tool in the early and timely diagnosis of severe neonatal conditions. Nevertheless, it is still not universally used in Latin America and work was needed to identify protocols. The SpO₂ screening technique is very easy to perform, and should be performed in all apparently healthy newborns between 12–48 h after birth (see below) or before discharge. It should be done by placing a sensor in the palm of the right hand (pre-ductal) and then another in one of the lower limbs (post-ductal). SpO₂ readings are taken and recorded from the two sites, one after the other (it is not necessary to use two monitors simultaneously). Screening has to be done with both pre- and post-ductal measurements because some heart defects with obstruction of the left output tract may not be diagnosed when performing a single post-ductal measurement.

The published evidence is clear in relation to the quality of the signal. The SIBEN consensus concludes that evaluating the quality of the signal is fundamental to being able to interpret that the SpO₂ readings are correct. Therefore, the screening must be performed with a SpO₂ monitor that functions in low perfusion states and is not subject to motion artefact.

4.2. Clinical Protocol

Based on the SIBEN clinical consensus, it is recommended that this SpO₂ screening method (pre and post ductal) be performed in all healthy newborns between 12 and 24 h of life, or before discharge home if the discharge is prior to that age. If the first pre- and post-ductal SpO₂ measurements are both 95–100% with <3% difference between them, the evaluation is normal and the newborn has a negative screening test. If the first measurement is positive/abnormal (SpO₂ 90–95% and/or difference >2%) and the infant looks healthy, the pre- and post-ductal measurements must be repeated once more, according to the protocol chosen by SIBEN, described in Figure 1 below. In infants with clinical symptoms or when SpO₂ is <90%, prompt admission to NICU and further evaluation should be initiated without delay.

SCREEN ALL HEALTHY NEWBORN INFANTS WITH PRE AND POST-DUCTAL MEASUREMENTS AT 12–24 H OF AGE (or before discharge, whichever comes first)

RESULTS:

o   Normal (negative) screen: One time SpO₂ ≥ 95% hand AND foot AND <3% difference
o   Abnormal (positive) screen: One time SpO₂ < 90% hand OR foot: evaluate/admit quickly
o   Abnormal (positive) screen: Any time an infant is symptomatic

When to repeat evaluation in 15–30, 60 min:

✓   SpO₂ 90–94% hand OR foot if newborn is asymptomatic and appears healthy
✓   Difference in SpO₂ between post and pre-ductal values is >2% (either one higher than the other one) if newborn is asymptomatic and appears healthy
✓   If on repeat SpO₂ ≥ 95% hand AND foot AND <3% difference: normal (negative) screen
✓   If on repeat SpO₂ 90–94% hand OR foot or >2% difference: abnormal (positive) screen

---

Figure 1. Screening protocol-algorithm recommended by SIBEN.

A second measurement is only done if the first one is positive (abnormal) and if the infant continues to appear completely healthy. If the infant has any clinical signs, they should be admitted, as would any sick neonate for any other reason. The second evaluation should be done 15–30 min after the first in order to reduce delay. Furthermore, if the infant was sound asleep during the first evaluation, they should be alert for the second. If the second measurement is normal, the test is considered normal, that is to say that the screening is negative. If first and second evaluations are positive, and/or if the infant has any clinical signs, immediate admission to NICU is recommended. If the infant appears healthy, they should be carefully assessed as described below.

4.3. What to Do with a Neonate Who Appears Clinically Healthy but Has Abnormal or Positive SpO_2?

Do not ignore the test and humbly accept that we may be wrong in our clinical assessment. It is necessary to evaluate quickly, in a detailed and complete approach, every newborn who has an abnormal test result with SpO_2. The absence of a murmur, normal blood pressure, or the presence of normal femoral pulses do not rule out a critical congenital heart disease. In addition, in infectious conditions or other hypoxemic conditions there will be no heart murmur and the other parameters may well be normal initially. If the diagnosis is not clear, other studies should be carried out for timely diagnosis, including frequent or continuous assessment of pre- and post-ductal SpO_2. According to the clinical suspicion, a complete diagnostic approach and may include complete blood count, cultures, blood gases, and chest X-rays. Some will require an echocardiogram, and in some it will be necessary to immediately start an infusion of prostaglandin to maintain patency of the ductus arteriosus.

4.4. Concept of False Positive and False Negative Screening

As mentioned, an infant with a positive screening test has one $SpO_2 < 90\%$ or two consecutive tests with SpO_2 90–95% and/or pre-post ductal difference >2%. A false positive result is when the infant is found NOT to have CCHD. This occurrence is extremely rare (<0.1%) if the screening method and protocol are followed rigorously—although it may be up to 1% [22]. If the evaluation with SpO_2 is done before 12 h of age there are slightly more false positives but diagnosis of infectious and respiratory causes of hypoxemia are more common. A false negative is when the evaluation with SpO_2 is normal (negative screening) but the infant is actually found hours or days later to actually have CCHD. As it can be easily understood, a false negative would be a significant issue. Most studies indicate that the most frequently undiagnosed lesions are left sided obstructed lesions with obstruction to the outflow of the aorta (e.g., coarctation of the aortic arch, hypoplastic left heart, aortic stenosis) which are not necessarily associated with hypoxemia. False negatives can also occur when not using appropriate technology. The use of the preductal and postductal saturation difference and the perfusion index improve detection, but they are not infallible either.

4.5. Altitude and Neonatal SpO_2 Screening

This is a topic that was addressed extensively, including physiology and alveolar gas equation. SIBEN's consensus found that, on average, SpO_2 values are not different in the first 12–24 h of life in infants born at less than 2500 m (about 8200 feet) above sea level. Therefore, if screening is done as mentioned and at the age recommended here, the values for positive and negative results could be kept the same. The issue is that the mean normal SpO_2 is a bit lower at higher altitude (93–96%) but with larger standard deviations. Therefore, some totally normal babies can have SpO_2 of 91–94% at >2700 m above sea level. So, more detailed observation would be recommended for asymptomatic infants, exercising caution and avoidance of aggressive investigations in order to prevent increasing the number of false positives. Still, exact cut-off points in moderate and high altitudes are not precisely known to adequately balance sensitivity with false positive rates.

4.6. Care of the Family with an Abnormal or Positive Screening

In the first hours after birth, various events generate great emotional tension. Health care providers should make an effort to decrease this by all possible means. Families should always actively participate in the care of their newborn infant and they should also be involved during SpO_2 screening. As this can be stressful for some parents, every effort should be made so that they clearly understand what is being done to their babies and why. Studies have shown that parents who have been well informed are mostly satisfied with the SpO_2 screening test and have perceived the screening as valuable test to detect sick babies. In addition, parents of neonates who had a false positive result did not show greater anxiety than those with negative or normal screenings [23].

It is recommended that parents of apparently normal newborns receive written information on the SpO_2 screening test. This written information must be accompanied by clear verbal information and clarification of any doubts that may have arisen with the information received. It is also recommended that the screening is performed with the parents present. In the face of a positive result, appropriate information and support is essential throughout.

5. Summary and Discussion

We have reviewed the evidence in a formal process of clinical consensus and presented the available data that demonstrates that early evaluation with pulse oximetry in apparently healthy newborns does easily detect asymptomatic newborns with severe health conditions, such as critical congenital heart disease, respiratory disorders, neonatal sepsis, persistent pulmonary hypertension, and other hypoxemic pathologies. The objective of implementing systematic protocols in clinical practice for the screening of all newborns by early pulse oximetry is to detect pathologies with early hypoxemia and to perform a therapeutic approach without delays. The consensus group of SIBEN, concludes that adequate early monitoring of SpO_2 in apparently healthy newborns is useful for early detection of several neonatal conditions which evidence has shown that the diagnosis is sometimes untimely or late. It was estimated that about 2000 neonates died or were diagnosed late each year in the US, and that around 300,000 babies per year die worldwide because of this. The number of undiagnosed cases in developing countries is higher than in developed nations and it is estimated that less than half of the cases of CCHD are diagnosed in the first week of life. The prenatal diagnosis of CCHD can improve perinatal outcomes for certain lesions [54,55]. Recent evidence shows that CCHD detection has progressively increased from 2006 to 2012, but also that prenatal detection is highly variable in different countries [56]. In some cases, the diagnosis of fetal CCHD is made to later see that the newborn is healthy. Repeated prenatal ultrasounds are much more difficult and costly than simple SpO_2 screening. Early diagnosis of CCHD in postnatal life significantly decreases morbidity and mortality rates [24].

The effectiveness of screening is also shown in recent publications on home births in The Netherlands [58], as well as other very comprehensive reviews [59–61]. Adding detailed physical examination to early evaluation with SpO_2 increases significantly early diagnosis of hypoxemic neonatal conditions. SIBEN underscores that neonatal screening with SpO_2 for the specific diagnosis of early CCHD does not, of course, replace prenatal detection or clinical examination but is a very useful complement. Accurate prenatal ultrasound, physical examination, and SpO_2 screening may increase CCHD detection rates to more than 90–95%. One of SIBEN's recommendations is that, at the beginning of this screening program each center must use a clearly defined protocol (as described previously) and at least one quality indicator e.g., performing a random evaluation every 1–2 weeks of the number of babies with screening indication (infants that should have been evaluated) and verified that the program has been met 100% of the time. If this is not the case, processes need to be improved in order to meet the objective of the evaluation and detection of all newborn infants. The quality indicators are not only for CCHD but also for early detection of respiratory or infectious conditions. Physicians should be aware that, even though the combination of early detection with pulse oximetry with other methods of evaluation reduces errors and diagnostic errors, some babies can still be discharged without proper diagnosis.

Early detection of CCHD and hypoxemic neonatal conditions not only reduces the suffering of children and families, but it can also reduce associated costs and long-term neurological compromise by not delaying admission to a specialized care unit. This is also associated with significant reductions in mortality, better surgical outcomes, less prolonged ventilation, and diminished potential developmental problems. For all of the above, actively addressing the neonatal screening of CCHD and neonatal hypoxemic conditions can achieve a significant improvement in the quality and safety of health care, as well as cost savings. In addition, and of significant importance, the screening with pulse oximetry in the newborn has been shown to detect hypoxemia in newborns with severe conditions other than CCHD—such as respiratory problems, sepsis, and persistent pulmonary hypertension.

We conclude, together with many other authors, that significant deaths and morbidity can be avoided or significantly reduced if hospitals adopt SpO_2 screening for early and timely detection of CCHD and other hypoxemic conditions [46,57–62]. Its implementation will benefit many newborns in Latin America, where it is estimated that 60% of neonatal deaths are preventable [63,64].

Author Contributions: Both authors contributed equally in the research and writing of the manuscript

References

1.   Bernier, P.L.; Stefanescu, A.; Samoukovic, G.; Tchervenkov, C.I. The challenge of congenital heart disease worldwide: Epidemiologic and demographic facts. *Semin. Thorac. Cardiovasc. Surg. Pediatr. Card. Surg. Annu.* **2010**, *13*, 26–34. [CrossRef] [PubMed]
2.   Reller, M.D.; Strickland, M.J.; Riehle-Colarusso, T.; Mahle, W.T.; Correa, A. Prevalence of congenital heart defects in metropolitan Atlanta, 1998–2005. *J. Pediatr.* **2008**, *153*, 807–813. [CrossRef] [PubMed]
3.   Hoffman, J.I.E.; Kaplan, S. The incidence of congenital heart disease. *J. Am. Coll. Cardiol.* **2002**, *39*, 1890–1900. [CrossRef]
4.   Van der Linde, D.; Konings, E.E.M.; Slager, M.A.; Witsenburg, M.; Helbin, W.A.; Takkenberg, J.J.M.; Roos-Hesselink, J.W. Birth Prevalence of Congenital Heart Disease Worldwide: A Systematic Review and Meta-analysis. *J. Am. Coll. Cardiol.* **2011**, *58*, 2241–2247. [CrossRef] [PubMed]
5.   Oster, M.; Lee, K.; Honein, M.; Riehle-Colarusso, T.; Shin, M.; Correa, A. Temporal trends in survival among infants with critical congenital heart defects. *Pediatrics* **2013**, *131*, e1502–e1508. [CrossRef] [PubMed]
6.   Chang, R.K.; Gurvitz, M.; Rodriguez, S. Missed diagnosis of critical congenital heart disease. *Arch. Pediatr. Adolesc. Med.* **2008**, *162*, 969–974. [CrossRef] [PubMed]
7.   GBD 2013 Mortality and Causes of Death Collaborators. Global, regional, and national age-sex specific all-cause and cause-specific mortality for 240 causes of death, 1990–2013: A systematic analysis for the Global Burden of Disease Study 2013. *Lancet* **2015**, *385*, 117–171.
8.   Hoffman, J.I.E. The global burden of congenital heart disease. *Cardiovasc. J. Afr.* **2013**, *24*, 141–145. [CrossRef] [PubMed]
9.   Kuehl, K.S.; Loffredo, C.A.; Ferencz, C. Failure to diagnose congenital heart disease in infancy. *Pediatrics* **1999**, *103*, 743–747. [CrossRef] [PubMed]
10. Meberg, A.; Lindberg, H.; Thaulow, E. Congenital heart defects: The patients who die. *Acta Paediatr.* **2005**, *94*, 1060–1065. [CrossRef] [PubMed]
11. Ailes, E.C.; Honein, M.A. Estimated Number of Infants Detected and Missed by Critical Congenital Heart Defect Screening. *Pediatrics* **2015**, *135*, 1000–1008. [CrossRef] [PubMed]
12. De-Wahl Granelli, A.; Wennergren, M.; Sandberg, K.; Mellander, M.; Bejlum, C.; Inganäs, L.; Eriksson, M.; Segerdahl, N.; Agren, A.; Ekman-Joelsson, B.M.; et al. Impact of pulse oximetry screening on the detection of duct dependent congenital heart disease: A Swedish prospective screening study in 39,821 newborns. *BMJ* **2009**, *338*, a3037. [CrossRef] [PubMed]

13. Ewer, A.K.; Middleton, L.J.; Furmston, A.T.; Bhoyar, A.; Daniels, J.P.; Thangaratinam, S.; Deeks, J.J.; Khan, K.S.; PulseOx Study Group. Pulse oximetry as a screening test for congenital heart defects in newborn infants (PulseOx): A test accuracy study. *Lancet* **2011**, *378*, 785–794. [CrossRef]

14. Hu, X.J.; Ma, X.J.; Zhao, Q.M.; Yan, W.L.; Ge, X.L.; Jia, B.; Liu, F.; Wu, L.; Ye, M.; Liang, X.C.; et al. Pulse Oximetry and Auscultation for Congenital Heart Disease Detection. *Pediatrics* **2017**, *140*, e20171154. [CrossRef] [PubMed]

15. Kemper, A.R.; Mahle, W.T.; Martin, G.R.; Cooley, W.C.; Kumar, P.; Morrow, W.R.; Kelm, K.; Pearson, G.D.; Glidewell, J.; Grosse, S.D.; et al. Strategies for Implementing Screening for Critical Congenital Heart Disease. *Pediatrics* **2011**, *128*, 1259–1267. [CrossRef] [PubMed]

16. Frank, L.H.; Bradshaw, E.; Beekman, R.; Mahle, W.T.; Martin, G.R. Critical Congenital Heart Disease Screening Using Pulse Oximetry. *J. Pediatr.* **2012**, *162*, 445–453. [CrossRef] [PubMed]

17. Glidewell, J.; Olney, R.S.; Hinton, C.; Pawelski, J.; Sontag, M.; Wood, T.; Kucik, J.E.; Daskalov, R.; Hudson, J. Centers for Disease Control and Prevention (CDC). State Legislation, Regulations, and Hospital Guidelines for Newborn Screening for Critical Congenital Heart Defects—United States, 2011–2014. *Morb. Mortal. Wkly. Rep.* **2015**, *64*, 625–630.

18. Thangaratinam, S.; Brown, K.; Zamora, J.; Khan, K.S.; Ewer, A.K. Pulse oximetry screening for critical congenital heart defects in asymptomatic newborn babies: A systematic review and meta-analysis. *Lancet* **2012**, *379*, 2459–2464. [CrossRef]

19. Sola, A.; Fariña, D.; Mir, R.; Garrido, D.; Pereira, A.; Montes Bueno, M.T.; Lemus, L. y Colaboradores del Consenso Clínico SIBEN. In *Detección Precoz con Pulsioximetría de Enfermedades que Cursan con Hipoxemia Neonatal*; EDISIBEN: Asunción, Paraguay, 2016; ISBN 978-1-5323-0369-2.

20. Roberts, T.E.; Barton, P.M.; Auguste, P.E.; Middleton, L.J.; Furmston, A.T.; Ewer, A.K. Pulse oximetry as a screening test for congenital heart defects in newborn infants: A cost-effectiveness analysis. *Arch. Dis. Child.* **2012**, *97*, 221–226. [CrossRef] [PubMed]

21. Peterson, C.; Grosse, S.D.; Oster, M.E.; Olney, R.S.; Cassell, C.H. Cost-effectiveness of routine screening for critical congenital heart disease in US newborns. *Pediatrics* **2013**, *132*, e595–e603. [CrossRef] [PubMed]

22. Oster, M.E.; Aucott, S.W.; Glidewell, J.; Hackell, J.; Kochilas, L.; Martin, G.R.; Phillippi, J.; Pinto, N.M.; Saarinen, A.; Sontag, M.; et al. Lessons Learned From Newborn Screening for Critical Congenital Heart Defects. *Pediatrics* **2016**, *137*, e20154573. [CrossRef] [PubMed]

23. Powell, R.; Pattison, H.M.; Bhoyar, A.; Furmston, A.T.; Middleton, L.J.; Daniels, J.P.; Ewer, A.K. Pulse oximetry screening for congenital heart defects in newborn infants: An evaluation of acceptability to mothers. *Arch. Dis. Child. Fetal Neonatal Ed.* **2013**, *98*, F59–63. [CrossRef] [PubMed]

24. Abouk, R.; Grosse, S.D.; Ailes, E.C.; Oster, M.E. Association of US State Implementation of Newborn Screening Policies for Critical Congenital Heart Disease With Early Infant Cardiac Deaths. *JAMA* **2017**, *318*, 2111–2118. [CrossRef] [PubMed]

25. Sola, A.; Urman, J. *Cuidados Intensivos Neonatales: Fisiopatología y Terapéutica*; Científica Interamericana: Buenos Aires, Argentina, 1987; ISBN 9509428078, 9789509428072.

26. Sola, A.; Rogido, M. *Cuidados Neonatales*; Científica Interamericana: Buenos Aires, Argentina, 2000; Volume 2, ISBN 89872427570-4.

27. Zhang, L.; Mendoza-Sassi, R.; Santos, J.C.; Lau, J. Accuracy of symptoms and signs in predicting hypoxaemia among young children with acute respiratory infection: A meta-analysis. *Int. J. Tuberc. Lung Dis.* **2011**, *15*, 317–325. [PubMed]

28. Niermeyer, S.; Yang, P.; Shanmina; Drolkar; Zhuang, J.; Moore, L.G. Arterial oxygen saturation in Tibetan and Han infants born in Lhasa, Tibet. *N. Engl. J. Med.* **1995**, *333*, 1248–1252. [CrossRef] [PubMed]

29. Laman, M.; Ripa, P.; Vince, J.; Tefuarani, N. Can clinical signs predict hypoxaemia in Papua New Guinean children with moderate and severe pneumonia? *Ann. Trop. Paediatr.* **2005**, *25*, 23–27. [CrossRef] [PubMed]

30. Dawson, A.L.; Cassell, C.H.; Riehle-Colarusso, T.; Grosse, S.D.; Tanner, J.P.; Kirby, R.S.; Watkins, S.M.; Correia, J.A.; Olney, R.S. Factors associated with late detection of critical congenital heart disease in newborns. *Pediatrics* **2013**, *132*, e604–e611. [CrossRef] [PubMed]

31. Dawson, J.; Ekström, A.; Frisk, C.; Thio, M.; Roehr, C.C.; Kamlin, C.O.; Donath, S.M.; Davis, P.G.; Giraffe Study Group. Assessing the tongue colour of newly born infants may help predict the need for supplemental oxygen in the delivery room. *Acta Paediatr.* **2015**, *104*, 356–359. [CrossRef] [PubMed]

32. Sola, A.; Chow, L.; Rogido, M. Pulse oximetry in neonatal care in 2005. A comprehensive state of the art review. *An. Pediatr. (Barc)* **2005**, *62*, 266–281. [CrossRef] [PubMed]

33. Barker, S.J. The effects of motion and hypoxemia upon the accuracy of 20 pulse oximeters in human volunteers. *Sleep* **2001**, *24*, A406–A407.

34. Hay, W.; Rodden, D.; Collins, S.; Melaria, D.; Hale, K.; Faushaw, L. Reliability of conventional and new pulse oximetry in neonatal patients. *J. Perinatol.* **2002**, *22*, 360–366. [CrossRef] [PubMed]

35. Sola, A. Monitorización biofísica y saturometría. In *Cuidados Neonatales*, 3rd ed.; Edimed: Buenos Aires, Argentina, 2011; ISBN 8963252767-5.

36. Sola, A.; Golombek, S.; Montes Bueno, M.T.; Lemus, L.; Zuluaga, C.; Domínguez, F.; Baquero, H.; Young Sarmiento, A.E.; Natta, D.; Rodriguez Perez, J.M.; et al. Safe oxygen saturation targeting and monitoring in preterm infants: Can we avoid hypoxia and hyperoxia? *Acta Paediatr.* **2014**, *103*, 1009–1018. [CrossRef] [PubMed]

37. Dawson, J.A.; Vento, M.; Finer, N.N.; Rich, W.; Saugstad, O.D.; Morley, C.J.; Davis, P.G. Managing oxygen therapy during delivery room stabilization of preterm infants. *J. Pediatr.* **2012**, *160*, 158–161. [CrossRef] [PubMed]

38. Davis, P.G.; Dawson, J.A. New concepts in neonatal resuscitation. *Curr. Opin. Pediatr.* **2012**, *24*, 147–153. [CrossRef] [PubMed]

39. Niermeyer, S.; Andrade-M, M.P.; Vargas, E.; Moore, L.G. Neonatal oxygenation, pulmonary hypertension, and evolutionary adaptation to high altitude (2013 Grover Conference series). *Pulm. Circ.* **2015**, *5*, 48–62. [CrossRef] [PubMed]

40. Hill, C.M.; Baya, A.; Gavlak, J.; Carroll, A.; Heathcote, K.; Dimitriou, D.; L'Esperance, V.; Webster, R.; Holloway, J.; Virues-Ortega, J.; et al. Adaptation to Life in the High Andes: Nocturnal Oxyhemoglobin Saturation in Early Development. *Sleep* **2016**, *39*, 1001–1008. [CrossRef] [PubMed]

41. Diaz, G.; Sandoval, J.; Sola, A. *Hipertensión Pulmonar en Niños*; Distribuna: Bogotá, Colombia, 2011; ISBN 9789588379357.

42. Sendelbach, D.M.; Jackson, G.L.; Lai, S.S.; Fixler, D.E.; Stehel, E.K.; Engle, W.D. Pulse oximetry screening at 4 h of age to detect critical congenital heart defects. *Pediatrics* **2008**, *122*, e815–e820. [CrossRef] [PubMed]

43. Ewer, A.K. Evidence for CCHD screening and its practical application using pulse oximetry. *Early Hum. Dev.* **2014**, *90*, S19–S21. [CrossRef]

44. Ewer, A.K. Pulse oximetry screening: Do we have enough evidence now? *Lancet* **2014**, *30*, 725–726. [CrossRef]

45. Ewer, A.K. Pulse oximetry screening for critical congenital heart defects. Should it be routine? *Arch. Dis. Child. Fetal Neonatal Ed.* **2014**, *99*, F93–F95. [CrossRef] [PubMed]

46. Ewer, A.K. Review of pulse oximetry screening for critical congenital heart defects. *Curr. Opin. Cardiol.* **2013**, *28*, 92–96. [CrossRef] [PubMed]

47. Zhao, Q.; Ma, Z.; Ge, Z.; Liu, F.; Yan, W.L.; Wu, L.; Ye, M.; Liang, X.C.; Zhang, J.; Gao, Y.; et al. Pulse oximetry with clinical assessment to screen for congenital heart disease in neonates in China: A prospective study. *Lancet* **2014**, *384*, 747–754. [CrossRef]

48. Singh, A.; Rasiah, S.V.; Ewer, A.K. The impact of routine predischarge pulse oximetry screening in a regional neonatal unit. *Arch. Dis. Child. Fetal Neonatal Ed.* **2014**, *99*, F297–302. [CrossRef] [PubMed]

49. Piasek, C.Z.; Van Bel, F.; Sola, A. Perfusion index in newborn infants: A noninvasive tool for neonatal monitoring. *Acta Paediatr.* **2014**, *103*, 468–473. [CrossRef] [PubMed]

50. Granelli, A.; Ostman-Smith, I. Noninvasive peripheral perfusion index as a possible tool for screening for critical left heart obstruction. *Acta Paediatr.* **2007**, *96*, 1455–1459. [CrossRef] [PubMed]

51. Ewer, A.K.; Furmston, A.T.; Middleton, L.J.; Deeks, J.J.; Daniels, J.P.; Pattison, H.M.; Powell, R.; Roberts, T.E.; Barton, P.; Auguste, P.; et al. Pulse oximetry as a screening test for congenital heart defects in newborn infants: A test accuracy study with evaluation of acceptability and cost-effectiveness. *Health Technol. Assess.* **2012**, *16*, 1–184. [CrossRef] [PubMed]

52. Ewer, A.K. How to develop a business case to establish a neonatal pulse oximetry screening programme for screening of congenital heart defects. *Early Hum. Dev.* **2012**, *88*, 915–919. [CrossRef] [PubMed]

53. De Wahl Granelli, A.; Mellander, M.; Sunnegårdh, J.; Sandberg, K.; Ostman-Smith, I. Screening for duct-dependant congenital heart disease with pulse oximetry: A critical evaluation of strategies to maximize sensitivity. *Acta Paediatr.* **2005**, *94*, 1590–1596. [CrossRef] [PubMed]

54. Tworetzky, W.; McElhinney, D.B.; Reddy, V.M.; Brook, M.M.; Hanley, F.L.; Silverman, N.H. Improved surgical outcome after fetal diagnosis of hypoplastic left heart syndrome. *Circulation* **2001**, *103*, 1269–1273. [CrossRef] [PubMed]

55. Bonnet, D.; Coltri, A.; Butera, G.; Fermont, L.; Le Bidois, J.; Kachaner, J.; Sidi, D. Detection of transposition of the great arteries in fetuses reduces neonatal morbidity and mortality. *Circulation* **1999**, *99*, 916–918. [CrossRef] [PubMed]

56. Quartermain, M.D.; Pasquali, S.K.; Hill, K.D.; Goldberg, D.J.; Huhta, J.C.; Jacobs, J.P.; Jacobs, M.L.; Kim, S.; Ungerleider, R.M. Variation in Prenatal Diagnosis of Congenital Heart Disease in Infants. *Pediatrics* **2015**, *136*, e378–385. [CrossRef] [PubMed]

57. Narayen, I.C.; Blom, N.A.; Bourgonje, M.S.; Haak, M.C.; Smit, M.; Posthumus, F.; van den Broek, A.J.; Havers, H.M.; te Pas, A.B. Pulse Oximetry Screening for Critical Congenital Heart Disease after Home Birth and Early Discharge. *J. Pediatr.* **2016**, *170*, 188–192. [CrossRef] [PubMed]

58. De-Wahl Granelli, A.; Meberg, A.; Ojala, T.; Steensberg, J.; Oskarsson, G.; Mellander, M. Nordic pulse oximetry screening—Implementation status and proposal for uniform guidelines. *Acta Paediatr.* **2014**, *103*, 1136–1142. [CrossRef] [PubMed]

59. Narayen, I.C.; Blom, N.A.; Ewer, A.K.; Vento, M.; Manzoni, P.; Te Pas, A.B. Aspects of pulse oximetry screening for critical congenital heart defects: How, when and why? *Arch. Dis. Child. Fetal Neonatal Ed.* **2016**, *101*, F162–167. [CrossRef] [PubMed]

60. Lakshminrusimha, S.; Sambalingam, D.; Carrion, V. Universal pulse oximetry screen for critical congenital heart disease in the NICU. *J. Perinatol.* **2014**, *34*, 343–344. [CrossRef] [PubMed]

61. Teitel, D. Recognition of Undiagnosed Neonatal Heart Disease. *Clin. Perinatol.* **2016**, *43*, 81–98. [CrossRef] [PubMed]

62. Ravert, P.; Detwiler, T.L.; Dickinson, J.K. Mean oxygen saturation in well neonates at altitudes between 4498 and 8150 feet. *Adv. Neonatal Care* **2011**, *11*, 412–417. [CrossRef] [PubMed]

63. Sandoval, N. Cardiopatías congénitas en Colombia y en el mundo. *Rev. Colomb. Cardiol.* **2015**, *22*, 1–2. [CrossRef]

64. Reducing Neonatal Mortality and Morbidity in Latin America and The Caribbean. An Interagency Strategic Consensus. Available online: http://resourcecentre.savethechildren.se/sites/default/files/documents/2729 (accessed on 30 January 2018).

23

Lessons Learned from Pompe Disease Newborn Screening and Follow-up

Tracy L. Klug [1,*], Lori B. Swartz [1], Jon Washburn [2], Candice Brannen [2] and Jami L. Kiesling [1]

[1]   Missouri Department of Health and Senior Services, P.O. Box 570, Jefferson City, MO 65102-0570, USA

[2]   Baebies, Inc., P.O. Box 14403, Durham, NC 27709, USA

*   Correspondence: tracy.klug@health.mo.gov

Abstract: In 2015, Pompe disease became the first lysosomal storage disorder to be recommended for universal newborn screening by the Secretary of the U.S. Department of Health and Human Services. Newborn screening for Pompe has been implemented in 20 states and several countries across the world. The rates of later-onset disease phenotypes for Pompe and pseudodeficiency alleles are higher than initially anticipated, and these factors must be considered during Pompe disease newborn screening. This report presents an overview of six years of data from the Missouri State Public Health Laboratory for Pompe disease newborn screening and follow-up.

Keywords: Pompe disease; newborn screening; follow-up; pseudodeficiency

1. Introduction

Pompe disease, also called glycogen storage disease type II, is a rare genetic disorder in which variants in the glucosidase alpha acid gene (gene abbreviation: *GAA*) result in low levels of acid alpha-glucosidase enzyme (enzyme abbreviation: GAA) and consequent accumulation of glycogen in various tissues of the body [1,2]. The build-up of glycogen damages muscles throughout the body, most notably the heart and skeletal muscle, and leads to general muscle weakness, breathing problems, and feeding difficulties. The onset and severity of disease symptoms vary widely based on the precise *GAA* variant(s) inherited [3]. The most severe phenotype, the classical infantile form, is clinically apparent in the first two months of life, causes cardiomyopathy, and is typically fatal in the first year of life [4]. The nonclassical infantile form of Pompe disease typically presents in the first year of life, progresses more slowly than the classical infantile onset form, and typically leads to respiratory failure without cardiomyopathy and death in later childhood. Later-onset forms of Pompe disease, with onset ranging from infantile to early adulthood, are also possible and progress at a variable rate [3].

Targeted enzyme-replacement therapy (ERT) for Pompe disease can effectively slow disease progression by providing sufficient enzyme to degrade glycogen [5]. Because ERT has the greatest benefit if started prior to the onset of symptoms [6] and individuals with Pompe disease are typically asymptomatic at birth, newborn screening for Pompe disease has been recommended by the Secretary of the U.S. Department of Health and Human Services [7] to identify children at risk for Pompe disease as early as possible.

The Missouri State Public Health Laboratory (MSPHL) initiated universal newborn screening for Pompe disease in January 2013, following guidance set by House Bill 716, the Brady Alan Cunningham Act [8]. This bill was signed into law in 2009 and mandated the expansion of newborn screening to include Pompe disease and several other lysosomal storage disorders (LSDs). This manuscript summarizes how MSPHL has refined its Pompe newborn screening protocols over the first six years in practice and highlights important findings through the follow-up program.

2. Materials and Methods

On 16 October 2012, MSPHL received a waiver from the Missouri Department of Health and Senior Services' Institutional Review Board, as implementation of LSD screening did not meet the IRB definition of research. MSPHL utilizes digital microfluidic fluorometry (DMF) (SEEKER; Baebies, Inc., Durham, NC) for Pompe disease screening [9–11]. Decreased enzyme activity of acid α-glucosidase (GAA) indicates an increased risk for Pompe disease. MSPHL initially established cutoffs based on the enzyme activity of diagnostic samples from patients with Pompe disease, which were provided by the Missouri genetic referral centers. These samples included newborn and nonnewborn samples from patients with infantile Pompe as well as later-onset Pompe. As more data was collected from routine newborn screening for Pompe, cutoffs were refined to better reflect newborn enzyme activity levels. As depicted in Figure 1, samples with measured enzyme activity above the instrument cutoff are presumed to be normal and no further testing is performed. For any samples with measured activity below the instrument cutoff, testing is repeated in duplicate and the average of the three values is calculated and used to assess risk. If the average value is below the referral cutoff, the baby is referred to a genetic referral center for evaluation and diagnostic confirmatory testing. If the average value is below the borderline cutoff but above the referral cutoff, an additional newborn screening sample is requested to repeat the dried blood spot (DBS) screening test. If the average value is above the borderline cutoff, the sample is presumed normal.

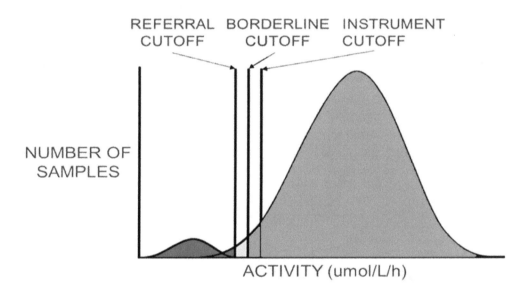

Figure 1. Representative depiction of the distribution of acid alpha-glucosidase (GAA) enzyme activity (low to high) in newborns. The small population to the left of the referral cutoff (depicted in red) indicates the high risk patient population that is referred for confirmatory testing. The large distribution to the right of the borderline cutoff (depicted in green) indicates the presumed normal population, who require no further action. As with many other newborn screening assays, there is an area of overlap between the affected and normal populations (indicated in yellow).

The cutoffs initially established by MSPHL did not account for age of the baby at sample collection, but after gathering population data over time, it was apparent that GAA enzyme activities decreased with the age of the newborn at the time of sample collection and that age-related cutoffs should be utilized. New cutoffs for samples from newborns >14 days of age at collection were implemented in mid-2013 and further refined as more data were collected and analyzed. MSPHL also discovered that lysosomal enzyme activities were affected by seasonal variability. Enzyme activities were reduced during the summer months, causing an increase in false positive referrals. After observing this trend, MSPHL implemented cutoff adjustments between winter and summer to reduce unnecessary referrals. Because four lysosomal enzymes are measured simultaneously with the DMF method, MSPHL leverages all four lysosomal enzyme results to ascertain sample quality. If multiple lysosomal enzyme activities are below their respective cutoffs, the sample is considered to have compromised quality and an additional newborn screening sample is requested. Whereas many other screening programs base GAA cutoffs on the percent of the daily mean or median, MSPHL has found that with the relatively small number of births per day in Missouri, fixed cutoffs that can be modified seasonally are more effective.

Because the need for second-tier testing for some LSDs was unrecognized when MSPHL began screening and there were no established second-tier testing options available at the time, MSPHL did not employ second-tier testing for Pompe disease. All presumptive positive screens were referred to a genetic referral center for diagnostic testing. In Missouri, there are four such centers to accept these patient referrals, and referrals are made based on predetermined geographic boundaries. The diagnostic testing performed for a presumptive positive patient is dependent on the referred condition; for Pompe disease, this testing may include leukocyte GAA enzyme activity, creatine kinase (CK) enzyme activity, urinary glucotetrasaccharide (HEX4), targeted gene sequencing, and cardiac evaluation. Additional testing may include quantification of lactic acid dehydrogenase (LDH), CK-MB (an isoenzyme of creatine kinase that is found mostly in the heart), liver enzymes (AST and ALT), and/or brain natriuretic peptide (BNP). While confirmatory testing for Pompe disease follows a general protocol, the procedure for each patient is highly dependent on the specific clinical presentation.

The predicted onset—infantile or late—is made during the time of confirmatory testing based on biochemical test results, imaging, clinical presentation including presence of cardiomyopathy, and variant analysis. Table 1 outlines the criteria used by the Missouri follow-up program to determine disease status. These are the general guidelines; the final classification is made by the follow-up team based on evaluation of all of the clinical information. Following a confirmation of infantile onset Pompe disease, treatment with enzyme replacement therapy is typically initiated as quickly as possible; in patients with a diagnosis of later-onset Pompe, treatment with ERT is typically delayed until the onset of symptoms or laboratory results consistent with progression of disease are observed.

Table 1. Missouri Newborn Screening Follow-Up Criteria for Pompe Disease.

Newborn Assessment	Classical Infantile	NonClassical Infantile	Later Onset	Genotype of Unknown Significance	Pseudodeficiency	Carrier
GAA enzyme activity	Absent or within affected range	Within affected range	Decreased	Decreased	Decreased	Decreased or normal
HEX4	Elevated	Elevated or WNL	WNL	WNL	WNL	WNL
Creatine Kinase (& other labs as indicated)	Elevated	Elevated or WNL	WNL	WNL	WNL	WNL
Chest x-ray, EKG, Echo	Abnormal	Mild abnormalities or WNL	WNL	WNL	WNL	WNL
Variant analysis	-Two pathogenic variants -One pathogenic variant and one or more VUS -Two VUS	-Two pathogenic variants -One pathogenic variant and one or more VUS -Two VUS	-Two pathogenic variants -One pathogenic variant and one or more VUS -Two VUS	-One infantile variant and one or more VUS -One late onset variant and one or more VUS -Two or more VUS	-Two pseudodeficiency alleles	-One pathogenic variant -May or may not be in combination with pseudo alleles
Clinical presentation	Muscle weakness, poor muscle tone, feeding issues, cardio-myopathy present	Muscle weakness or WNL	WNL at birth	WNL at birth	WNL at birth	WNL at birth

Abbreviations: WNL = within normal limits; VUS = variant(s) of unknown significance.

3. Results

3.1. Screening Results

In the first six years of LSD screening (January 2013 through December 2018), MSPHL tested approximately 467,000 newborns, of which 274 screened positive based on decreased GAA activity. Results of confirmatory testing for these specimens are presented in Table 2.

Table 2. Results of Confirmatory Pompe Testing.

Total Screened	~467,000
Screen Positives	274
Confirmed Disorders	46
Infantile Onset Pompe Disease	10
Later-onset Pompe Disease	36
Genotypes of Unknown Significance	8
Pseudodeficiencies	53
Carriers	65
Normal	97
Lost to Follow-up	5
Positive Predictive Value (PPV)	17.1%
False Positive Rate (FPR)	0.05%

Ten newborns were found to have infantile Pompe disease, and 36 were found to have later-onset Pompe disease. Eight newborns were found to have genotypes of unknown significance (GUS), and 51 newborns that screened positive were found to have pseudodeficiency variants. The false positive rate (FPR—0.05%) and the positive predictive value (PPV—17.1%) for the Pompe assay is comparable to published prospective screening results for GAA without the use of second-tier screening [12] and for other newborn screening tests in general [13].

Each genetic referral center was contacted to request follow-up information for newborns diagnosed with Pompe disease or a genotype of unknown significance. For each case, the referral center was asked to provide variant information and biochemical or other diagnostic test results. Additionally, referral centers were surveyed with specific questions about the current developmental status of each patient remaining in active follow-up. This survey collected binary responses (e.g., improved/unchanged/worsening) for symptoms in the following categories: cardiac, myopathy/hypotonia, respiratory, feeding, hearing, overall development, and laboratory test results (normal/abnormal).

Data from confirmatory testing for newborns confirmed with Pompe disease (infantile and later-onset) as well as newborns with genotypes of unknown significance was compiled (Table 3).

Table 3. Confirmatory Test Results for Patients with Pompe Disease or Genotypes of Unknown Significance (GUS).

Disease Classification	HEX4 (nmol/mol Creatinine)			Creatine Kinase (U/L)		
	n (Data Reported)	Median	Range	*n* (Data Reported)	Median	Range
Classical Infantile	7 (7)	22.7	13.4–38.6	7 (7)	662	466–3537
Nonclassical Infantile	3 (3)	5	3.7–25.2	3 (2)	416	398–435
Later-onset	36 (26)	4.65	2.3–12.3	36 (25)	127	50–466
GUS	8 (5)	6.6	2.3–7	8 (7)	87	71–203
Normal Range	<20 nmol/mol creatinine			<305 U/L		

3.2. Confirmed Positive Pompe Patients

3.2.1. Infantile Onset

Ten newborns were found to have infantile onset Pompe disease, with seven considered "classical" and three considered "nonclassical". Classical infantile Pompe is differentiated from nonclassical infantile Pompe by the presence of hypertrophic cardiomyopathy at birth. Of the classical infantile onset patients, all seven received testing for urine HEX4 and CK. Six (86%) had elevated HEX4 and seven (100%) had elevated CK activity. Six cases received a cardiac workup including EKG and echocardiogram; all six cases (100%) showed evidence of cardiomyopathy. The seventh case that did not receive a cardiac workup was diagnosed via amniocentesis, and had extremely elevated HEX4 and CK levels. All seven newborns began treatment with enzyme replacement therapy (ERT) at ages ranging from four days to one month. One of these patients was CRIM-negative and thus underwent immunosuppressive therapy prior to receiving ERT.

Three newborns were diagnosed with nonclassical infantile onset Pompe disease. Two of the three newborns were from the same family (separate births); both newborns were compound heterozygotes for the severe c.525DelT variant and the common later-onset c.-32-13T>G variant. These two newborns had normal HEX4 levels but mildly elevated CK. While the first newborn's HEX4 and cardiac workup were normal, the patient's liver enzymes (AST and ALT) were abnormal, CK-MB and LDH were elevated, and the newborn was failing to thrive. This newborn was initiated on enzyme replacement therapy at 29 days of age. The second newborn also had normal HEX4 but showed mild concentric left ventricular hypertrophy and elevated LDH. This newborn began treatment with ERT at 1 month of age. The third newborn with nonclassical infantile onset Pompe disease had significantly elevated HEX4 and CK. This newborn was compound heterozygous for the c.2560C>T variant, which is commonly associated with classical infantile onset Pompe disease and the c.2236T>C variant, which is a less common missense variant. This newborn began ERT at 1 month of age.

3.2.2. Later-Onset

Through screening, 36 newborns were identified and subsequently diagnosed with later-onset Pompe disease. Of these, 35 newborns received tests for HEX4 only ($n = 7$), CK only ($n = 9$), or both ($n = 19$). All newborns that received testing had normal results for HEX4 and six (21%) had mildly elevated CK. Ten of the newborns were found to have abnormal results for some combination of liver enzymes, LDH, CK-MB, and/or BNP.

Sixteen newborns received cardiac testing including a combination of chest x-ray, EKG, and echocardiogram—of which 15 were within normal limits. The other newborn in this group had an abnormal ECG with concern for right ventricular or biventricular hypertrophy. This newborn was compound heterozygous for the c.2560C>T variant and the c.-32-13T>G variant. During follow-up testing, this newborn exhibited worsening cardiomyopathy and hypotonia as well as abnormal labs; the newborn began ERT at 13 months of age.

3.2.3. Genotypes of Unknown Significance

Eight newborns were found to have genotypes of unknown significance. All eight received testing for either HEX4 only ($n = 1$), CK only ($n = 3$), or both ($n = 4$); all results were normal. Additionally, three of the newborns received an EKG and echocardiogram; these results were also normal. The genotypes of these eight patients were all different, and four of the eight had at least three detected variants. Two of these newborns remain in active follow-up and neither has begun to show clinical manifestations of Pompe disease. For two others, follow-up was deemed unnecessary unless clinical concerns arose, and the remaining four cases were lost to follow-up.

3.2.4. Pseudodeficiencies

Through screening, 53 newborns were found to have GAA pseudodeficiency. Three common GAA pseudodeficiency variants were represented in the Missouri population: c.1726G>A, c.2065G>A, and c.271G>A, including the common c.1726G>A/c.2065G>A haplotype. In total, the incidence of pseudodeficiency homozygotes or compound heterozygotes was 1:8811 (0.01%).

3.2.5. Other Results

Sixty five newborns were found through confirmatory testing to be heterozygous for a pathogenic variant, likely pathogenic variant, or variant of unknown significance. Additionally, 97 newborns were classified as normal due to normal confirmatory enzyme activities.

3.3. Current Follow-up Status

Of the 54 newborns identified with infantile onset or later-onset Pompe disease, or a genotype of unknown significance, 59% (32/54) remain in active follow-up with the genetic referral centers. This includes 7/10 infantile onset cases, 23/36 later-onset cases, and 2/8 with genotypes of unknown significance.

All ten patients with infantile onset Pompe disease—seven classical and three nonclassical—initiated enzyme replacement therapy at ages between four days and one month. Four of the classical infantile onset cases remain in active follow-up (two of the patients have moved out of the state and one is deceased). Cardiac symptoms (hypertrophic cardiomyopathy) have improved in all four active cases (4/4). In three of the cases, myopathy/hypotonia, growth, respiratory symptoms, hearing, feeding, and overall development have improved or remained unchanged since the initiation of ERT. In the remaining case, in which the patient has been receiving ERT for approximately 5.5 years, myopathy and hypotonia have worsened, hearing loss has occurred, and overall development has slowed.

All three of the newborns with nonclassical infantile onset remain in active follow-up. Cardiac symptoms, hypotonia, respiratory, hearing, feeding, and development status are unchanged in all three cases. In one case, ERT was discontinued within the first year of life due to infusion-related reactions. A desensitization protocol was attempted and unsuccessful. This patient is still followed closely and continues to have normal labs, normal growth, and no pulmonary concerns.

Of the 23 later-onset cases that are still in active follow-up, the status of 20/23 is unchanged and ERT has not been administered. In one case, cardiac symptoms improved without the aid of ERT; in another case, both cardiac symptoms and myopathy improved without ERT. In the final case, hypotonia worsened on follow-up and labs were abnormal, which resulted in the introduction of ERT at 13 months of age.

4. Discussion

4.1. Screening Results

Through nearly 6 years of prospective testing, Missouri screened approximately 467,000 newborns for GAA activity; as a result of this screening, 46 newborns were diagnosed with Pompe disease, including 10 with infantile onset Pompe disease. From the evidence report compiled in 2013 by the Condition Review Workgroup of the Advisory Committee on Heritable Diseases in Newborn and Children (ACHDNC), the incidence of Pompe disease in the United States was estimated at 1:28,000, with approximately 28% of the cases (1:100,000) presenting in the first 12 months of life (infantile onset) [4]. Missouri's screening program identified a higher than expected overall rate of Pompe disease (1:10,152) and infantile Pompe disease (1:46,700), with a slightly lower than expected percentage of cases diagnosed with infantile onset (22%).

The Missouri newborn screening laboratory overcame several challenges during the first months of screening for Pompe. As the first U.S. state to screen for Pompe, there was limited data available for the laboratory to reference when determining preliminary cutoffs, specifically for demographic variables. For example, the laboratory implemented age-related cutoffs for GAA activity after approximately four months of live screening when it was observed that median GAA activity decreases by more than 30% from birth to the 14th day of life. The decrease in median enzyme activity as a function of age at sample collection is illustrated in Figure 2. After implementation of age-related thresholds, the retest and false positive rates for the assay both decreased.

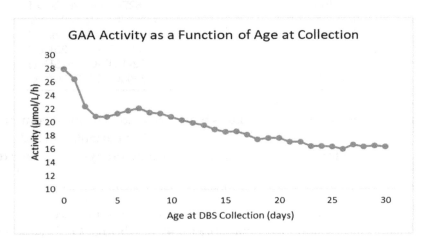

Figure 2. GAA enzyme activity decreases during the first 30 days of life. GAA enzyme activity data (Y axis) from this chart includes average screening results from 338,743 full-term newborns (>38 weeks gestational age) prospectively screened at MSPHL. Age at DBS sample collection (X axis) was rounded down to the nearest full day.

Similarly, the laboratory began to utilize the activity of all tested lysosomal enzymes as a measure of sample quality. This was beneficial with leukodepleted samples; since lysosomal enzymes in blood are predominantly present in white cells, activity of all lysosomal enzymes can be decreased in leukodepleted samples. Evaluation of all lysosomal enzymes is also useful during periods of high temperature and humidity. During the summer months, lysosomal enzymes may be denatured during extended exposure to elevated heat and humidity. Beginning the first summer following the start of screening, MSPHL has used all lysosomal enzyme activities as an indicator of sample quality and considers results that were abnormal for multiple lysosomal enzymes to be inconclusive, thereby requiring only a repeat/second newborn screen. The laboratory also adjusts the cutoffs during the summer months to account for the decrease in activity.

Comparison of HEX4 and CK, two diagnostic tests that are completed during the Pompe follow-up protocol, shows a correlation between disease severity and HEX4 and CK levels. The classical infantile onset patients all displayed elevated HEX4 and CK, while the nonclassical infantile and later-onset patients had results within the normal limits or mildly elevated results. Although CK activity for the nonclassical infantile cases was only mildly elevated, these cases were significantly elevated (median = 416) relative to the later-onset group (median = 126).

4.2. Variant Frequencies

4.2.1. Infantile and Later-Onset Variants

Of the 10 newborns diagnosed with infantile onset Pompe through screening, a total of 13 different variants were identified. Specific variant information is presented in Table 4. The c.525DelT variant was the most common infantile onset variant in this cohort, as was found in 3/10 cases, including two newborn family members prospectively identified through screening. The c.1447G>A, c.1802C>T, c.2560C>T, c.-32-13T>G, and exon 18 deletions were found in two patients each.

Table 4. Variants Identified in Infantile Pompe Disease Patients through Prospective Screening.

Diagnosis	Variants
Classical Infantile	c.1548G>A/del exon 18
Classical Infantile	c.1447G>A/c.2560C>T
Classical Infantile	c.670C>T/c.2481+31Del
Classical Infantile	c.525DelT/c.1447G>A
Classical Infantile	c.1827C>G/c.2662G>T
Classical Infantile	c.1802C>T/c.1802C>T
Classical Infantile	c.947A>G/del exon 18
Nonclassical Infantile	c.-32-13T>G/c.525DelT
Nonclassical Infantile	c.-32-13T>G/c.525DelT
Nonclassical Infantile	c.2560C>T/c.2236T>C

Of the later-onset patients, 36 different variants were detected. The most common variant detected was the c.-32-13T>G variant, which was found in 66.7% (24/36) patients, including 10 homozygotes. The c.841C>T variant was also found as part of a compound heterozygote in four different patients.

4.2.2. Pseudodeficiency

The frequency of pseudodeficiency variants was also evaluated. Of the 53 cases classified as pseudodeficiencies, variant information was available for 49 newborns. Of these 49 newborns, 48 (98%) had the common c.1726G>A/c.2065G>A pseudodeficiency haplotype. Two newborns also possessed the c.271G>A pseudodeficiency variant; one newborn was homozygous for this allele, and one newborn possessed this allele as a compound heterozygote with the c.1726G>A/c.2065G>A haplotype. When evaluating the ethnicities of the pseudodeficiency cases, 43 (88%) of the 49 cases with available variant information reported the newborn's ethnicity on the sample collection form as either "Asian", "Pacific Islander", or multiethnic including at least one of those two groups. These pseudodeficiency variants have previously been reported at high prevalence in the Asian population [14,15], and the results of screening in Missouri indicate that the vast majority of GAA pseudodeficiency cases are of Asian ethnicity. Based on the 2010 U.S. Census [16], 2.0% of Missouri's population is of Asian ethnicity, which is significantly below the U.S. average of 5.6%; other U.S. states or territories with a higher population proportion of Asian ethnicity may encounter higher rates of pseudodeficiency.

4.3. Current Follow-up Status

Fifty nine percent of newborns with Pompe disease or genotypes of unknown significance have maintained active follow-up after the initial diagnosis. All infantile onset patients remain in active follow-up with the exception of two families that no longer reside in the state; however, the proportion of later-onset patients and patients with genotypes of unknown significance that maintain active follow-up is far lower (23 of 36 later-onset, 64%, remain active; 2 of 8, 25%, GUS remain active).

Of the 10 infantile onset cases diagnosed, all 10 started enzyme replacement therapy. Nine of the infantile cases were CRIM-positive. Eight of ten have improved or unchanged symptoms, with one case of worsening hypotonia after more than 5 years on ERT, and another discontinuing ERT after less than one year following development of infusion-related reactions. Both of the newborns with worsening symptoms or adverse reactions were CRIM-positive. The CRIM-negative newborn has moved out of state and is no longer in active follow up in Missouri. One of the later-onset cases has developed symptoms consistent with Pompe disease and has initiated treatment; as this patient was 13 months of age at initiation of treatment, it reinforces that patients with later-onset Pompe disease may develop symptoms and require intervention with ERT in early childhood.

5. Conclusions

The Missouri newborn screening program continues to operate the longest continuous Pompe screening program in the United States and has screened approximately 467,000 newborns during its first six years of screening. Pompe screening has been very successful as 46 patients (approximately 1:10,000) have been diagnosed with Pompe disease, including 10 children (1:46,700) with infantile onset disorder. MSPHL also detected several common pseudodeficiency variants through screening, which caused an increased false positive rate. Implementation of second-tier testing would improve the FPR and PPV, as these pseudodeficiency variants are prevalent in the state's population; Missouri is currently evaluating options to implement second-tier testing for Pompe as well as use of postanalytical tools. Through analysis of screening results, the laboratory found that GAA activity decreases from birth to the 14th day of life and requires age-related cutoffs for the most appropriate risk assessment. MSPHL also found that testing for multiple lysosomal enzymes can aid in the determination of sample quality, as the lysosomal enzyme activities can be decreased in leukodepleted samples or in samples that are exposed to elevated heat and humidity.

To date, 11 patients (10 with infantile onset, 1 with later-onset) have begun treatment with enzyme replacement therapy through the screening and follow-up program. Early initiation of ERT has led to normal development and cardiac improvement for the majority of the infantile onset Pompe disease cases, and only one patient has discontinued ERT due to infusion-related reactions. Additionally, the presence of a patient with diagnosed later-onset disease that has already begun ERT offers a case study that later-onset disease may still present in infancy or early childhood.

Author Contributions: Conceptualization, J.L.K. and L.B.S.; formal analysis, T.L.K. and J.W.; investigation, T.L.K.; resources, J.L.K. and L.B.S.; data curation, L.B.S.; writing—original draft preparation, T.L.K. and J.W.; writing—review and editing, T.L.K., J.L.K., L.B.S., J.W., and C.B.; supervision, J.L.K. and T.L.K. All authors have read and agree to the published version of the manuscript.

Acknowledgments: Special thanks to the Missouri Genetic Referral Centers (Cardinal Glennon Children's Hospital, Children's Mercy Hospital, St. Louis Children's Hospital, and University of Missouri Healthcare Children's Hospital) for providing follow-up and confirmatory data for these cases.

References

1. Pompe, J.C. Over idiopathische hypertrophie van het hart. *Ned. Tijdschr. Geneeskd* **1932**, *76*, 304–311.
2. Bischoff, G. Zum klinischen Bild der Glykogen-Speicherungskrankheit (Glykogenose). *Z. Kinderheilkd.* **1932**, *52*, 722–726. [CrossRef]
3. Kishnani, P.S.; Beckemeyer, A.A.; Mendelsohn, N.J. The new era of Pompe disease: Advances in the detection, understanding of the phenotypic spectrum, pathophysiology, and management. *Am. J. Med. Genet. Part C Semin. Med. Genet.* **2012**, *160C*, 1–7. [CrossRef] [PubMed]
4. Kemper, A.R.; Comeau, A.M.; Prosser, L.A.; Green, N.S.; Tanksley, S.; Goldenberg, A.; Weinreich, S.; Ojodu, J.; Lam, M.K.K. Evidence Report: Newborn Screening for Pompe Disease by The Condition Review Workgroup: Chair Condition Review Workgroup. Available online: https://www.hrsa.gov/sites/default/files/hrsa/advisory-committees/heritable-disorders/rusp/previous-nominations/pompe-external-evidence-review-report-2013.pdf (accessed on 16 December 2019).
5. Kishnani, P.S.; Corzo, D.; Leslie, N.D.; Gruskin, D.; van Der Ploeg, A.; Clancy, J.P.; Parini, R.; Morin, G.; Beck, M.; Bauer, M.S.; et al. Early treatment with alglucosidase alfa prolongs long-term survival of infants with pompe disease. *Pediatr. Res.* **2009**, *66*, 329–335. [CrossRef] [PubMed]
6. Yang, C.-F.; Yang, C.C.; Liao, H.-C.; Huang, L.-Y.; Chiang, C.-C.; Ho, H.-C.; Lai, C.-J.; Chu, T.-H.; Yang, T.-F.; Hsu, T.-R.; et al. Very Early Treatment for Infantile-Onset Pompe Disease Contributes to Better Outcomes. *J. Pediatr.* **2016**, *169*, 174–180. [CrossRef] [PubMed]
7. Discretionary Advisory Committee on Heritable Disorders in Newborns DACHDNC Letter on the Addition of Pompe Disease to the Recommended Uniform Screening Panel. Available online: https://www.hrsa.gov/sites/default/files/hrsa/advisory-committees/heritable-disorders/reports-recommendations/letter-to-sec-pompe.pdf (accessed on 16 December 2019).

8.   HB716|Missouri 2009|Establishes the Brady Alan Cunningham Newborn Screening Act Which Adds Certain Lysosomal Storage Diseases to the List of Required Newborn Screenings|TrackBill. Available online: https: //trackbill.com/bill/missouri-house-bill-716-establishes-the-brady-alan-cunningham-newborn-screening-act-which-adds-certain-lysosomal-storage-diseases-to-the-list-of-required-newborn-screenings/40648/ (accessed on 16 December 2019).

9.   Hopkins, P.V.; Campbell, C.; Klug, T.; Rogers, S.; Raburn-Miller, J.; Kiesling, J. Lysosomal storage disorder screening implementation: Findings from the first six months of full population pilot testing in Missouri. *J. Pediatr.* **2015**, *166*, 172–177. [CrossRef] [PubMed]

10.   Hopkins, P.V.; Klug, T.; Vermette, L.; Raburn-Miller, J.; Kiesling, J.; Rogers, S. Incidence of 4 lysosomal storage disorders from 4 years of newborn screening. *JAMA Pediatr.* **2018**, *172*, 696–697. [CrossRef] [PubMed]

11.   Sista, R.S.; Wang, T.; Wu, N.; Graham, C.; Eckhardt, A.; Winger, T.; Srinivasan, V.; Bali, D.; Millington, D.S.; Pamula, V.K. Multiplex newborn screening for Pompe, Fabry, Hunter, Gaucher, and Hurler diseases using a digital microfluidic platform. *Clin. Chim. Acta* **2013**, *424*, 12–18. [CrossRef] [PubMed]

12.   Burton, B.K.; Charrow, J.; Hoganson, G.E.; Waggoner, D.; Tinkle, B.; Braddock, S.R.; Schneider, M.; Grange, D.K.; Nash, C.; Shryock, H.; et al. Newborn Screening for Lysosomal Storage Disorders in Illinois: The Initial 15-Month Experience. *J. Pediatr.* **2017**, *190*, 130–135. [CrossRef] [PubMed]

13.   Kwon, C.; Farrell, P.M. The magnitude and challenge of false-positive newborn screening test results. *Arch. Pediatr. Adolesc. Med.* **2000**, *154*, 714–718. [CrossRef] [PubMed]

14.   Chiang, S.C.; Hwu, W.L.; Lee, N.C.; Hsu, L.W.; Chien, Y.H. Algorithm for Pompe disease newborn screening: Results from the Taiwan screening program. *Mol. Genet. Metab.* **2012**, *106*, 281–286. [CrossRef] [PubMed]

15.   Kumamoto, S.; Katafuchi, T.; Nakamura, K.; Endo, F.; Oda, E.; Okuyama, T.; Kroos, M.A.; Reuser, A.J.J.; Okumiya, T. High frequency of acid α-glucosidase pseudodeficiency complicates newborn screening for glycogen storage disease type II in the Japanese population. *Mol. Genet. Metab.* **2009**, *97*, 190–195. [CrossRef] [PubMed]

16.   2010 Census Data|Office of Administration. Available online: https://oa.mo.gov/budget-planning/demographic-information/2010-census-data (accessed on 16 December 2019).

24

Is Newborn Screening the Ultimate Strategy to Reduce Diagnostic Delays in Pompe Disease? The Parent and Patient Perspective

Raymond Saich *, Renee Brown, Maddy Collicoat, Catherine Jenner, Jenna Primmer, Beverley Clancy, Tarryn Holland and Steven Krinks

Australian Pompe Association Inc., Kellyville, NSW 2155, Australia; Renee@australianpompe.org.au (R.B.); Maddy@australianpompe.org.au (M.C.); Catherine@australianpompe.org.au (C.J.); Jennaprimmer1@bigpond.com (J.P.); Beverley@australianpompe.org.au (B.C.); tarryn_80@hotmail.com (T.H.); stevenkrinks@msn.com (S.K.)
* Correspondence: Raymond@australianpompe.org.au;

Abstract: Pompe disease (PD) is a rare, autosomal-recessively inherited deficiency in the enzyme acid α-glucosidase. It is a spectrum disorder; age at symptom onset and rate of deterioration can vary considerably. In affected infants prognosis is poor, such that without treatment most infants die within the first year of life. To lose a baby in their first year of life to a rare disease causes much regret, guilt, and loneliness to parents, family, and friends. To lose a baby needlessly when there is an effective treatment amplifies this sadness. With so little experience of rare disease in the community, once a baby transfers to their home they are subject to a very uncertain and unyielding diagnostic journey while their symptomology progresses and their health deteriorates. With a rare disease like PD, the best opportunity to diagnose a baby is at birth. PD is not yet included in the current newborn screening (NBS) panel in Australia. Should it be? In late 2018 the Australian Pompe Association applied to the Australian Standing committee on Newborn Screening to have PD included. The application was not upheld. Here we provide an overview of the rationale for NBS, drawing on the scientific literature and perspectives from The Australian Pompe Association, its patients and their families. In doing so, we hope to bring a new voice to this very important debate.

Keywords: Pompe disease; newborn screening; diagnosis; infantile onset Pompe disease; late onset Pompe disease; patient perspective

1. Introduction

Pompe disease (PD), also known as glycogen storage disease II or acid maltase deficiency, is a rare, progressively debilitating lysosomal storage disorder. It is named after Joannes Cassianus Pompe, who first described a case of idiopathic hypertrophy of the heart in a 7-month old infant in the Netherlands in 1932, noting massive vacuolar glycogen accumulation not only in the heart but in all tissues examined [1].

Affected patients have an autosomal-recessively inherited deficiency in the enzyme acid α-glucosidase (GAA, also called acid maltase). This deficiency leads to accumulation of glycogen in multiple tissues, especially in the skeletal muscles, heart, and liver [2]. These glycogen deposits disrupt muscle cell architecture and function, causing progressive motor, respiratory, and cardiac dysfunction. While both genders are equally affected, PD is a spectrum disorder in which the age at symptom onset and rate of deterioration can vary considerably.

The clinical impact of PD is determined primarily by the amount of residual GAA enzyme activity. Enzyme activity is absent or minimal (<3%) in infantile-onset disease (IOPD), but may be reduced to varying degrees (3%–30%) in those with juvenile-onset (JOPD) or late-onset disease (LOPD) [3]. A lower residual enzyme activity level is associated with earlier onset, more severe disease, faster progression, worse prognosis and a shorter survival time [4]. In IOPD clinical symptoms typically become apparent within the first few months of life; prognosis is poor such that without treatment most infants die within the first year of life [5].

The rarity of PD combined with a variety of overlapping clinical signs and symptoms hamper its diagnosis and the initiation of therapy [6–8]. Such delays have a significant negative impact on patients and their families. Recent research has shown that newborn screening (NBS) appears to be better at identifying PD cases than does clinical examination, especially for classical IOPD [9]. Is NBS the ultimate strategy to reduce diagnostic delays in PD? Here we provide an overview of the rationale for NBS, drawing on the scientific literature and including perspectives from patients and their families. In doing so, we hope to bring a new voice to this very important debate.

2. Diagnostic Delay

Diagnostic delay is common in PD, and it exists across the disease spectrum [8]. Data from the Pompe Registry has found the diagnostic gap to be shortest (average 1.4 months; range: 0.0–13.9 months) in patients with classic IOPD and longest in patients with JOPD (average 12.6 years; range: 0.0–60.0 years). Delays are also significant for LOPD (average 6.0 years; range: 0.0–49.8 years) [8]. Within Australia, IOPD diagnosis can occur within a few months of initial symptom onset, but diagnostic delays of up to 7 months have been reported in the literature [10].

The impact of this delay is such that for many patients, health and functional status is often already severely impaired at the time of their diagnosis. Analysis of data from 53 patients (age range 0–64 years) has shown that at the time of diagnosis [11]:

- Classic IOPD patients—cardiac function, hearing, muscle strength and motor development were all impaired, one in three (36%) required supplemental oxygen and two in three (64%) required nasogastric tube feeding;
- LOPD patients—advanced muscle weakness and impaired respiratory function were present, causing varying degrees of handicap, and respiratory support (14% of adults) and use of a wheelchair (7% of adults) were required.

2.1. Barriers to Timely Diagnosis—Australian Perspectives

Although not specific to PD, prompt diagnosis of rare diseases can have many important positive ramifications. Prompt diagnosis facilitates access to appropriate treatment, it can help parents to better understand their child's condition and explain it to others, it may reduce the burden of blame parents feel and it may alleviate some of the stress of the unknown [12].

Australian research (Table 1) has highlighted a lack of screening tests and limited knowledge amongst healthcare professionals as key barriers to diagnostic delays in rare diseases, with the authors calling for more educational support and wider access to a multi-disciplinary team approach to patient care [13]. Australian pediatric research has shown that more than half of the children with a rare disease were not diagnosed until after referral to a clinical specialist in a large metropolitan pediatric hospital [12], confounding the diagnostic delay.

Table 1. Australian survey data: Diagnostic delays are common in rare diseases.

Age Group	Results	Reference
Adults	Time to diagnosis: • 1 year in 51.2% of cases • ≥5 years in 30.0% of cases Number of doctors seen to get confirmed diagnosis: • 1–2 in 33.7% of cases • 3–5 in 37.4% of cases • ≥6 in 28.8% of cases Number with at least one incorrect diagnosis: • 45.9% of cases	Molster, 2016 [13]
Children	Time to diagnosis: • 1 year in 59.8% of cases • ≥3 years in 8.0% of cases Number of doctors seen to get confirmed diagnosis: • 1–2 in 12.5% of cases • 3–5 in 41.8% of cases • ≥6 in 27.7% of cases Number with at least one incorrect diagnosis: • 27.3% of cases	Zurynski, 2017 [12]

Key Considerations:

• Receiving a diagnosis of a rare disease is a life-changing event; delays in receiving a diagnosis are associated with anxiety, stress, symptomatic worsening, inappropriate use of resources and lack of access to appropriate support and care;
• Health professional education is needed to increase awareness of rare diseases and improve the diagnostic process;
• Resources, including access to multi-disciplinary care teams, are needed to support the requirements of people newly diagnosed with rare diseases.

Specialist referral is reported as a pivotal step in obtaining a clinical diagnosis of rare diseases in Australia [12]. In accordance with this, a recent European survey exploring diagnostic odyssey in PD found that circuitous involvement of several healthcare professionals increased the diagnostic delay of IOPD by 200% compared to direct referral to a specialist center [14].

Australians living in rural and remote areas have additional diagnostic barriers, confounded by lack of proximity and timely access to such specialist healthcare providers. In such cases, the typical care pathway involves multiple steps—initial parental recognition that something is not right with their baby, general practitioner (GP) acknowledgement, and referral to a pediatrician—before the child can be seen in a specialist center. This stepwise approach can take a minimum of 3 months and can place a significant financial and psychosocial burden on the family. Some babies survive the time it takes to confirm a diagnosis, but many do not.

2.2. Diagnostic Delays—Australian IOPD Experiences

In the case of PD, the presenting symptoms are diverse and not likely to be suggestive of this diagnosis unless another family member or relative has already been diagnosed [15]. A high index of clinical suspicion is needed to ensure that patients are appropriately examined and tested. A doctor with intimate experience in the diagnosis or management of PD may be more likely to recognize symptoms in an undiagnosed patient; unfortunately very few doctors will have seen a PD patient in Australia. Testing for PD is a relatively simple procedure that can be undertaken in a few days.

Clinician awareness of, and increased vigilance for, the early symptoms of PD are therefore also important contributory factors to timely diagnosis [10].

A particular case in point is that of NP (Figure 1). NP was born 4–6 weeks prematurely; whilst he developed normally at first, early symptomology became apparent within the first few months of his life. Hypotonia, dysphagia, and developmental delays resulted in the family GP diagnosing failure to thrive at age 2 months and NP was placed on a wait-list for pediatrician referral. At age 6 months, not having seen the pediatrician, NP contracted a viral infection. He was hospitalized initially in a regional hospital 58 km from home and transferred 2 days later to the main tertiary hospital, 168 km away. Upon being admitted to the tertiary hospital blood samples were taken and sent interstate (to South Australia) and overseas (to the USA) for analysis. Ten days later the results were returned and NP was formally diagnosed with IOPD. The extent of physical damage sustained to his body during the time to diagnosis was such that NP was unable to survive, passing away aged 32 months.

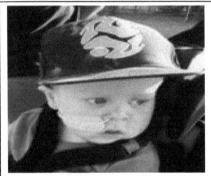

"With the logistical issues from living in a rural area, despite a known family history of PD, it still took more than 7 months to get a diagnosis of IOPD. He never regained movement in his legs and did not fully recover from the viral infection. He always had breathing difficulties and respiratory infections. The heartbreak at the loss of such a young life after undergoing months of uncertainty is difficult to comprehend, particularly given that earlier diagnosis would have enabled him to have access to treatment and potentially provided a better long-term outlook."

NP diagnosed at age 7 months.

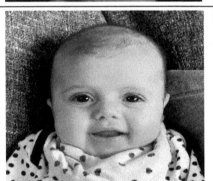

"She had been a more sleepy baby than our first and we put it down to jaundice but then she was slow to put on weight and fell behind in some key markers at maternal health appointments. The maternal health nurse noticed her shallow breathing at around 9 weeks; I took her hospital they put it down to suspected bronchiolitis and we stayed the night for monitoring. At the next weeks' appointment, the pediatrician picked up that the hospital chest X-ray showed her heart was enlarged. We then saw a pediatric cardiologist who diagnosed her with hypertrophic cardiomyopathy and the concern was to why at a young age she has this and the reasons being life threatening. We then sought further advice from the hospital team and they ran a series of tests after she was admitted at around 12 weeks of age and she never left. We anxiously waited for test results, which validated one of the worst outcomes of Infantile Pompe. It all happened so quickly and she passed away at 14 weeks old, just 99 days. We had never heard of this disease and have no family history on either side of the condition."

LC diagnosed at age 12 weeks.

Figure 1. Parents' perspectives on Australian infantile-onset disease (IOPD) diagnostic experiences. In lieu of patient informed consent, photographs and comments have been provided by, and reproduced with permission from, the parents of these two children both of whom were deceased at the time the paper was written.

In the last 5 years, the Australian Pompe Association is aware of at least four infants passing away in their first few months of life. These include a baby girl (LC, Figure 1), who was diagnosed at age 12 weeks and three baby boys the youngest of whom died at age 15 weeks. A further two young children, one of whom was diagnosed at age 3 months and died at 19 months and the other who was diagnosed at 9 months and died at 24 months, both had commenced enzyme replacement therapy (ERT) but experienced substantial immune responses [10].

3. What Do We Know about NBS for PD?

The overarching aim of any NBS program is to improve early identification of patients with treatable genetic metabolic disorders diseases in order to confirm diagnosis and initiate management to improve overall health outcomes [16]. Since the initiation of NBS for phenylketonuria, the criteria published by Wilson and Junger in 1968 have provided guiding principles to determine which conditions should be added to the panel [17]. These criteria include availability of a suitable screening test, an effective treatment, an early onset form of the disease that would be debilitating if not treated soon after birth, and consideration of overall cost-effectiveness [18].

Population NBS for PD was first implemented in Taiwan in 2005. A decade later, in 2015, it was added to the USA Department of Health and Human Services-endorsed Recommended Uniform Screening Panel (RUSP) [19]. As of November 2019, implementation has occurred in 23 states and a further 9 states are actively pursuing implementation or conducted pilot studies [20]. Including Taiwan, an estimated 239,333,512 people benefit from the protection of NBS for PD. Pilot NBS studies have also been conducted in Austria, Italy, Hungary, and Japan [21]. Whilst establishment of these programs is challenging and controversial, key driving factors include [19]:

- The development of promising new treatment options;
- Advances in screening technology;
- Advocacy by special interest groups.

3.1. Benefits of NBS for PD

3.1.1. Reduced Diagnostic Odyssey in IOPD

The primary benefit of NBS for PD is the potential to identify patients before symptoms arise, enabling timely initiation of therapy before irreversible damage occurs. Babies with IOPD identified via NBS would be eligible to receive treatment at around 22 days of life, compared to 4 or 5 months of age when relying on symptom-based referral and subsequent diagnosis [8].

Research based on using different decision-analytic models has demonstrated NBS to be superior to clinical examination in identifying IOPD cases, with a significant, positive impact on projected health outcomes [9]. Identifying 40 cases of IOPD via NBS would avert 13 (range 8–19) deaths and 26 (range 20–28) cases of ventilator dependence amongst babies surviving to 36 months of age, assuming all children were treated with ERT. The authors compared their analysis to available real-world data from infants who had undergone NBS for PD in the USA pilot studies at that time, noting that this data supported their models and indicated that the number of cases likely to be detected would be at the upper range of these predictions [9].

3.1.2. Greater Knowledge of Reproductive Risk

At present PD is carried undetected in the community. While patients who have a family history of PD are cognizant of its impact, for many patients there is no such history and a diagnosis of PD can devastate these unexpecting families. NBS provides secondary benefits that positively impact these families, and the wider community, by creating an opportunity to inform about reproductive risks [22]. Early diagnosis of LOPD enables these patients to make better-informed choices regarding future family planning. In addition, a positive NBS screen can be the stepping-stone to identifying reproductive risks in the parents before the birth of a second child. NBS will provide recourse to advice and options, and with knowledge comes informed choices.

Clear frameworks would need to be established to ensure patients and their families are closely followed-up and provided with access to genetic counseling. Equipping key healthcare providers, such as the GP, with information about carrier results and their reproductive implications may help to facilitate parents' understanding of their child's NBS results.

3.1.3. Improved Understanding of the True Prevalence of PD

PD has been thought of as a rare genetic metabolic disease; estimates vary but the literature generally states an incidence of approximately 1 in 40,000 births, of which one-third are infants with IOPD. The Australian Pompe Association membership register does not reflect these IOPD numbers. The youngest treated child currently listed in the Australian Pompe Association membership register is 5 years old; the group is aware of a younger child, aged 4 years, who is diagnosed but not a currently registered member of the Association.

Published Australian data from the mid-1990s estimated an incidence of 1 in 201,000, a prevalence of 1 in 146,000 and a carrier frequency of 1 in 191,000 [23]. No breakdown on the type of PD was provided. As part of reforms into the Government-funded Life Saving Drug Program, a protocol has been established to review the prevalence of PD in Australia based on literature and other published data sources [24]. Data from this review are not yet available, but it is recognized that it will be limited by the availability and incompleteness of identified datasets.

NBS for PD provides a means to help better quantify the true prevalence of this disease. The number of PD cases identified in NBS programs are summarized in Table 2 [21]. These data demonstrate that NBS is finding up to twice the number of cases than were previously thought to exist, underscoring the immense difficulty in diagnosing this condition based on clinical symptomology alone.

Table 2. Results from newborn screening (NBS) programs for Pompe disease (PD). Adapted from Bodamer 2017 [21].

Country and Region	Sample Size	Total Cases of IOPD	Total Cases of LOPD	Prevalence
Taiwan	473,738	9	19	1/16,919
Austria *	34,736	0	4	1/8684
Italy *	3403	0	0	-
Hungary *	40,024	7	2	1/4400
USA (State):				
Illinois *	166,463	2	9	1/15,133
Missouri	269,500	4	20	1/11,229
Washington *	154,544	0	5	1/31,000
New York	390,000	1	30	1/165,000

* Pilot studies.

It is possible that in Australia alone up to two or more babies may die every year without ever having been diagnosed with their underlying IOPD; with these deaths being registered instead as cardiomyopathy or other symptoms of unknown cause. Importantly, the diverse origins of the Australian population may alter the prevalence of PD in the community, but a true understanding of this will not be known without including PD in the national NBS program or, at the very least, investing in a pilot NBS study.

3.2. What Have We Learnt from Current PD NBS Programs?

NBS for PD was first piloted in Taiwan in 2005 and introduced into the Taiwan NBS panel in 2007 [25]. Modification of methodology and systems over time has resulted in a substantial shortening of time to first diagnosis from 19 to 9 days and the time to first treatment initiation from 26 days to 1 day after IOPD confirmation.

Many factors can influence an individual's response to treatment with ERT, including their age and the extent of preexisting pathology [26]. Experience in Taiwan shows that the sooner ERT is commenced, the better the results are [27]. Commencing ERT even a few days earlier can lead to better patient outcomes [28]. For example, 100% of the patients identified through NBS in Taiwan who were initiated on ERT at 6–34 days, and treated for a median of 63 months, remained ventilator-free and have been able to meet age-specific developmental milestones, such as normal independent walking age [29]. By comparison, studies assessing the long-term outcomes of IOPD patients in countries that do not have NBS (including the UK, Germany, the Netherlands, and Italy) report that a substantial number (27%–40%) of children pass away within the first years of life despite ERT [30].

The Taiwanese experience demonstrates that earlier intervention with ERT in IOPD cases can have a positive impact by reducing the future burden of this disease. Moreover, the Erasmus university PD variant database (http://www.pompevariantdatabase.nl/pompe_mutations_list.php?orderby=aMut_ID1) provides data linking the progression and outcomes of over 860 patients with their genetic errors. If genetic sequencing is included as part of NBS confirmatory protocols, this information provides an opportunity to better understand the mutation and to more clearly predict the outcome for the patient.

On this basis, we are of the opinion that the costs of early identification via NBS and early initiation of ERT treatment could be offset by the potential for improved patient quality of life, reduced disease-related disability (such as reduced need for ventilatory support) and reduced associated costs. However, we are unable to support this with hard data at present. Importantly, we remain cognizant that that the current treatment for PD is a first generation product. With considerable research underway for second generation ERT and the potential of gene therapy, the current challenge is to keep Pompe babies as well as possible with the technology available today until a cure is available tomorrow.

3.3. Impact on Immunomodulation Protocols

The development of high and sustained antibody titers (HSAT) is most often associated with IOPD patients who are cross-reactive immunological material negative (CRIM-negative) leading to the recommendation that these patients receive prophylactic immunomodulatory therapy [31]. Whilst ERT has improved clinical outcomes for many patients with PD, there is a risk of developing anti-drug antibodies. HSAT can be associated with worse clinical outcomes. Prophylactic and therapeutic immunomodulation reduce antibody levels, but questions remain as to optimal timing and protocols [32]. HSAT has also been observed in some CRIM-positive patients, raising questions as to how to determine which of these patients should also receive prophylactic immunomodulation [26].

Initiating ERT within the first month of life has not been shown to prevent HSAT [26]. However, experience from Japan, not undertaken in the context of a NBS setting, suggests that early initiation of ERT in the pre-symptomatic period may prevent the progression of IOPD and reduce the likelihood of anti-drug antibody production [33]. These authors suggested that starting ERT before the immune system had matured might have enabled natural immune tolerance. Further research is clearly needed in this area, but this finding opens up possibilities of additional benefits for NBS beyond diagnosis and treatment initiation, because earlier treatment may modify the need for and extent of immunomodulatory approaches.

3.4. Weighing Prognostic Uncertainty against Informed Decision Making

3.4.1. False Positives

Identification of false positive and subsequent prognostic uncertainty is always going to be a core consideration with any NBS program. The extensive Taiwanese experience reports a false positive rate of 0.02% in IOPD targets and 0.01% in IOPD/LOPD targets. Similarly low false positive rates of 0.04% (38.3 per 100,000) and 0.05% (53.2 per 100,000) have been reported from pilot NBS programs in Missouri and Illinois [17] and in a Japanese feasibility study (false positives 0.3%, 2/530) [34].

The literature demonstrates that while prognostic uncertainty does cause heightened anxiety amongst parents in the short-term, there are no documented long-term harms [35]. Options are available to mitigate the issues surrounding identification of false-positives. For example, integrating tandem mass spectrometry with multivariate pattern recognition software to determine which patients warrant second-tier confirmatory testing has been evaluated in the USA with good results, significantly reducing the false-positive rate [36]. The investigators involved in the New York State pilot NBS program suggest the use of second-tier molecular analysis to reduce the burden of referral in screen-positive infants [37]. With their long history of experience in NBS for PD, Taiwanese experts also suggest a second-tier test to reduce the rate of false-positives and facilitate referral of true positives [38].

3.4.2. Early Identification of LOPD

Given that PD is a spectrum disorder, NBS also has the potential for identifying babies with LOPD, noting that their clinical symptomology would not manifest until later in life. Current estimates of the Australian Pompe Association would suggest that if Australia first-tier testing of dry blood spot samples were to take place, for every IOPD case identified there would also be 6 LOPD cases identified. This brings with it several ethical questions surrounding when to start treatment and the burden placed on the patient and their family in terms of waiting for symptoms to appear [39,40].

In the Taiwanese NBS program, 473,738 newborns were screened and 19 LOPD cases had been identified by 2011; 6 (32%) of these patients had commenced ERT between the ages of 1.5–36 months [25]. All 6 patients showed abnormalities with glycogen storage prior to commencing treatment; currently, aged 8–13 years, they have met normal developmental milestones. The remaining 13 patients have not been treated and continue to develop normally, likely representing a milder phenotype [25]. This experience suggests that close monitoring of symptoms and timely ERT initiation, in combination with genetic counseling, education and support should form key aspects in the long-term care of less severe LOPD patients identified through NBS. The ultimate aim being to minimize early medicalization of children while at the same time providing robust protocols to assure the appropriate provision of available treatments.

Aside from treatment and care considerations, there are many positives that must also be considered in the early detection of LOPD cases. These include the ability to learn more about the natural history of the disease and to better As we enter the 2020s equip individuals to make informed choices later in life regarding family planning issues, as discussed above.

The humanistic burden of LOPD is high [41]. Misdiagnosis further impacts this, in terms of costs to the healthcare system incurred as a result of multiple tests and medications being tried without treating the underlying cause and to the patient in terms of ongoing uncertainty, dealing with symptoms and never being quite sure if they would have a better quality life now had they been diagnosed earlier. Early diagnosis of LOPD enables more timely management and may help prevent complications and improve outcomes now that therapy is available [42].

Consider a patient in their 30–40s with mild symptomology. The differential diagnosis for PD is so wide that confirmation of diagnosis may take several years (estimates are in the range of 5–8 years). Importantly anecdotal experience dictates that diagnosis frequently comes after a crisis or other major life event, such as after childbirth, creating additional complexity to what is already a potentially difficult situation.

Without NBS, LOPD patients may go for many years endeavoring to find a diagnosis. The Community loses so much through the cost of unnecessary health care visits while patients struggle for years to find a diagnosis for the want of a simple test at birth that would have alerted the parents or the patient. From a patient's perspective a key advantage to early identification of LOPD via NBS is that it vastly reduces their personal diagnostic journey. In the words of an Australian PD patient, diagnosed in 2010 after a 13-year diagnostic journey:

"There is much that needs to be done to help people with rare diseases, particularly around raising awareness to the public and also medical professionals in order for early diagnosis and also correcting misdiagnosis to occur. Had I been diagnosed even in 1997 when I was 17 and received treatment as soon as it became available perhaps my life would be very different today."

4. Specific Considerations for NBS in the Australian Setting

4.1. Current NBS Policies and Processes

Within Australia, NBS is offered free of charge, and, although not compulsory, participation is high [43]. Australian NBS programs began with screening for phenylketonuria (1967), followed by the addition of congenital hypothyroidism (1977), cystic fibrosis (1981 in New South Wales, 1999 in all other states) and galactosemia (early 1980s). In the late 1990s with advances in technology the list has expanded to include around 25 different disorders [44]. There had been a long silence, with no new conditions added for over 17 years, until the recent initiation of two pilot studies in New South Wales, for primary immune deficiency and spinal muscular atrophy.

All NBS services are coordinated from five centralized screening laboratories (one each in New South Wales, Queensland, South Australia, Victoria, and Western Australia). However, prior to 2018, specific program policies and which conditions to include were individually decided by each state jurisdiction. This has now been replaced with a National Policy Framework, which is accessible via the internet (http://www.cancerscreening.gov.au/internet/screening/publishing.nsf/Content/newborn-bloodspot-screening) [45]. This framework unites these programs for the first time since their inception over 50 years ago. Importantly, it provides a nationally agreed vision and way of working and outlines what will be needed to ensure the ongoing success of the NBS program in Australia; noting that state and territory governments will have the final responsibility for adding the condition in their jurisdictions.

As part of this framework, there is now a national evidence-based process to evaluate proposals to include new conditions in the NBS program [45]. This framework requires the provision of published evidence to support the condition proposed, the test that will be used and the availability and efficacy of treatment such that decisions to include new conditions can be made in line with agreed criteria. These criteria include consideration of (1) whether there is benefit to the baby from early diagnosis of conditions screened, (2) whether the benefit is reasonably balanced against any harms and costs, (3) the availability of a reliable test suitable for newborn bloodspot screening and (4) the availability of a satisfactory system in place to deal with diagnostic testing and follow-up care of babies with abnormal screening results.

The National Policy Framework sets out a step-wise decision-making pathway to carefully evaluate all applications [45]. Following a request to include a new condition in the NBS program and assessment of the available evidence, the possible outcomes include a recommendation to screen, a recommendation to conduct a pilot study, a recommendation to review at a later point in time and a recommendation not to screen.

4.2. Application to Include PD in the NBS

On the basis of the criteria set out in the new NBS National Policy Framework, the Australian Pompe Association took the initiative to submit an application to add IOPD to the NBS program. An initial application was submitted in 2018 but was not reviewed; it was then resubmitted in November 2018 to meet the timelines for a 2019 meeting and decision.

As part of its submission, the Australian Pompe Association calculated that the cost of first-tier dry blood spot testing for PD would be $8.78, amounting to approximately AUD$2.7 million each year, assuming an estimated total birth rate of 310,000 per annum and testing via established tandem mass spectrometry methods. However, recognized additional cost considerations included the need for each State/Territory to purchase a new mass spectrometer because current facilities are believed to be at capacity, funding for additional staff to manage this workload, the establishment and provision of genetic counseling services and costs incurred in second-tier confirmatory testing.

A key consideration of the application was its focus on IOPD, given that this has the most benefit to be gained by minimizing the diagnostic delay. It was hoped that, at the very least, this application would have been seen as a positive step forward and enable a pilot program to be implemented. A pilot program to evaluate first-tier testing has been developed but not implemented due to lack of funding and clinical resources. Such a program would help to define the prevalence of PD in Australia, enable evaluation of the optimal methodology for measuring GAA activity, and better inform costs and resourcing needs for NBS. In addition, it would aid in establishing post-testing diagnostic and confirmatory protocols and procedures for managing JOPD, LOPD, and patients with pseudodeficiency alleles that can lead to false positives.

After consideration by the Standing Committee on Screening, the application has not progressed to a more detailed review. The primary reasons for this being limited longitudinal evidence of survival improvements in treated IOPD patients as a result of identification via NBS and concerns regarding the negative impact of identifying patients at risk of developing LOPD. To a large extent, as has been discussed in this paper, literature providing answers to these concerns is becoming more readily available.

The rapid pace at which new data are emerging, coupled with the increase in uptake of NBS in developed countries like the USA, underscores the drive of the clinical, research and patient communities to provide earlier diagnosis and better outcomes for PD patients and their families. The Australian Pompe Association is encouraged by this and will seek to resubmit its nomination for adding IOPD to the Australian NBS program in the future.

4.3. Access to Current Therapies in Australia

Australia has an established and advanced program for the treatment of rare diseases, the Life Saving Drugs program (LSDP) was established in the mid-1990s and provides people with rare and life-threatening disease with access to medicines that are not listed on the Pharmaceutical Benefits Scheme. Currently 10 conditions are supported by the program, and of the treatments available alglucosidase alfa (Myozyme®) is subsidized for the treatment of IOPD, JOPD, and LOPD.

The LSDP requires that patients meet specific conditions to obtain access to treatment; including initial and ongoing eligibility criteria, and that they undergo annual reviews. Clear protocols are in place for diagnosing the disease and for its ongoing management, including starting and stopping treatment.

The decision by the Australian government to fund treatment through the LSDP is an example to all countries for programs to establish treatment for minority patient groups who face the challenge of living with a rare disease. Treatment is expensive. The only currently approved treatment is ERT and a recent review of the economic costs of PD has established that while available data demonstrate a high cost to patients and healthcare systems, there are substantial gaps in the literature [46]. It is hoped that as new treatment options became available, and competitive interest develops, production methodology will become more cost effective enabling the overall cost of ERT treatment to decline.

4.4. Potential Impact of Future Therapies

Prior to 2006, the only therapy available to patients with PD was palliative. ERT, the only currently available treatment for PD, has been very successful; it can extend the lifespan of babies born with IOPD and stabilize disease progression in patients with LOPD. However, it does not represent a cure. Research continues with many potential avenues including investigations into other therapies such as immune modulation, upregulation of receptor expression, second-generation recombinant ERT, chaperone therapy, substrate reduction therapy, and gene therapy [47]. Recent reviews provide up-to-date information of the available data for these potential new therapies [48,49].

Amongst these therapies, the prospect of gene therapy is of great interest. Currently several biotechnology companies are actively developing gene therapies for PD, while some therapies are still in preclinical development, other have entered early phase clinical trials [48]. Gene therapy has the potential to enable sustained enzyme supply after a single medical intervention; by enabling the patient to produce his or her own enzyme it will vastly change the way in which PD is managed.

As we enter the 2020s, for the first time in 56 years we have an opportunity to significantly reduce the suffering, distress and despair that a diagnosis of PD brings. NBS combined with the potential for gene therapy provides hope that in the not too distant future such patients will be able to say 'Yes I had PD as a baby, but I am fine now thanks to my early detection and treatment'.

5. Conclusions

NBS has emerged over the past decade as an important contributor to more timely diagnosis and treatment of PD, particularly for babies with IOPD who would otherwise not survive and pass away with their true diagnosis undocumented. Early diagnosis and early access to treatment are pivotal to optimal clinical outcomes.

Australia is not alone in not yet having an NBS program for PD. Here, as in many other countries, the current scenario for patients with PD involves a lengthy diagnostic journey and belated commencement of treatment; in the case of IOPD often after considerable damage has already occurred. NBS facilitates earlier diagnosis and treatment access in a disease in which this timing is absolutely crucial. Identifying and treating IOPD earlier can make a difference between survival and death, between positive outcomes and severe disability. Existing NBS programs have demonstrated the ability to improve patients' lives. Thus, despite its challenges, these positives greatly outweigh the negatives. While we have not had a positive outcome from our application, we hope that by taking the initiative to submit a proposal to include IOPD on the Australian NBS program it will encourage other groups elsewhere to be proactive in investigating and utilizing whatever systems are available in their countries to make similar applications.

The Pompe patient community, both in Australia and around the globe, is highly supportive of NBS [50]. Much headway has been made in ensuring that this patient voice is heard by medical specialists, scientific researchers and industry. Now it is time that this voice is also heard by the regulator to ensure equal and equitable access to NBS and the many benefits it can bring to the lives of PD patients and their families.

Author Contributions: Conceptualization, R.S.; writing—original draft preparation, R.S. with assistance from Hazel Palmer (see below); writing—review and editing, R.S., R.B., M.C., C.J., J.P., B.C., T.H., and S.K.; funding acquisition, R.S. All authors have read and agreed to the published version of the manuscript.

Acknowledgments: The authors acknowledge professional writing assistance provided by Hazel Palmer MSc, ISMPP CMPP™ (Scriptix Pty Ltd., Freshwater, NSW, 2096 Australia) in the preparation of this manuscript. The authors thank Bevan Sweerts, Anthony Earp and Jana Chromika, non-author reviewers and employees of SANOFI-GENZYME AUSTRALIA PTY LTD, for their insightful suggestions and comments.

References

1. Pompe, J.C. Over idiopatische hypertrophie van het hart. *Ned. Tijdschr. Geneeskd.* **1932**, *76*, 304.
2. Angelini, C.; Nascimbeni, A.C.; Semplicini, C. Therapeutic advances in the management of Pompe disease and other metabolic myopathies. *Ther. Adv. Neurol. Disord.* **2013**, *6*, 311–321. [CrossRef] [PubMed]
3. Lim, J.A.; Li, L.; Raben, N. Pompe disease: From pathophysiology to therapy and back again. *Front. Aging Neurosci.* **2014**, *6*, 177. [CrossRef] [PubMed]
4. Herzog, A.; Hartung, R.; Reuser, A.J.; Hermanns, P.; Runz, H.; Karabul, N.; Gökce, S.; Pohlenz, J.; Kampmann, C.; Lampe, C.; et al. A cross-sectional single-centre study on the spectrum of Pompe disease, German patients: Molecular analysis of the GAA gene, manifestation and genotype-phenotype correlations. *Orphanet J. Rare Dis.* **2012**, *7*, 35. [CrossRef] [PubMed]
5. Kemper, A.R.; Comeau, A.M.; Green, N.S.; Goldenberg, A.; Ojodu, J.; Prosser, L.A.; Tanksley, S.; Weinreich, S.; Lam, K.K. *The Condition Review Workgroup. Evidence Report: Newborn Screening for Pompe Disease*; US Department of Health and Human Services: Rockville, MD, USA, 2013. Available online: http://www.hrsa.gov/advisorycommittees/mchbadvisory/heritabledisorders/nominatecondition/reviews/pompereport2013.pdf (accessed on 18 November 2019).

6. Kishnani, P.S.; Steiner, R.D.; Bali, D.; Berger, K.; Byrne, B.J.; Case, L.E. Pompe disease diagnosis and management guideline. *Genet. Med.* **2006**, *8*, 267–288. [CrossRef]

7. Toscano, A.; Montagnese, F.; Musumeci, O. Early is better? A new algorithm for early diagnosis in late onset Pompe disease (LOPD). *Acta Myol.* **2013**, *32*, 78–81.

8. Kishnani, P.S.; Amartino, H.M.; Lindberg, C.; Miller, T.M.; Wilson, A.; Keutzer, J. Timing of diagnosis of patients with Pompe disease: Data from the Pompe registry. *Am. J. Med. Genet. A* **2013**, *161A*, 2431–2443. [CrossRef]

9. Prosser, L.A.; Lam, K.K.; Grosse, S.D.; Casale, M.; Kemper, A.R. Using Decision Analysis to Support Newborn Screening Policy Decisions: A Case Study for Pompe Disease. *MDM Policy Pract.* **2018**, *3*. [CrossRef]

10. Owens, P.; Wong, M.; Bhattacharya, K.; Ellaway, C. Infantile-onset Pompe disease: A case series highlighting early clinical features, spectrum of disease severity and treatment response. *J. Paediatr. Child Health* **2018**, *54*, 1255–1261. [CrossRef]

11. Rigter, T.; Weinreich, S.S.; van El, C.G.; de Vries, J.M.; van Gelder, C.M.; Gungor, D.; Reuser, A.J.J.; Hagemans, M.L.C.; Cornel, M.C.; van der Ploeg, A.T.; et al. Severely impaired health status at diagnosis of Pompe disease: A cross-sectional analysis to explore the potential utility of neonatal screening. *Mol. Genet. Metab.* **2012**, *107*, 448–455. [CrossRef]

12. Zurynski, Y.; Deverell, M.; Dalkeith, T.; Johnson, S.; Christodoulou, J.; Leonard, H.; Elliott, E.J. Australian children living with rare diseases: Experiences of diagnosis and perceived consequences of diagnostic delays. *Orphanet J. Rare Dis.* **2017**, *12*, 68. [CrossRef] [PubMed]

13. Molster, C.; Urwin, D.; Di Pietro, L.; Fookes, M.; Petrie, D.; van der Laan, S.; Dawkins, H. Survey of healthcare experiences of Australian adults living with rare diseases. *Orphanet J. Rare Dis.* **2016**, *11*, 30. [CrossRef] [PubMed]

14. Lagler, F.B.; Moder, A.; Rohrbach, M.; Hennermann, J.; Mengel, E.; Gökce, S.; Hundsberger, T.; Rösler, K.M.; Karabul, N.; Huemer, M.; et al. Extent, impact, and predictors of diagnostic delay in Pompe disease: A combined survey approach to unveil the diagnostic odyssey. *JIMD Rep.* **2019**, *49*, 89–95. [CrossRef] [PubMed]

15. Di Iorio, G.; Cipullo, F.; Stromillo, L.; Sodano, L.; Capone, E.; Farina, O. S1.3 Adult-onset Pompe disease. *Acta Myol.* **2011**, *30*, 200–202.

16. Burton, B.K.; Kronn, D.F.; Hwu, W.-L.; Kishnani, P.S. The Initial Evaluation of Patients After Positive Newborn Screening: Recommended Algorithms Leading to a Confirmed Diagnosis of Pompe Disease. *Pediatrics* **2017**, *140*, S14. [CrossRef] [PubMed]

17. Millington, D.S.; Bali, D. Current state of the art of newborn screening for lysosomal storage disorders. *Int. J. Neonatal Screen.* **2018**, *4*, 24. [CrossRef]

18. Millington, D.S. The Role of Technology in Newborn Screening. *N. C. Med. J.* **2019**, *80*, 49–53. [CrossRef]

19. Baker, M.; Griggs, R.; Byrne, B.; Connolly, A.M.; Finkel, R.; Grajkowska, L.; Haidet-Phillips, A.; Hagerty, L.; Ostrander, R.; Orlando, L.; et al. Maximizing the Benefit of Life-Saving Treatments for Pompe Disease, Spinal Muscular Atrophy, and Duchenne Muscular Dystrophy Through Newborn Screening: Essential Steps. *JAMA Neurol.* **2019**, *76*, 978–983. [CrossRef]

20. Newborn Screening Technical Assistance and Evaluation Program (NewSTEPs). *Disorders Screening Status Map New Steps: US National Newborn Screening Resource Center*; Association of Public Health Laboratories: Silver Spring, MD, USA. Available online: https://www.newsteps.org/resources/newborn-screening-status-all-disorders (accessed on 20 November 2019).

21. Bodamer, O.A.; Scott, C.R.; Giugliani, R. Newborn Screening for Pompe Disease. *Pediatrics* **2017**, *140*, S4. [CrossRef]

22. Bombard, Y.; Miller, F.A.; Hayeems, R.Z.; Avard, D.; Knoppers, B.M. Reconsidering reproductive benefit through newborn screening: A systematic review of guidelines on preconception, prenatal and newborn screening. *Eur. J. Hum. Genet.* **2010**, *18*, 751–760. [CrossRef]

23. Meikle, P.J.; Hopwood, J.J.; Clague, A.E.; Carey, W.F. Prevalence of lysosomal storage disorders. *JAMA* **1999**, *281*, 249–254. [CrossRef] [PubMed]

24. Health Consult. Review of Life Saving Drugs Program Medicines: Pompe Disease. In *Final Review Protocol*; Australian Government Department of Health: Canberra, Australia, 2019. Available online: https://www1.health.gov.au/internet/main/publishing.nsf/Content/E959F2C329B6255ACA258308001F0EE1/$File/Review-Protocol-for-Pompe-disease.pdf (accessed on 20 November 2019).

25. Chien, Y.H.; Hwu, W.L.; Lee, N.C. Newborn screening: Taiwanese experience. *Ann. Transl. Med.* **2019**, *7*, 281. [CrossRef] [PubMed]

26. Desai, A.K.; Kazi, Z.B.; Bali, D.S.; Kishnani, P.S. Characterization of immune response in Cross-Reactive Immunological Material (CRIM)-positive infantile Pompe disease patients treated with enzyme replacement therapy. *Mol. Genet. Metab. Rep.* **2019**, *20*, 100475. [CrossRef] [PubMed]

27. Chien, Y.H.; Hwu, W.L.; Lee, N.C. Pompe disease: Early diagnosis and early treatment make a difference. *Pediatr. Neonatol.* **2013**, *54*, 219–227. [CrossRef]

28. Yang, C.F.; Yang, C.C.; Liao, H.C.; Huang, L.Y.; Chiang, C.C.; Ho, H.C.; Lai, C.J.; Chu, T.H.; Yang, T.F.; Hsu, T.R.; et al. Very Early Treatment for Infantile-Onset Pompe Disease Contributes to Better Outcomes. *J. Pediatr.* **2016**, *169*, 174–180. [CrossRef]

29. Chien, Y.H.; Lee, N.C.; Chen, C.A.; Tsai, F.J.; Tsai, W.H.; Shieh, J.Y.; Huang, H.J.; Hsu, W.C.; Tsai, T.H.; Hwu, W.L.; et al. Long-term prognosis of patients with infantile-onset Pompe disease diagnosed by newborn screening and treated since birth. *J. Pediatr.* **2015**, *166*, 985–991. [CrossRef]

30. Hahn, A.; Schänzer, A. Long-term outcome and unmet needs in infantile-onset Pompe disease. *Ann. Transl. Med.* **2019**, *7*, 283. [CrossRef]

31. Desai, A.K.; Li, C.; Rosenberg, A.S.; Kishnani, P.S. Immunological challenges and approaches to immunomodulation in Pompe disease: A literature review. *Ann. Transl. Med.* **2019**, *7*, 285. [CrossRef]

32. Poelman, E.; Hoogeveen-Westerveld, M.; van den Hout, J.M.P.; Bredius, R.G.M.; Lankester, A.C.; Driessen, G.J.A.; Kamphuis, S.S.M.; Pijnappel, W.W.M.; van der Ploeg, A.T. Effects of immunomodulation in classic infantile Pompe patients with high antibody titers. *Orphanet J. Rare Dis.* **2019**, *14*, 71. [CrossRef]

33. Matsuoka, T.; Miwa, Y.; Tajika, M.; Sawada, M.; Fujimaki, K.; Soga, T.; Tomita, H.; Uemura, S.; Nishino, I.; Fukuda, T.; et al. Divergent clinical outcomes of alpha-glucosidase enzyme replacement therapy in two siblings with infantile-onset Pompe disease treated in the symptomatic or pre-symptomatic state. *Mol. Genet. Metab. Rep.* **2016**, *9*, 98–105. [CrossRef]

34. Oda, E.; Tanaka, T.; Migita, O.; Kosuga, M.; Fukushi, M.; Okumiya, T.; Osawa, M. Newborn screening for Pompe disease in Japan. *Mol. Genet. Metab.* **2011**, *104*, 560–565. [CrossRef] [PubMed]

35. Goldenberg, A.J.; Comeau, A.M.; Grosse, S.D.; Tanksley, S.; Prosser, L.A.; Ojodu, J.; Botkin, J.R.; Kemper, A.R.; Green, N.S. Evaluating Harms in the Assessment of Net Benefit: A Framework for Newborn Screening Condition Review. *Matern. Child Health J.* **2016**, *20*, 693–700. [CrossRef] [PubMed]

36. Minter Baerg, M.M.; Stoway, S.D.; Hart, J.; Mott, L.; Peck, D.S.; Nett, S.L.; Eckerman, J.S.; Lacey, J.M.; Turgeon, C.T.; Gavrilov, D.; et al. Precision newborn screening for lysosomal disorders. *Genet. Med.* **2018**, *20*, 847–854. [CrossRef] [PubMed]

37. Wasserstein, M.P.; Caggana, M.; Bailey, S.M.; Desnick, R.J.; Edelmann, L.; Estrella, L.; Holzman, I.; Kelly, N.R.; Kornreich, R.; Kupchik, S.G.; et al. The New York pilot newborn screening program for lysosomal storage diseases: Report of the First 65,000 Infants. *Genet. Med.* **2019**, *21*, 631–640. [CrossRef] [PubMed]

38. Chiang, S.C.; Chen, P.W.; Hwu, W.L.; Lee, A.J.; Chen, L.C.; Lee, N.C.; Chiou, L.Y.; Chien, Y.H. Performance of the Four-Plex Tandem Mass Spectrometry Lysosomal Storage Disease Newborn Screening Test: The Necessity of Adding a 2nd Tier Test for Pompe Disease. *Int. J. Neonatal Screen.* **2018**, *4*, 41. [CrossRef]

39. Van El, C.G.; Rigter, T.; Reuser, A.J.; van der Ploeg, A.T.; Weinreich, S.S.; Cornel, M.C. Newborn screening for pompe disease? A qualitative study exploring professional views. *BMC Pediatr.* **2014**, *14*, 203. [CrossRef]

40. Wilcken, B. Newborn Screening for Lysosomal Disease: Mission Creep and a Taste of Things to Come? *Int. J. Neonatal Screen.* **2018**, *4*. [CrossRef]

41. Schoser, B.; Bilder, D.A.; Dimmock, D.; Gupta, D.; James, E.S.; Prasad, S. The humanistic burden of Pompe disease: Are there still unmet needs? A systematic review. *BMC Neurol.* **2017**, *17*, 202. [CrossRef]

42. Reardon, K.; McKelvie, P. 090 The expanding clinical phenotype of late onset pompe disease: A multi-system disorder. *JNNP* **2018**, *89*. [CrossRef]

43. Royal Australian Collge of General Practitioners. *Genomics in General Practice*; RACGP: East Melbourne, Australia, 2018; Available online: https://www.racgp.org.au/download/Documents/Guidelines/Genomics-in-general-practice.pdf (accessed on 20 November 2019).

44. O'Leary, P.; Maxwell, S. Newborn bloodspot screening policy framework for Australia. *Australas. Med. J.* **2015**, *8*, 292–298. [CrossRef]

45.   White, C. *Newborn Bloodspot Screening Working Group: Newborn Bloodspot Screening National Policy Framework*; Australian Government Department of Health: Canberra, Australia, 2018. Available online: http://www.cancerscreening.gov.au/internet/screening/publishing.nsf/Content/newborn-bloodspot-screening (accessed on 5 December 2019).

46.   Schoser, B.; Hahn, A.; James, E.; Gupta, D.; Gitlin, M.; Prasad, S. A Systematic Review of the Health Economics of Pompe Disease. *Pharm. Open* **2019**, *3*, 479–493. [CrossRef] [PubMed]

47.   Kishnani, P.S.; Beckemeyer, A.A. New therapeutic approaches for Pompe disease: Enzyme replacement therapy and beyond. *Pediatr. Endocrinol. Rev.* **2014**, *12*, 114–124. [PubMed]

48.   Ronzitti, G.; Collaud, F.; Laforet, P.; Mingozzi, F. Progress and challenges of gene therapy for Pompe disease. *Ann. Transl. Med.* **2019**, *7*, 287. [CrossRef] [PubMed]

49.   Salabarria, S.M.; Nair, J.; Clement, N.; Smith, B.K.; Raben, N.; Fuller, D.D.; Byrne, B.J.; Corti, M. Advancements in AAV-mediated Gene Therapy for Pompe Disease. *J. Neuromuscul. Dis.* **2019**. [CrossRef]

50.   House, T.; O'Donnell, K.; Saich, R.; Di Pietro, F.; Broekgaarden, R.; Muir, A.; Schaller, T. The role of patient advocacy organizations in shaping medical research: The Pompe model. *Ann. Transl. Med.* **2019**, *7*, 293. [CrossRef]

Permissions

List of Contributors

Valentine Brousse and Mariane De Montalembert
Department of General Pediatrics and Pediatric Infectious Diseases, Sickle Cell Disease Reference Center, Necker-Enfants Malades Hospital, Assistance Publique-Hôpitaux de Paris (AP-HP), Université de Paris, 75005 Paris, France

Cécile Arnaud and Françoise Bernaudin
Department of Pediatrics, Sickle Cell Disease Reference Center, CHIC Hospital, Université de Paris-Est Créteil, 94000 Créteil, France

Emmanuelle Lesprit and Béatrice Quinet
Department of Pediatrics, Sickle Cell Disease Reference Center, Trousseau Hospital, Assistance Publique-Hôpitaux de Paris (AP-HP), 75012 Paris, France

Marie-Hélène Odièvre
Department of Pediatrics, Louis Mourier Hospital, Assistance Publique-Hôpitaux de Paris (AP-HP), 92700 Colombes, France

Cécile Guillaumat
Department of Pediatrics, Centre Hospitalier Sud Francilien, 91100 Corbeil-Essonne, France

Gisèle Elana
Sickle Cell Disease Unit, Sickle Cell Disease Reference Center, University Hospital of Martinique, 97261 Fort De France, Martinique, France

Marie Belloy
Department of Pediatrics, Robert Ballanger Hospital, 93600 Aulnay Sous Bois, France

Nathalie Garnier
Department of Pediatric Onco-Hematology, Institut d'Hématologie et d'Oncologie Pédiatrique, 69008 Lyon, France

Corinne Pondarre
Department of Pediatrics, Sickle Cell Disease Reference Center, CHIC Hospital, Université de Paris-Est Créteil, 94000 Créteil, France
Department of Pediatric Onco-Hematology, Institut d'Hématologie et d'Oncologie Pédiatrique, 69008 Lyon, France

Abdourahim Chamouine
Department of Pediatrics, Mamoudzou Hospital, 97600 Mayotte, France

Cécile Dumesnil
Department of Pediatric Onco-Hematology, Charles Nicolle Hospital, 76600 Rouen, France

Nathalie Couque
Biochemistry and Molecular Biology Laboratory, Robert Debré Hospital, Assistance Publique-Hôpitaux de Paris (AP-HP), 75019 Paris, France

Emmanuelle Boutin
Department of Public Health And Biostatistics, Henri Mondor Hospital, Assistance Publique-Hôpitaux de Paris (AP-HP), 94010 Créteil, France

Josiane Bardakjian
Department of Biochemistry and Genetics, Henri Mondor Hospital, Assistance Publique-Hôpitaux de Paris (AP-HP), 94010 Créteil, France

Fatiha Djennaoui
Clinical Research Unit, Albert Chenevier Hospital, 94010 Créteil, France

Ghislaine Ithier and Malika Benkerrou
Sickle Cell Disease Reference Center, Robert Debré Hospital, Assistance Publique-Hôpitaux de Paris (AP-HP), 75019 Paris, France

Isabelle Thuret
Department of Pediatric Onco-Hematology, Thalassemia Reference Center, Timone Enfant Hospital, Assistance Publique-Hôpitaux de Marseille (AP-HM), 13005 Marseille, France

Frank-Thomas Riede and Christian Paech
Department of Paediatric Cardiology, Heart Centre, University of Leipzig, 04289 Leipzig, Strümpellstr. 39, Germany

Thorsten Orlikowsky
Department of Neonatology, University Childrens Hospital Aachen, 52072 Aachen, Pauwelsstr. 30, Germany

William Walsh
Department of Pediatrics, Vanderbilt University Medical Center, Nashville, TN 37232, USA

Jean A. Ballweg
Department of Pediatrics, University of Nebraska Medical Center, Nashville, TN 37232, USA

Virginie Scotet
Inserm, University of Brest, EFS, UMR 1078, GGB, F-29200 Brest, France

Hector Gutierrez
Department of Pediatrics, University of Alabama at Birmingham, Birmingham, AL 35233, USA

Philip M. Farrell
Departments of Pediatrics and Population Health Sciences, University of Wisconsin School of Medicine and Public Health, Madison, WI 53705, USA

Michael Angastiniotis
Thalassemia International Federation, Strovolos 2083, Nicosia, Cyprus

Stephan Lobitz
Department of Pediatric Oncology/Hematology, Kinderkrankenhaus Amsterdamer Straße, 50735 Cologne, Germany

Olaf Sommerburg
Division of Pediatric Pulmonology & Allergy and Cystic Fibrosis Center, Department of Pediatrics III, University of Heidelberg, Im Neuenheimer Feld 430, D-69120 Heidelberg, Germany
Translational Lung Research Center Heidelberg (TLRC), Member of the German Center for Lung Research (DZL), Im Neuenheimer Feld 350, D-69120 Heidelberg, Germany

Jutta Hammermann
Pediatric Department, University Hospital of Dresden, Fetscherstr. 74, D-01307 Dresden, Germany

Lutz Naehrlich
Department of Pediatrics, Justus-Liebig-University Giessen, D-35392 Giessen, Germany

Martin Kluckow
Department of Neonatal Medicine, Royal North Shore Hospital and University of Sydney, Sydney, NSW 2065, Australia

Zoltan Lukacs and Paulina Nieves Cobos
Newborn Screening and Metabolic Diagnostics Unit, Hamburg University Medical Center, 20251 Hamburg, Germany

Petra Oliva, Jacob Scott, Thomas P. Mechtler and David C. Kasper
ARCHIMED Life Science GmbH, 1110 Vienna, Austria

Maddalena Martella, Giampietro Viola, Silvia Azzena, Sara Schiavon, Giuseppe Basso, Raffaella Colombatti and Laura Sainati
Dipartimento di Salute della Donna e del Bambino, Università di Padova, 35128 Padova, Italy

Andrea Biondi and Paola Corti and Nicoletta Masera
Dipartimento di Pediatria, Università di Milano-Bicocca-Fondazione MBBM, San Gerardo Hospital, 20900 Monza, Italy

Béatrice Gulbis, Anne-Sophie Adam and Frédéric Cotton
Department of Clinical Chemistry, LHUB-ULB, Université Libre de Bruxelles (ULB) 322, Rue Haute, 1000 Brussels, Belgium

Phu-Quoc Lê and Alina Ferster
Department of Hemato-Oncology Hôpital Universitaire des Enfants Reine Fabiola, Université Libre de Bruxelles (ULB) 15, av. J.J. Crocq, 1020 Brussels, Belgium

Olivier Ketelslegers and Jean-Marc Minon
Department of Laboratory Medicine CHR de la Citadelle, 1, Boulevard de la 12ème Ligne, 4000 Liège, Belgium

Marie-Françoise Dresse
Department of Pediatric, University Hospital Liège, CHR de la Citadelle, 1, Boulevard de la 12ème Ligne, 4000 Liège, Belgium

François Boemer and Vincent Bours
Department of Human Genetics CHU Sart Tilman, Université de Liège (ULg) Domaine Universitaire du Sart Tilmant Bâtiment 35-B, 4000 Liège, Belgium

Takaaki Sawada, Jun Kido and Kimitoshi Nakamura
Department of Pediatrics, Graduate School of Medical Sciences, Kumamoto University, Kumamoto 860-8556, Japan

Jane Chudleigh
School of Health Sciences, City, University of London, London EC1V 0HB, UK

Hao Tang, Lisa Feuchtbaum, Stanley Sciortino, Jamie Matteson, Deepika Mathur, Tracey Bishop and Richard S. Olney
Genetic Disease Screening Program, California Department of Public Health, 850 Marina Bay Parkway, MS 8200, USA

Holly Chinnery
Faculty of Sports, Health and Applied Science, St Mary's University, London TW1 4SX, UK

Yvonne Daniel
Viapath, Guy's & St Thomas Hospital, London SE17EH, UK

Charles Turner
WellChild Laboratory, Evelina London Children's Hospital, London SE17EH, UK

Lisa A. Wandler and Gerard R. Martin
Children's National Heart Institute, Washington, DC 20010-2970, USA

Jennifer Knight-Madden, Lesley King and Monika Asnani
Caribbean Institute for Health Research—Sickle Cell Unit, The University of the West Indies, Mona, Kingston 7, Jamaica

Ketty Lee
Laboratory of Molecular Genetics, Academic Hospital of Guadeloupe, 97159 Pointe-à-Pitre, Guadeloupe

Narcisse Elenga
Referral Center for Sickle Cell Disease, Department of Pediatric Medicine and Surgery, Andrée Rosemon General Hospital, 97306 Cayenne, French Guiana, France

Beatriz Marcheco-Teruel
National Center of Medical Genetics, 11300 La Habana, Cuba

Ngozi Keshi
Paediatric Department, Scarborough General Hospital, 00000 Scarborough, Tobago

Maryse Etienne-Julan
Sickle Cell Disease Unit, Sickle Cell Disease Reference Center, University Hospital of Pointe-à-Pitre/Abymes, BP 465 Pointe-à-Pitre, Guadeloupe, France
Referral Center for Sickle Cell Disease, Sickle Cell Unit, Academic Hospital of Guadeloupe, 97159 Pointe-à-Pitre, Guadeloupe, France

Marc Romana
UMR Inserm 1134 Biologie Intégrée du Globule Rouge, Inserm/Université Paris Diderot—Université Sorbonne Paris Cité/INTS/Université des Antilles, Hôpital Ricou, Academic Hospital of Guadeloupe, 97159 Pointe-à-Pitre, Guadeloupe
Laboratoire d'Excellence du Globule Rouge (Labex GR-Ex), PRES Sorbonne, 75015 Paris, France

Marie-Dominique Hardy-Dessources
UMR Inserm 1134 Biologie Intégrée du Globule Rouge, Inserm/Université Paris Diderot—Université Sorbonne Paris Cité/INTS/Université des Antilles, Hôpital Ricou, Academic Hospital of Guadeloupe, 97159 Pointe-à-Pitre, Guadeloupe
Laboratoire d'Excellence du Globule Rouge (Labex GR-Ex), PRES Sorbonne, 75015 Paris, France
Caribbean Network of REsearchers on Sickle Cell Disease and Thalassemia, UMR Inserm 1134, Hôpital Ricou, Academic Hospital of Guadeloupe, 97159 Pointe-à-Pitre, Guadeloupe

Anne Munck
Hopital Necker Enfants-Malades, AP-HP, CF centre, Université Paris Descartes, 75015 Paris, France

Roshan B. Colah, Pallavi Mehta and Malay B. Mukherjee
ICMR-National Institute of Immunohaematology, KEM Hospital Campus, Mumbai 400012, India

Baba P.D. Inusa
Department Evelina Children's Hospital, Guy's and St Thomas' NHS Foundation Trust, London SE1 7EH, UK

Kofi A. Anie
Department of Haematology and Sickle Cell Centre, London North West University Healthcare NHS Trust and Imperial College, London NW10 7NS, UK

Andrea Lamont
Department of Implementation Science, University of South Carolina, Columbia, SC 29208, USA

Livingstone G. Dogara and Ifeoma Ijei
Department of Haematology, School of Medicine, Kaduna State University, Barau Dikko Teaching Hospital, Kaduna 800212, Nigeria

Bola Ojo
Sickle Cell Cohort Research Foundation, WUSE Zone II, Abuja 70032, Nigeria

Wale Atoyebi
Department of Haematology, Oxford University Hospitals NHS Foundation Trust, Oxford OX3 9DU, UK

Larai Gwani
Kaduna State Assembly Office, Kaduna 800212, Nigeria

Esther Gani
Library Department, Kaduna State University, Kaduna 800241, Nigeria

Lewis Hsu
Department of Pediatric Hematology-Oncology, University of Illinois at Chicago, Chicago, IL 60612, USA

Shu-Chuan Chiang and Kai-Ling Chang
Department of Medical Genetics, National Taiwan University Hospital, Taipei 100, Taiwan

Yin-Hsiu Chien, Ni-Chung Lee and Wuh-Liang Hwu
Department of Medical Genetics, National Taiwan University Hospital, Taipei 100, Taiwan
Department of Pediatrics, National Taiwan University Hospital, Taipei 100, Taiwan

Augusto Sola
Professor of Pediatrics and Neonatology, Medical Executive Director of SIBEN, Wellington, FL 33414, USA

Sergio G. Golombek
President of SIBEN, Professor of Pediatrics and Clinical Public Health, New York Medical College, 40 Sunshine Cottage RD, Valhalla, NY 10595, USA

Attending Neonatologist, Maria Fareri Children's Hospital at Westchester Medical Center, 100 Woods Road, Valhalla, NY 10595, USA

Tracy L. Klug, Lori B. Swartz and Jami L. Kiesling
Missouri Department of Health and Senior Services, Jefferson City, MO 65102-0570, USA

Jon Washburn and Candice Brannen
Baebies, Inc., Durham, NC 27709, USA

Raymond Saich, Renee Brown, Maddy Collicoat, Catherine Jenner, Jenna Primmer, Beverley Clancy, Tarryn Holland and Steven Krinks
Australian Pompe Association Inc., Kellyville, NSW 2155, Australia

Index

Printed in the USA
CPSIA information can be obtained
at www.ICGtesting.com
JSHW051409091023
49903JS00006B/348